Handbook of
Pediatric
Dentistry

W9-CFI-775

Editors

Angus C Cameron
BDS (Hons) MDSc (Syd) FRACDS

Specialist, Paediatric Dentistry
Westmead Hospital

Clinical Senior Lecturer, Paediatric Dentistry
The University of Sydney

Visiting Specialist
Royal Alexandra Hospital for Children
Westmead
Sydney
Australia

Richard P Widmer
BDSc (Hons) MDSc (Melb) FRACDS

Head of Unit
Paediatric Dentistry
Westmead Hospital

Adjunct Associate Professor
Paediatric Dentistry
The University of Sydney

Head of Dentistry
Royal Alexandra Hospital for Children
Westmead
Sydney
Australia

Mosby London • Philadelphia
St Louis • Sydney • Tokyo

Publisher:
Jill Northcott

Development Editor:
Gillian Harris

Project Manager:
Peter Harrison

Production:
Siobhan Egan

Design:
Greg Smith

Layout:
Rob Curran

Cover Design:
Greg Smith

Illustration Management:
Lynda Payne

Illustration:
Sue Tyler

Index:
Dr Laurence Errington

Printed by Grafos S.A. Arte sobre papel, Barcelona, Spain.

Published by Mosby, an imprint of Mosby International Ltd
Lynton House, 7–12 Tavistock Square, London WC1H 9LB, UK.

ISBN 0 7234 3068 3

A CIP catalogue record for this book is available from the British Library. Library of Congress Cataloging-in-Publication data has been applied for.

Text set in Octavo Light 9.75 on 12 pt.

The authors and editors have attempted to reflect in this book the most up-to-date treatment approaches adopted in current paediatric dentistry. However, neither they nor the publishers can accept responsibility for any treatment errors, omissions or any consequences which may arise from the use of the information provided. Readers are strongly advised to use this book in the setting of current accepted standards of clinical care. They should also check carefully the stated precautions and directions for use supplied by manufacturers of dental materials or medications. Please note that the inclusion or omission of specific dental materials or pharmaceuticals does not imply that the authors or the publishers advocate or reject the use of those products.

Contents

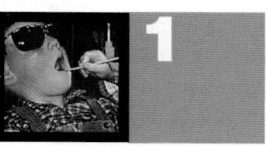

13
Child management

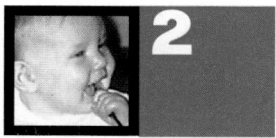

39
Fluoride modalities

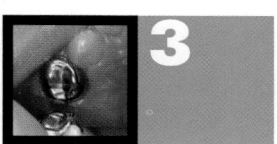

55
Dental caries and restorative paediatric dentistry

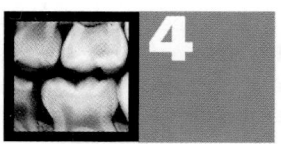

83
Pulp therapy for primary teeth

Contents

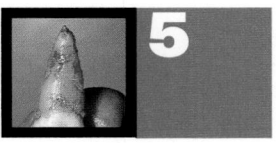
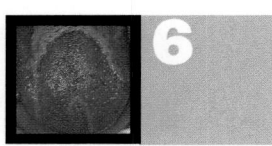
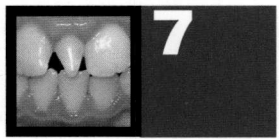
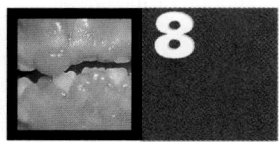

Contents

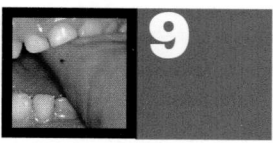
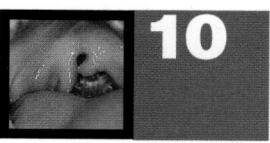
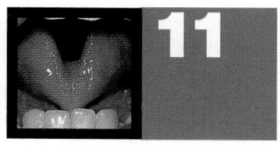
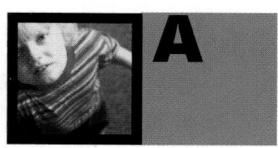

Foreword

Handbooks on paediatrics and, more recently, paediatric dentistry have been produced for some years now by paediatric hospitals and departments of paediatric dentistry in Australia, to assist trainee staff with ready-reference access to advice on common paediatric problems.

This new, more comprehensive publication is the outcome of an enthusiastic response to the first Handbook of Paediatric Dentistry from the Department of Paediatric Dentistry at Westmead Hospital Dental Clinical School and the University of Sydney, edited by Angus Cameron and Richard Widmer. In this new publication there are additional contributions from members of the Australasian Academy of Paediatric Dentistry and the Australian and New Zealand Society of Paediatric Dentistry. The authors have added many colour plates and tables and high-quality colour illustrations of dental abnormalities, which are important adjuncts to the written descriptions of disorders and facilitate diagnosis.

Most orofacial disorders in children have a developmental basis. Lesions or conditions may be present at birth, or become evident soon after. They may appear, change character or arrest and regress (or disappear) as growth proceeds. Certain diseases are inherited and others may be acquired from parents, siblings or other children, but for many orofacial disorders the aetiology is still unknown. Although we may not yet know the precise cause of many conditions, we do know how to manage them—often in close cooperation with our paediatric medical and surgical colleagues. This handbook sets out in concise form the essentials of management of children with, for example, oral and dental trauma, dental caries, oral infections, cardiac disease, endocrine, haematological and oncological disorders. The management of children who have received organ transplants is also covered.

Dental practitioners and students need information on all these areas of dental care for children on a daily basis. This handbook provides the basic information necessary in a clear and readily retrievable form, at the same time providing guidance on the most appropriate texts or journals where more detailed information may be found.

Roger K Hall OAM
Foundation President
Australasian Academy of Paediatric Dentistry
and Director
Department of Dentistry
Royal Children's Hospital
Melbourne
Australia

Foreword

For some time we have recognised that oral health for infants, children and adolescents plays a very important part in the overall health of children. Even though there has been remarkable progress in the promotion of oral health it will be some time before oral diseases are wholly eradicated and most likely this will never occur. Those diseases known as caries and periodontal disease remain in varying degrees throughout the world. It is therefore extremely important that all dentists be prepared to deal with the most common oral problems encountered in the paediatric population. Also, as in all clinical specialties, new advances are made almost daily and it is difficult for the student or practitioner to keep abreast of these changes.

Both the busy practitioner and dental student frequently require a quick reference to a topic, a clinical procedure, or to an oral finding. However, although there are many excellent textbooks in paediatric dentistry, it may not always be easy to find the information required.

It is the intent of this handbook to provide the practitioner and dental student with an easily available and readable source of information for dealing with a specific clinical problem, or to assist in diagnosing a clinical finding. The editors are respected faculty members in the Department of Paediatric Dentistry at the Westmead Hospital Dental Clinical School in Sydney, and have used their departmental handbook as a framework for developing this book. The publication of the handbook utilizing colour photographs provides a level of excellence in paediatric dentistry to which all choosing to care for paediatric patients can aspire. In addition, the editors have called upon their colleagues in the Australasian Academy of Paediatric Dentistry to provide contributions, giving the handbook an even broader perspective and scope.

Although many departments of paediatric dentistry across the world have handbooks, I know of none that is as extensive or as well done as this one. I find the information to be contemporary in its scope and comprehensive in its presentation. It is not meant to cover all topics or conditions that might be encountered in paediatric dentistry but to provide a foundation for the practitioner in those conditions most commonly seen in paediatric patients. The editors hope that in those very complex cases that are beyond the scope of this handbook, practitioners will call upon their colleagues in paediatric dentistry to assist them in management and treatment.

The handbook is written in an outline fashion, which allows for quick reference and easy reading; it is also profusely supplemented with colour photographs which aid greatly in the understanding of conditions. The appendices are lengthy and provide the reader with information that is often difficult to find and which can, therefore, be overlooked.

I congratulate the authors, Drs Cameron and Widmer, for their vision in taking departmental notes out of the classroom and organizing them into a handbook version that is now available to the entire profession. This achievement will further promote the importance of oral health care for all paediatric patients and increase the availability of professional care.

Arthur J Nowak MD
Professor
Departments of Paediatric Dentistry and Paediatrics
Colleges of Dentistry and Medicine
University of Iowa
USA

Preface

For many years, dentists treating children were seen only to be fixing the little holes, in little teeth, of little people: a rather narrow and mechanistic view. We regard these restorative aspects of treating children as 'paedodontics', and the term 'paediatric dentistry' to more properly express the broad scope of child dental health, the basis of most specialist work.

We have perceived the need for a paediatric dentistry handbook, specialising in the important but often hard-to-find information about current paediatric dental practice. Children are not little adults; and as more children with chronic disease are being managed away from major paediatric centres, it is important for general dental practitioners to have access to the knowledge available in such centres. It is not the role of the specialist paediatric dentist to manage every medically compromised or difficult child. Indeed, it is our belief that the majority of these children can be safely and successfully managed in most general practices. On the other hand, the general practitioner must also know when it is appropriate to refer those children who require acute care and be aware of the facilities provided by modern paediatric hospitals.

This new appearance of the handbook has been a collaborative effort by members of the Australasian Academy of Paediatric Dentistry and a wide range of specialists involved in paediatric care. It has been designed for dental undergraduate students and is also intended as a chairside reference for general practitioners. It provides a unique compilation of modern diagnostic and treatment philosophies, not only from Australasia, but also from diverse world opinions. It has furthermore been written with our medical colleagues in mind to provide them with appropriate information on contemporary paediatric dental care and to aid in the diagnosis of orofacial pathology.

The authors have sought to provide the most up-to-date information about the clinical practice of paediatric dentistry. They have made every effort to identify, acknowledge and obtain appropriate permission for the reuse of published material.

Angus Cameron and Richard Widmer
Westmead
Sydney
Australia

April 1997

Acknowledgements

The editors are extremely grateful for the support of all those involved in the teaching of paediatric dentistry thoughout Australia and New Zealand and the members of the Australasian Academy of Paediatric Dentistry. The list of contributors reflects the depth of experience in child dental care that has been gathered to complete this publication and we would like to thank all those who have been intimately involved, or who have offered advice. We would especially like to thank the staff of Westmead Hospital, in particular Mrs Frances Porter and Mrs Maggie Melink for their invaluable secretarial efficiency and patience.

The quiet support and encouragement of our families must not go unmentioned and, finally, we would like to thank our child patients, with whose care we are entrusted. They give us wonder as we watch them grow, give us joy in our daily work, and give us the motivation for our endeavours.

List of contributors

Paul Abbott
BDSc (WA) MDS (Adel) FRACDS
(Endo)
Specialist Endodontist,
Melbourne, Victoria
Senior Lecturer,
University of Western Australia,
Australia

Michael Aldred
BDS (Wales) PhD (Wales) FDS
RCS (Eng) MRCPath GradCertEd
(QUT)
Professor in Oral Biology,
Centre for Molecular and
Cellular Biology,
The University of Queensland,
Australia

Louise Brearley Messer
BDSc LDS MDSc (Melb) PhD
(Minn)
Eldston Storey Professor of Child
Dental Health,
The University of Melbourne
Adjunct Professor, Pediatric
Dentistry, University of Minnesota,
USA

Roland Bryant
MDS (Syd) PhD FRACDS
Professor of Conservative
Dentistry,
The University of Sydney,
Australia

Santo Cardaci
BDSc Hons (WA) MDSc (Adel)
FRACDS
Specialist Endodontist, Perth, WA
Australia

Peter J Cooper
BSc MB ChB MRCP (UK)
Paediatric Respiratory Physician,
Royal Alexandra Hospital for
Children, Westmead
Australia

Bernadette Drummond
BDS (Otago) PhD FRACDS
Senior Lecturer and Head,
Department of Community Dental
Health,
The University of Otago,
New Zealand

John Fricker
BDS MDSc (Syd) Grad Dip Adult
Ed FRACDS
Specialist Orthodontist, Canberra,
ACT Visiting Dental Officer
(Paediatric Dentistry),
Westmead Hospital,
Australia

Peter Gregory
BDSc MDSc (WA) FRACDS
Specialist Paediatric Dentist,
Visiting Paedodontist, Princess
Margaret Hospital for Children,
Perth, WA
Clinical Lecturer,
The University of Western
Australia,
Australia

Roger K Hall
OAM MDSc (Melb) FRACDS FICD
Director, Department of Dentistry,
Royal Children's Hospital,
Melbourne
Senior Associate,
The University of Melbourne,
Australia

Kerrod Hallett
BDSc (Hons) MDSc (Qld) FRACDS
Consultant Paediatric Dentist,
Royal Children's Hospital,
Herston, Queensland,
Australia

Fiona Heard
BDSc (Melb) LDS MDSc (Syd)
FRACDS
Specialist Endodontist,
Sydney, NSW
Visiting Dental Officer,
Westmead Hospital,
Australia

Justine Hemmings
B App Sc (Speech Path)
Senior Speech Pathologist, Royal
Alexandra Hospital for Children,
Westmead,
Australia

David Isaacs
MB BChir MD MRCP FRACP
Associate Professor and Head,
Department of Immunology,
Royal Alexandra Hospital for
Children,
Westmead,
Australia

Tissa Jayasekera
MDSc (Melb) MDS (Syd) FRACDS
Specialist Orthodontist, Bendigo,
Victoria
Visiting Dental Officer (Paediatric
Dentistry), Westmead Hospital,
Australia

Timothy Johnston
BDSc (WA) MDSc (Melb)
Specialist Paediatric Dentist, Perth,
Western Australia,
Australia

Allison Kakakios
MB BS (Hons) FRACP
Staff Specialist, Paediatric
Immunology,
Royal Alexandra Hospital for
Children, Westmead,
Australia

Nicky Kilpatrick
BDS (Birm) PhD (Newcastle)
FDSRCPS
Senior Lecturer and Head of
Discipline, Paediatric Dentistry,
The University of Sydney,
Australia

Nigel King
BDS Hons (Lond) MSc Hons
(Lond) PhD (Hong Kong) LDSRCS
(Eng) FHKAM
Reader, Department of Children's
Dentistry and Orthodontics,
Prince Phillip Dental Hospital,
The University of Hong Kong

Linda Kingston
B App Sci (Speech Path)
Senior Speech Pathologist, Royal
Alexandra Hospital for Children,
Westmead,
Australia

Peter King
MDS (Syd)
Head of Unit, Community Dental
Health,
Westmead Hospital Dental Clinical
School,
Australia

Judy Kirk
MB BS (Syd) FRACP
Staff Specialist Cancer Genetics
Medical Oncology,
Westmead Hospital,
Australia

Sandy Lopacki
MA (Speech Path) (Northwestern)
CCC-ASHA
Senior Speech Pathologist,
Westmead Hospital Dental
Clinical School,
Australia

James Lucas
MDSc (Melb) MS (LaTrobe)
FRACDS LDS
Deputy Director, Department of
Dentistry,
Royal Children's Hospital,
Melbourne,
Australia

Jane McDonald
MB BS (NSW) FANZCA
Visiting Medical Officer, Paediatric
Anaesthetics,
Westmead Hospital,
Australia

Daniel W McNeil
PhD
Associate Professor and Director
of Clinical Training, Department of
Psychology,
West Virginia University, West
Virginia, USA

Cheryl B McNeil
PhD
Assistant Professor, Department of
Psychology,
West Virginia University, West
Virginia, USA

Kareen Mekertichian
BDS (Hons) MDSc FRACDS
Specialist Paediatric Dentist,
Visiting Dental Officer (Paediatric
Dentistry), Westmead Hospital,
Australia

Stephen O'Flaherty
MB ChB FRACP FAFRM
Head, Department Paediatric
Rehabilitation,
Royal Alexandra Hospital for
Children, Westmead,
Australia

Christopher Olsen
MDSc (Melb) FRACDS
Senior Lecturer, Child Dental
Health, The University of
Melbourne
Paediatric Dentist, Royal Dental
Hospital, Melbourne,
Australia

Sarah Raphael
BDS (Adel) MDSc (Syd) FRACDS
Senior Registrar, Paediatric
Dentistry,
Westmead Hospital,
Australia

Tony Sandler
BDS (Witw) HD Dent (Witw)
Specialist Endodontist,
Perth, WA,
Australia

Kim Seow
BDS (Adel) MDSc (Qld) DDSc PhD
FRACDS
Associate Professor, Paediatric
Dentistry,
University of Queensland,
Queensland,
Australia

Margarita Silva
CD (Mexico) MS (Minn)
Specialist Paediatric Dentist,
Melbourne, Victoria,
Australia

Sarah Starr
BAppSci (Speech Path) Dip Health
Sci (Ed)
Senior Speech Pathologist, Royal
Alexandra Hospital for Children,
Westmead,
Australia

Neil Street
MB BS (NSW) MAppSci (UTS)
FANZCA
Staff Specialist, Paediatric
Anaesthetics,
Royal Alexandra Hospital for
Children,
Westmead,
Australia

Joe Verco
BDS (Adel) LDS (Vic) BSc Dent
(Hons) MDS FAAPD
Specialist Paediatric Dentist
Adelaide,
South Australia

Peter Wong
BDS (Hons) MDSc (Syd) FRACDS
Specialist Paediatric Dentist,
Canberra ACT,
Visiting Dental Officer (Paediatric
Dentistry), Westmead Hospital,
Australia

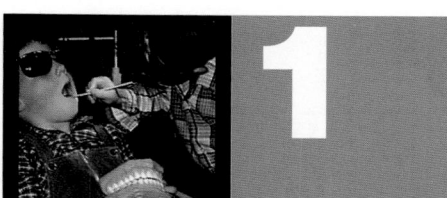

Child management

Contributors
Angus Cameron, Richard Widmer, Bernadette Drummond,
Daniel McNeil, Cheryl McNeil, Jane McDonald

History

A clinical history should be taken in a logical and systematic way for each patient and should be updated regularly. Thorough history-taking is time-consuming and requires practice. It is an opportunity to get to know the child and family. Furthermore, the history facilitates the diagnosis of many conditions even before the hands-on examination. Because there are often specific questions pertinent to the child's medical history that will be relevant to the management of children, it is desirablethat parents be present. The understanding of medical conditions that can compromise treatment is essential.

It is not the purpose of your examination to check merely for caries or periodontal disease, as the treatment of children in paediatric dentistry encompasses all areas of growth and development. Having the opportunity to see the child regularly, the dentist can often be the first to recognize significant disease and anomalies.

Current complaints
The history of any current problems should be carefully documented. This might include the nature, onset or type of pain, relieving and exacerbating factors, or lack of eruption of permanent teeth.

Past dental history
- Previous treatment—how the child has coped with other forms of treatment.
- Eruption times and dental development.
- What preventive treatment has been undertaken.

Past medical history
Medical history should be taken in a systematic fashion covering all system areas of the body. The major areas include:
- Cardiovascular system (e.g. cardiac lesions, blood pressure, rheumatic fever).
- Central nervous system (CNS) (e.g. seizures, cognitive delay).

- Endocrine system (e.g. diabetes).
- Gastrointestinal tract (e.g. liver, hepatitis).
- Respiratory tract (e.g. asthma, bronchitis, upper respiratory tract infections).
- Bleeding tendencies (include family history of bleeding problems).
- Urogenital system (renal disease, ureteric reflux).
- Allergies.
- Past operations or treatment/medications.

Pregnancy history
- Length of confinement.
- Birthweight.
- Antenatal and perinatal problems, especially during delivery.
- Prematurity and treatment in special or neonatal intensive-care nurseries.

Growth and development
In many countries, an infant record book is issued to parents to record postnatal growth and development, childhood illness and visits to health providers. Areas of questioning should include:
- Developmental milestones.
- Speech and language development.
- Motor skills.
- Socialization.

Current medical treatment
- Medications.
- Current treatments.
- Immunizations.

Family and social history
- Family history of serious illness.
- Family pedigree tree (see Appendix O).
- Schooling, performance in class.
- Speech and language problems.
- Pets/hobbies.

This last area is very useful in beginning to establish an interest and a rapport with the child. In asking questions and collecting information, it is important to use lay terminology. The distinction between rheumatic fever and rheumatism is often not understood and more specific questioning may be required. Furthermore, questions regarding family and social history must be neither offensive nor intrusive. An explanation of the need for this information is helpful and appropriate.

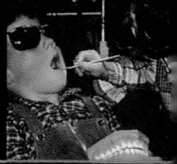

Examination

Extra-oral examination

The extra-oral examination should be one of general appraisal of the child's well-being. The dentist should observe the child's gait and the general interaction with his/her parents or peers in the surgery. An assessment of height and weight is useful and dentists should have a habit of routinely measuring both height and weight and plotting these measurements on a growth chart.

A general physical examination should be conducted. In some circumstances this may require examination of the chest, abdomen and extremities. Although this is often not common practice in a general-practice setting, there may be situations where this is required (i.e. checking for other injuries after trauma, assessing manifestations of syndromes or medical conditions).

Speech and language are also assessed at this stage (see Chapter 11). The clinician should check:

- Facial symmetry, dimensions and the basic orthodontic facial types.
- Eyes, including appearance of the globe, sclera, pupils and conjunctiva.
- Movements of the globe that may indicate squints or palsy.
- Skin colour and appearance.
- Temporomandibular joints.
- Cervical, submandibular and occipital lymph nodes.

Intra-oral examination

- Soft tissues including oropharynx and tonsils.
- Oral hygiene and periodontal status.
- Dental hard tissues.
- Occlusion and orthodontic relations.

Charting

Should be thorough and completed on a form similar to that illustrated in Appendix P.

Provisional diagnosis

A provisional diagnosis should be formulated for every patient. Whether this be caries, periodontal disease or, for example, aphthous stomatitis, it is important to make an assessment of the current conditions that are present. This will influence the ordering of special examinations and the final diagnosis and treatment planning.

Special examinations

Radiography

The prescription of radiographs needs to be specific to the individual. It should take into consideration such things as dental, family and social history.

The guidelines for prescribing radiographs in dental practice are shown in Table 1.1. The overriding principle in taking radiographs of children must be to minimize exposure to ionizing radiation consistent with the provision of the most appropriate treatment. Radiographs are essential for accurate diagnosis. If, however, the information gained from such an investigation does not influence treatment decisions, both the timing and the need for the radiograph should be questioned.

- Bite-wing radiographs.
- Periapical radiographs.
- Panoramic radiographs.
- Occlusal films.
- Extra-oral facial films (i.e. lateral ceph, Waters' projection).

It should be noted that the use of intensifying screens in extra-oral films, significantly reduces radiation dosage. As such, the use of a panoramic film in children is often more valuable than a full-mouth series.

Other imaging

There are many modern technologies available to the clinician and their applications can be a most valuable adjunct not only in the diagnosis of orofacial pathology, but also in the treatment of many conditions.

- Computerized axial tomography (CAT) with three-dimensional reconstruction.
- Magnetic resonance imaging (MRI).
- Nuclear medicine.
- Ultrasonography.

Pulp-sensibility (vitality) testing

- Thermal (i.e. carbon dioxide pencil).
- Electrical stimulation.
- Percussion.
- Mobility.
- Transillumination.

Blood investigations

- Full blood count with differential white-cell count.
- Clinical chemistry.

Microbiological investigations

- Culture of microorganisms and antibiotic sensitivity.
- Cytology.
- Serology.
- Direct and indirect immunofluorescence.

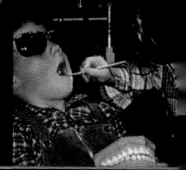

Patient	Child		Adolescent
	Primary dentition	Mixed dentition	

Table 1.1 Guidelines for prescribing radiographs

New patients

Patient	Child (Primary dentition)	Child (Mixed dentition)	Adolescent
All new patients to assess disease and growth and development	Bite-wings for closed contacts between posterior teeth. Panoramic film to assess other pathology or for growth and development.	Bite-wings and individualized examinations such as panoramic film to assess development and eruption of permanent teeth.	Individualized radiographic examinations with bite-wings and panoramic film.

Recall patients

Patient	Child (Primary dentition)	Child (Mixed dentition)	Adolescent
No clinical caries and low risk	If contacts can be visualized or probed, bite-wings may not be required, otherwise bite-wings at 12–24-month intervals.	One set of bite-wings once the first permanent molars have erupted.	Bite-wings every 18–36 months after the eruption of the second permanent molars up to age 20.
Clinical caries or high risk of disease	Bite-wings at 6–12-month intervals or until no new caries are evident over 12 months.		
Growth and development	Usually not required.	Individualized examination, based on anomaly or disease presence, with periapicals or panoramic film.	Panoramic or periapical films to assess position of third molars and other orthodontic considerations.

Anatomical pathology
- Histological examination of biopsy specimens.
- Hard-tissue sectioning (see diagnosis of enamel anomalies, Figure 7.11).
- Scanning and transmission electron microscopy (i.e. hair from children with ectodermal dysplasia Figure 7.1B).

Photography

Extra-oral and intra-oral photography provides an invaluable record of growing children. It is important as a legal document in cases of abuse or trauma, or as an aid in the diagnosis of anomalies or syndromes.

Diagnostic casts

Casts are essential in orthodontic or complex restorative treatment planning and in general record keeping.

Caries-activity tests

Although these are not definitive for individuals, they may be useful as an indicator of caries risk. Furthermore, the identification of defects in salivation in children with medical conditions may point to significant caries susceptibility.
- Diet history.
- Salivary flow rates.
- Salivary buffering capacity.

Definitive diagnosis

The final diagnosis is based on examination and history and determines the final treatment plan.

Assessment of disease risk

All children should have an 'assessment of disease risk' before the final treatment plan is determined. This is particularly important in the planning of preventive care for children with caries. This assessment should be based on:
- Past disease experience.
- Current dental status.
- Family history.
- Diet considerations.
- Oral hygiene.
- Concomitant medical conditions.
- Future expectations of disease activity.
- Social factors including recent migration, language barriers, and ethnic and cultural diversities can impact strongly on access to dental care and will therefore influence caries risk.

Low risk of disease
- No caries present.

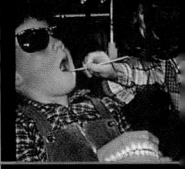

- Favourable family history (appropriate diet, dentally healthy siblings, good oral hygiene, motivated parents and caregivers).
- Access to community water fluoridation.

Moderate risk
- One or two new lesions per year.

High risk or future high risk
- Three or more new lesions per year.
- Beginning orthodontic treatment.
- Chronic illness or hospitalization.
- Medically compromised children.
- Social risk factors.

Treatment plan

1. Emergency care and relief of pain.
2. Preventive care.
3. Surgical treatment.
4. Restorative treatment.
5. Orthodontic treatment.
6. Extensive restorative or further surgical management.
7. Recall and review.

Clinical conduct

Infection control
It is now considered that 'universal precautions' are the expected standard of care in current paediatric dental practice. The principles of universal precautions involve:
- Prevention of contamination by strictly limiting and clearly identifying a 'zone of contamination'.
- The need for elimination of contamination should be minimal if this zone of contamination is observed.

Universal precautions regards every patient as being potentially infectious. Although it is possible to identify some patients who are known to be infectious, there are many others who have an unknown infectious state.

It is impossible to totally eliminate infection; thus, observing universal precautions is a sensible approach to minimizing the risk of cross-infection.

All children must be protected with safety glasses and clinicians must also wear protective clothing, eyeware, masks and gloves when treating patients.

Recording of clinical notes

Care must be taken when recording clinical information. Notes are legal documents and must be legible. Clinical notes should be succinct. Treatment planning should be conducted in each session so that at each subsequent appointment the clinician knows what work is planned. Furthermore, at the completion of the treatment for the day, a note should be made regarding the work to be done at the next visit.

Use of rubber dam

Wherever possible, rubber dam should be used for children. This may necessitate the use of local anaesthesia for the gingival tissues. When topical anaesthetics are used they must be given adequate time to work (i.e. at least 3 minutes). All rubber-dam clamps must have a tie of dental floss around the arch of the clamp to prevent accidental ingestion or aspiration.

Consent to treatment

There is often little provision in a dental file for a signed consent for dental treatment. The consent for a dentist to carry out treatment, be it cleaning of teeth or surgical extraction, is implied when the parent or guardian and child attends the surgery. It is incumbent upon the practitioner, however, to provide all the necessary information and detail in such a way as to enable 'informed consent'. This includes explaining the treatment using appropriate language to facilitate a complete understanding of proposed treatment plans.

It is important to record that the treatment plan has been discussed and that consent has been given for treatment. This consent would cover the period required to complete the work outlined. If there is any significant alteration to the original treatment plan (e.g. an extraction that was not previously anticipated) then consent should be obtained again from the parent or guardian and recorded in the file.

Generally, when undertaking clinical work on a child patient, it is good practice briefly to advise the parent or guardian at the commencement of the appointment what is proposed for that appointment. Also it is helpful to give the parent or guardian and child some idea of the treatment anticipated for the next appointment. This is especially relevant if a more invasive procedure such as local anaesthesia or removal of teeth is contemplated.

Non-pharmacological behaviour management

Promoting positive behaviour from children and adolescents in the dental surgery

Introduction This section is a practical guide for specific dental modes of interacting that can help produce positive and compliant behaviours in child and

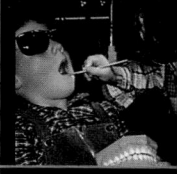

adolescent patients. These guidelines are based on research findings and principles from behavioural dentistry, as well as behavioural, developmental, child and paediatric psychology.

Much has been written about management of problem behaviour with a focus on the use of various techniques. This guide, however, emphasizes specific and mostly simple techniques that can be employed with almost all children and adolescents to enhance their comfort and cooperation in the dental surgery. The general idea is to use finesse instead of absolute control.

The perspective is that dentists, as integral members of the health-care team for children and adolescents, must have awareness of practical methods that they can use, based on a knowledge of psychological principles and issues of growth and development. The adage that 'children are not small adults' promotes the idea of special knowledge and behaviours that are important in caring for young dental patients. Dentists must have a knowledge base in child and adolescent medicine as well as in social and cultural factors affecting the health and behaviour of young people.

It is of the utmost importance that dental appointments in childhood and adolescence be positive, because research clearly shows that these early experiences have a strong effect on attendance in adulthood. Consequently, this section emphasizes the importance of the relationship between dentist and infant or child or adolescent patient. Interactions between dentist and parents or caregiver are also important because they are typically the most influential part of the child's life outside the surgery.

Developmental issues Working with children is different from working with adults. Children are not small adults and they are not all alike. Instead, children are in the process of developing language, intellect, motor skills and personalities. The rates at which specific abilities develop vary. To provide quality dental services to children it is necessary to have some basic knowledge of child development.

Piaget's four stages of intellectual development

Child development encompasses much more than a child's physical changes. It refers to a sequential unfolding of various abilities. Piaget hypothesized that:
- All children progress through the same sequence of cognitive stages.
- Children cannot reach a higher level of reasoning ability until they have mastered experiences in the previous stage (see Appendix K).

Understanding child temperament

There has been a long-standing discussion in child development literature about the degree to which a child's development is caused by 'nature' versus 'nurture'. Studies suggest that children do indeed enter the world with a characteristic temperament or personality that stays with them to some degree for the rest of their lives. Thomas and Chess (1977) suggested that there are three basic temperaments that influence later personality:

Easy temperament These children are viewed as being generally positive in mood. Their bodily functions are regular and they are considered adaptable and flexible. When problems occur they are expected to have a reaction of low or moderate intensity. Rather than withdrawing from new situations, the easy temperament child typically displays a positive approach.

Difficult temperament These children tend to have irregular body functions, such that they are slow to develop a daily pattern for sleeping, eating, and having bowel movements. In contrast to the easy temperament child, these infants often have an intense reaction to problems, have a tendency to withdraw from new situations, and have difficulty adapting to changes in their environment.

Slow to warm up temperament These children have a shy disposition. They tend to have a low activity level. Change is difficult for them as they are slow to adapt and respond negatively to novel situations. Their natural response to novelty is to withdraw and they respond to problems with a low intensity reaction.

Approximately 65% of infants can be categorized into one of these three categories. The remainder have a mixture of traits (Thomas and Chess, op. cit.).

Implications for dentists Dentists working with children must use different approaches and techniques depending upon the personality type of the child. Whereas an easy temperament child may be flexible enough to handle a quick change in plan, a slow to warm up child may need to be given a long time to adjust. Difficult children respond best to a dentist who provides a great deal of structure in a confident manner. The slow to warm up child needs the dentist to be patient, calm, and sensitive.

Developmental milestones

A dentist who is aware of children's abilities at various ages can use that information to communicate at the child's level and to have appropriate expectations for a particular child in the dental surgery. Therefore, it is helpful to become acquainted with certain developmental milestones in the life of the child. It is also important to realize that there is a great deal of variability regarding the ages at which children meet these milestones. As such, age ranges are used to describe the time when most children develop a certain ability.

Use of verbal and non-verbal communication to promote positive behaviour in children

- Respect.
- Show interest in the child as an individual.
- Share 'free information'.
- Give well-stated instructions.

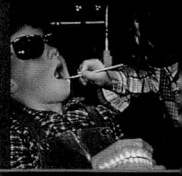

- Communicate at the child's level (Figure 1.1).
- Focus on the positive.
- Show ethnic, cultural, and gender sensitivity.

Physical structuring and timing during the dental visit

Setting the stage for positive behaviour In addition to communications from the dentist and dental staff, there are a number of aspects of the dental situation that can be arranged in such a way as to promote positive reactions in infants, children, and adolescents. The list below suggests practical guidelines for arranging the physical and social aspects of the dental appointment, as well as considerations of timing.

- Everyone in the surgery (dentist, auxiliary, parent) should be transmitting positive, comforting expectations to the patient.
- Use stimulating visual distracters in the surgery (child, adolescent-oriented posters).
- Have age-appropriate materials (safe toys, magazines) in the waiting room. Include materials for parents.
- Have toys available for younger children as distracters or tangible rewards.
- Greet child in the waiting room without a mask, and not wearing surgical garb.
- Pace procedures during the appointment, based on how the patient is coping, so that they are neither rushed nor bored.
- Inform and discuss with parent at conclusion of appointment.

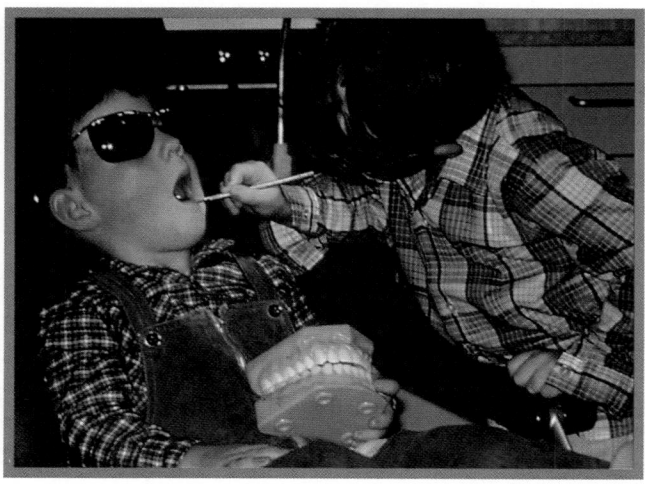

Figure 1.1 Giving children control in the dental surgery.

Presence or absence of family members in the surgery
- It is appropriate that parents are able to support their children during treatment.
- If parents are unable or unwilling to provide appropriate support, then it may be more desirable for them to wait outside the surgery. It is important to note that parental access to their children is never denied.
- When there are other siblings, who enjoy or readily cope with dental treatment, it is often helpful to use them as a model.

Transmission of emotion to the child or adolescent
- Children acquire some of their parents' fear and anxiety about dental treatment on both an acute and long-term basis.
- Emotion is transferred from parents, siblings, dentist and auxiliaries to the child, whose emotional state also impacts upon all of those persons.
- Dental staff who are calm and confident and use humour will promote positive experiences for their patients.

Physical proximity
- Initially work from in front, at eye level.
- Be aware of the child's 'intimate zone'. This zone is approximately 45 cm, but varies with different cultures. By necessity, the dentist must 'invade' this space, but frequent stopping between procedures allows the child some time for coping.

Timing
- It is best to introduce new procedures at an appropriate rate to avoid either rushing or boring the patient.
- Conducting less invasive procedures first will usually be more tolerable for the patient.

Stimulating and distracting objects and situations (Figure 1.2)
- Be aware of popular culture. In some settings, it is possible to have different areas of the surgery orientated to particular patient age ranges.
- An area might include puppets and pictures of colourful cartoon characters for children up to 8 years.
- For older children have wall posters of pop groups.
- Adolescents, like adults, are best treated in a modern, friendly environment.

Surgical clothing and instruments
- Never greet a child wearing a face mask and gloves.
- Explain the need for protective clothing.
- Familiarize children with appropriate instruments.

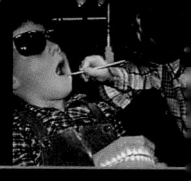

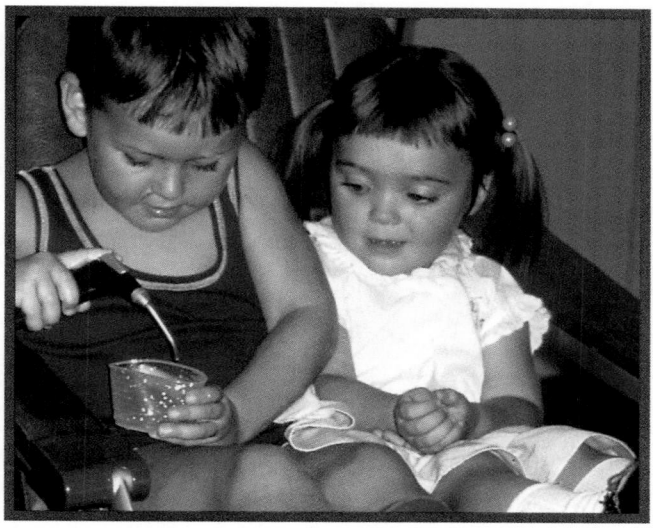

Figure 1.2 Involving children in their treatment. It is important to feel that the dental environment is non-threatening and safe, and can be a place for enjoyment.

Greetings in the waiting room

- It is ideal, particularly in initial meetings, for the dentist to greet the child and parent in the waiting area.
- An interview room or non-surgical environment is useful for new patients (Figures 1.3, 1.4 and 1.5).

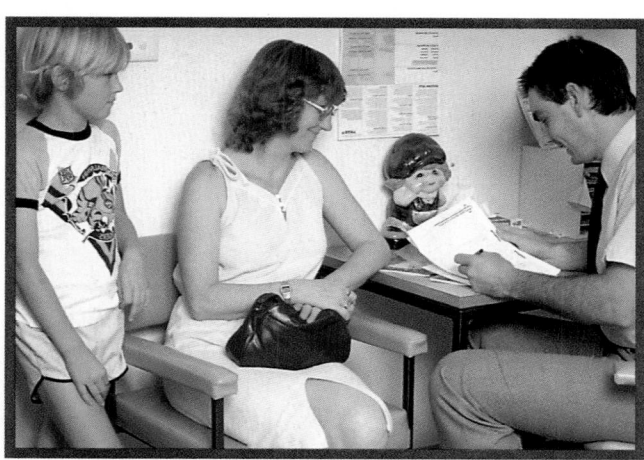

Figure 1.3 At the first visit, it is often good to see the child and parent away from the surgery. It provides an opportunity to talk with the child and establish a rapport.

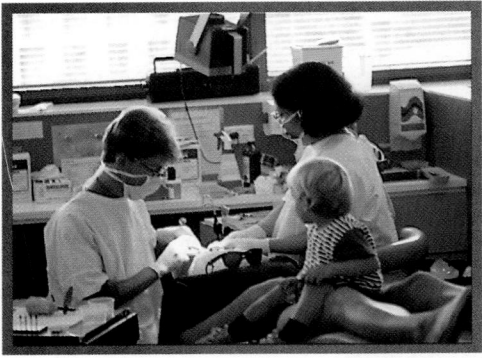

Figure 1.4 Introducing a child to the dental environment, part of familiarization.

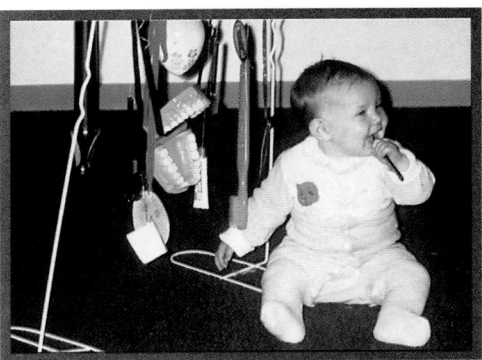

Figure 1.5 A dental mobile—every child should have one!

Talking with parents
- It is extremely helpful for the dentist to have a positive relationship with both children and their parents.
- Keep parents well informed.
- While asking for personal information always remember to involve the child in the discussion wherever appropriate.
- Be prepared to separate the child from the parent to discuss more sensitive issues. The chairside assistant can be asked to occupy the child, for example with a visit to the fish tank.

Special arrangements for first-time dental visits There are certain steps that are appropriate for an initial visit. In general, the pace of a first appointment is much slower. The emphasis is on educating the child, promoting comfort, and allowing the visit to be exciting and fun. Relatively simple and less invasive procedures are preferred.
- Use pre-appointment letters.
- Use an interview room for the initial contact.
- Introducing the child to the office, staff, and equipment and pointing out posters and other materials of interest in the treatment room can also be helpful.

Behavioural methods for reducing fear and pain-sensitivity
Table 1.2 identifies eight methods that can be employed across a variety of situations with children and adolescents of all ages. The particular uses depend on the patient's developmental age and personality, as well as on a variety of other factors such as the quality and depth of the dentist's relationship with the child or adolescent.

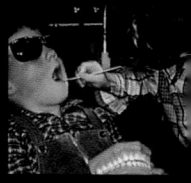

Table 1.2 Behavioural methods for removing anxiety	
Tell–Show–Do	Informing, then demonstrating, and finally performing part of a procedure
Playful humour	Using fun labels and suggesting use of imagination
Distraction	Ignoring and then directing attention away from a behaviour, thought, or feeling to something else
Positive reinforcement	Tangible or social reward in response to a desired behaviour
Modelling	Providing an example or demonstration about how to do
Shaping	Successive approximations to a desired behaviour
Fading	Providing external means to promote positive behaviour and then gradually removing the external control
Systematic desensitization	Reducing anxiety by first presenting an object or situation that evokes little fear, then progressively introducing stimuli that are more fear-provoking

Referring for possible mental health evaluation and care

When to refer
It is the role of the dentist to refer a child or family when there appear to be significant emotional or psychological issues. Even when those problems do not interfere with dental treatment it is the dentist's role, as a member of the health-care team, to identify possible psychopathologies and to refer for proper care.

Common reasons for referring a child or adolescent for mental health concerns
- Evidence of abuse or neglect (e.g. bruises, broken teeth, cigarette burns, inappropriate clothing for weather, severe hygiene problems, untreated breaks or sprains, etc.).
- Extremes of behaviour or emotion (i.e. dental phobia).
- Neurological signs or symptoms (i.e. possible seizure activity, tics).
- Severe developmental or cognitive delay (e.g. possible mental retardation, motor problems, feeding problems).
- Extremely poor parenting (i.e. sole use of excessive physical restraint and punishment).

To whom to refer

It is recommended that referrals for mental health concerns be made to psychologists, psychiatrists, or social workers. In a hospital setting, it is possible to refer to one of the available departmental services. In a dentist's private surgery, referrals can be made to professionals in private practice, community agencies, or hospitals. The following guidelines are suggested in selecting a specialty for referral.

Psychologists Refer in the case of abuse or neglect, extremes of behaviour, developmental or cognitive delay, or extremely poor parenting. When there is a need for sophisticated cognitive, personality, neuropsychological and/or behavioural assessment, referral to a psychologist is best as standardized psychometric tests are available for use. Psychologists can also provide individual child/adolescent, parent/child, and/or family therapy to address problems in the child/adolescent and family system.

Psychiatrists Refer when there are neurological signs or symptoms. When psychoactive medications may be needed, such as when a child demonstrates signs of psychosis, referral to a psychiatrist is most appropriate, as it is in cases in which there are complicating medical factors.

Social workers Refer for social problems, abuse or neglect. Referral to social workers is appropriate when there are existing social problems in the parents or family that require mobilization of community resources. Social workers know of, and help patients to use, available services in the community.

How to refer

It is acknowledged that suggesting mental-health care to parents can be an anxiety-provoking task for the dentist. Nevertheless, it is essential that such referrals are made, because the dentist is in a unique role as a health-care provider. If referrals are not made in a timely fashion then a condition can progress and worsen.
- Speak to the parents in a private setting, informing them of the signs or symptoms that are a cause for concern, without blaming or ascribing responsibility. When the parents understand the problems and your concern, referral to a specific professional or service can be made. It is often helpful to emphasize the good of the child and the need to address the problem for their proper development.
- Ensure that the parent and child or adolescent are aware of the referral and know the specialty of the referral. (It is not appropriate merely to describe the referral as 'to a doctor who will help your child'.) The dentist should also discuss the need for referral with the parent and child.
- Refer first to only one of the mental health specialties. If additional referral is necessary it can be arranged by the first referral source. In making the referral one can ask for feedback from the mental health professional after the appointment. If there is behavioural disruption in the surgery the mental health

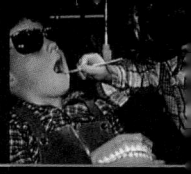

professional may have recommendations for management once the child or family has been evaluated.
- Mental health concerns are considered private by many individuals. Given this desire for privacy, releases to exchange relevant information, signed by a parent or guardian and the child if of an age to understand it, are required. Such a form can be signed in the dental surgery and sent to the mental health professional along with a request for feedback.

Pharmacological behaviour management

- Local anaesthesia (Table 1.3).
- Relative analgesia.
- Oral or rectal sedation.
- Intravenous sedation.
- General anaesthesia.

Local anaesthesia
Successful local anaesthesia depends on:
- Communication with the child.
- Good topical anaesthesia, allowing adequate time for it to act.
- Slow injection of warm solution.
- Avoid direct palatal injections—inject through the interdental papilla after adequate buccal infiltration:

2% lignocaine	=	20 mg/mL
2.2 mL/carpule	=	44 mg/carpule

Table 1.3 Maximum dosages for local anaesthetic agents

Anaesthetic agent	Name	Max. dose
2% lignocaine without vasoconstrictor	Xylocaine	3 mg/kg
2% lignocaine with 1:100 000 adrenaline	Nurocain	7 mg/kg
4% prilocaine plain	Citanest Plain	6 mg/kg
3% prilocaine with 0.03 IU/ml felypressin	Citanest	9 mg/kg
0.5% bupivacaine with 1:200 000 adrenaline	Marcain	2 mg/kg

A 20-kg child (approximately 5 years old) can tolerate a maximum dose of 2% lignocaine with vasoconstrictor of:
7 mg/kg × 20 kg = 140 mg. Equivalent of 3 carpules (6.6 mL).

Relative analgesia (nitrous oxide sedation)

Nitrous oxide sedation is of great benefit in relieving anxiety. It works well on children who are anxious but cooperative. An uncooperative child will often not allow the mask to be placed over the nose. It also requires a child of sufficient age to understand what is happening during the procedure. A trial appointment in order to estimate the correct dosage is beneficial.

Contraindications

- Upper airways obstruction.
- Children with psychoses.
- Pregnancy.
- Obstructive pulmonary disease.
- Malignant hyperthermia is not a contraindication to the use of N_2O.
- Pulse oximetry, although not mandatory, should be used if available.

Sedation

Pharmacological agents may be administered orally, nasally or rectally.

Oral sedation Oral sedation is frequently unreliable because of vomiting, gastric stasis and incomplete absorption. Overdosage cannot be reversed.

Rectal sedation Absorption is excellent by rectal administration. Although routinely performed in Scandinavia and Europe, rectal sedation is less commonly used in Australasia, the UK and the USA, probably because of cultural attitudes. It is, however, an excellent route for drug administration and probably provides the most reliable and controllable absorption.

Intravenous sedation Intravenous sedation has the advantage of the procedure being controllable and may be readily reversible, but as most children are frightened of needles it would seem an inappropriate form of drug administration in extremely anxious children.

- Drug cocktails should be avoided.

If facilities for general anaesthesia are not available, the following agents may be beneficial. In all cases, adequate facilities for recovery and observation must be present.

Medications

- Midazolam 0.2–0.5 mg/kg orally or rectally, or by intravenous or intramuscular injection. A short-acting benzodiazepine with rapid onset (15 minutes) and short half-life.

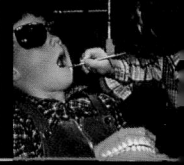

It may be given nasally where there is rapid absorption from the mucosa, although some of the agent finds its way into the nasopharynx and onto the tongue. The taste is extremely bitter. It appears absorption from oral ingestion is adequate.
- Diazepam   0.25–0.5 mg/kg intravenously, rectally or orally

A relatively long-acting but safe benzodiazepine with minimal CNS depression. It has an onset after about 60 minutes and a half-life of 36 hours.
- Fentanyl   1–2 µg/kg intravenously

For short procedures, such as the extraction of a single tooth or suturing of a laceration, fentanyl may be a useful analgesic.

General anaesthesia

Non-emergency general anaesthesia
The need for general anaesthesia represents the clinician's final solution to a child's dental problem. In most instances, a caring attitude in association with a period of familiarization will allow the child to be treated conservatively. It is assumed that the decision to arrange general anaesthesia is not taken lightly. The clinician must be certain about the need for the dental work that is planned. When deciding to use a general anaesthetic, the clinician must look at the whole picture.
- What is the dental condition?
    Is there gross dental caries?
    Does the child have a facial swelling?
    Is the child in pain?
- Is the treatment absolutely necessary?
- Could the patient be managed more conservatively?
    Has the child undergone a period of familiarization?
    Has there been a history of emotional trauma associated with the dental environment?

Certain clinical situations automatically indicate the need for a general anaesthesia.
- Multiple carious and abscessed teeth in very young children.
- Severe facial cellulitis.
- Facial trauma.

Often it is necessary for the patient to have several routine visits before the clinician can be sure that the dental work needs to be done; such visits also allow assessment of whether the child's behaviour precludes satisfactory completion of the work. In many instances, parents prevail upon the clinician to arrange general anaesthesia as soon as possible. This must be avoided because it is usually for the parents' convenience, not the child's benefit. The child must have a sensible treatment plan arranged. It should include home-care instruction (for the parents to help clean the child's teeth), dietician's referral, use of home fluorides and return visits. If, after seeing the child several times, the clinician feels that the child needs dental work, but is unmanageable, a general anaesthetic should be considered.

Consent forms

Consent for children less than 14 years old In children under 14 years of age, a 'Consent for Minor' form is completed. The parent or guardian must sign the form and a third party, usually the dentist, must witness the signature.

Consent for children 14–16 years of age Children aged 14–16 years must give their consent for the treatment to be performed. Although a 'responsible, informed child' can give this consent, the parent or guardian should also give consent and sign the Consent for Minor form. The dentist should witness the signatures.

Although there is no authoritative statement in law regarding consent for children under 16 years of age, common law dictates that:

'...as a matter of law the parents' right to determine whether or not their minor child below the age of 16 will have medical treatment terminates if and when their child achieves a sufficient understanding to enable him to understand fully what is proposed' (*Gillick v West Norfolk Area Health Authority [1986] AC 112, UK*).

Consent over 16 years A patient 16 years and over must consent for their own treatment and a Consent for Adult form is used.

Emergency treatment In emergency situations, dental treatment may be performed without the consent of the child or parent or guardian if, in the opinion of the practitioner, the treatment is necessary and a matter of urgency in order to save a child's life, or to prevent serious damage to the child's health. (Section 20B of the *Children [Care and Protection] Act [1987] NSW, Australia*)

Fortunately, there are few situations where this will occur in the dental environment, although situations do arise for those working in hospital settings. The overriding point is to 'do no harm'.

It is important that 'informed consent' be obtained. The clinician must carefully explain all the procedures planned using lay language as appropriate. All potential risks need to be mentioned and discussed. When completing the section on the nature of the operation, be specific, do not use abbreviations and include all procedures planned. Where appropriate use lay terminology to describe the operation.

Pre-anaesthetic assessment

A thorough medical history is required to eliminate any possible complications that may occur as a result of the anaesthetic. Most children with no medical complications can be assessed on the day of operation. Nonetheless, the anaesthetist should always be consulted before arranging an anaesthetic for any child with a significant disability. The anaesthetist will be concerned in particular about the following points:

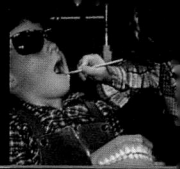

Past anaesthetic complications
- Vomiting.
- Allergic reactions.
- Intubation difficulties.
- Family history of death under anaesthesia.

Past medical history
- Asthma.
- Croup.
- Congenital cardiac disease.
- Suxamethonium apnoea. This results in postoperative apnoea caused by an inherited abnormality of cholinesterase. There is prolonged paralysis following a usual dose of suxamethonium.
- Syndromes of the head and neck.
- Malignant hyperpyrexia. This is a disease of muscle metabolism. Some anaesthetic drugs such as halothane and suxamethonium may trigger an increased metabolic rate and rhabdomyolysis. Malignant hyperpyrexia has a high mortality. Neuromuscular disorders, such as Duchenne muscular dystrophy and central-core disease are associated with an increased risk of malignant hyperpyrexia.
- Prematurity.

Medications
- Steroids.
- Bronchodilators.

Examination
- Temperature.
- Evidence of active upper respiratory tract infection (i.e. purulent rhinorrhoea).
- Airway assessment. Some syndromes are associated with micrognathia and present great difficulties in intubation (Pierre Robin syndrome, Treacher–Collins syndrome, mucopolysaccharidoses or children with cleft repairs or pharyngoplasty).
- Cardiovascular and respiratory status. Many innocent cardiac murmurs are detected by the anaesthetist during a routine pre-anaesthetic assessment. Asthma may be undiagnosed or improperly managed.
- Loose teeth.

Operating theatre environment
- Extremely anxious children should be allowed to wear their own clothes rather than being forced to change into theatre clothing. It is simple to change the child, if required, when asleep.
- Eutectic mixture of local anaesthetic cream should be placed on the back of the hand to allow the painless insertion of the canula or butterfly needle. This

mixture of 5% lignocaine and 5% prilocaine has revolutionized anaesthetic induction by allowing painless injection through the skin. It is essential that the cream is given at least 60 minutes to take effect.

- Anxiety is minimized by allowing the parent to be with the child during induction. It should be stressed, however, that this is for the benefit of the child and not the parent. There are some situations where this may not be possible because of the nature of the procedures, the cooperation of the parent, or the limitations of the individual operating theatre.
- Ideally, parents should be called into the recovery ward once the child has woken and is stable. Young children may be quite disoriented and unsettled as they are regaining consciousness and parents are often similarly upset at seeing their child in this state. It is important to be sympathetic to the parents' concerns and to reassure them that this is a normal response during emergence from anaesthesia and that the child will not remember the event.

Fasting instructions Fasting instructions must be given by the dentist.

Children 6 years and under
- No solids for 6 hours pre-operation.
- No breast milk for 4 hours pre-operation.
- No clear fluids for 2 hours pre-operation.

This effectively means, for a morning anaesthetic, that the child does not eat from midnight the night before, but the child may be given a small drink of water, or weak cordial up to 2 hours before the operation.

Child 6 years of age and older
- No solids or liquids for 6 hours pre-operation.

Overall, it is important to stress the need for strict adherence to these instructions, otherwise the anaesthetist may not go ahead with the anaesthetic, as failure to comply puts the patient at significant risk.

Categories of anaesthetic risk
American Society of Anaesthesiologists (ASA):

Class 1   Healthy patient.
Class 2   Mild to moderate systemic disease without significant limitations.
Class 3   Severe systemic disturbance with physical limitations.
Class 4   Life-threatening systemic disorder.
Class 5   Moribund patient not expected to survive >24 hours.
Class E   Emergency patient.

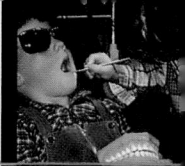

Suitability for day-stay anaesthetics (Figure 1.6)

Generally, patients graded as Class 3 ASA or greater are not suitable for day-stay general anaesthesia and require pre-operative admission. Children who automatically require pre-operative admission include those with:

- Cyanotic cardiac disease.
- Malignant hyperpyrexia risk.
- Severe asthma, with a history of more than one admission over the last 12 months.
- Diabetes.
- Coagulopathies.
- History of protracted postoperative vomiting.
- Any surgical procedure that will require extended postoperative care, especially those procedures that may interfere with the airway (i.e. floor of mouth swelling).

If there is any doubt as to the suitability of a general anaesthetic, then the anaesthetist and responsible paediatricians must be consulted with a thorough case work-up.

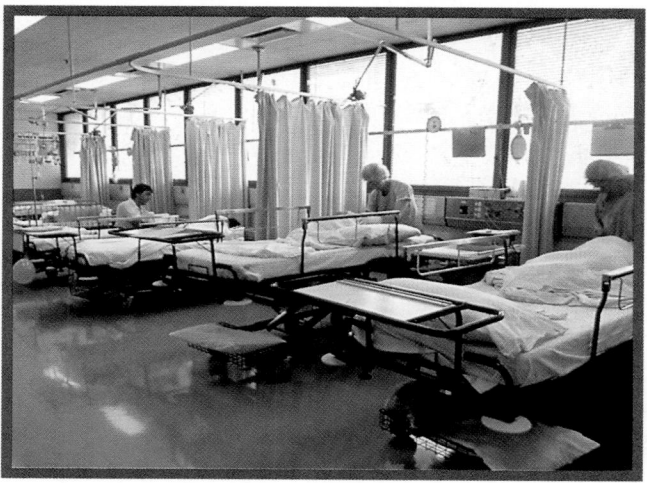

Figure 1.6 A day-stay recovery ward with one-to-one nursing care after general anaesthesia. Normal day-stay recovery is a minimum of 2 hours after the operation.

Handbook of Paediatric Dentistry

Ward instructions

Postoperative instructions and consultation notes in medical notes must be clear and legible. It is important for nursing staff to understand what procedures have been performed and by whom. They should also know whom to contact if complications arise.

An example of postoperative notes for a child admitted with a facial cellulitis is shown below.

1/1/96   **Paediatric Dentistry**

Extraction of teeth and drainage of facial abscess

Surgeon: A Cameron   *Assistant*: S Raphael

Anaesthetist: J McDonald

Extraction of teeth upper right primary first and second molars (Teeth 54, 55)

Buccal flap raised and drainage of abscess

Specimen for culture and sensitivity

Irrigation with 1% H_2O_2 and normal saline

Penrose drain inserted

3-0 Chromic gut

WARD

Benzylpenicillin 600 mg intravenously, four times a day, 1st dose given in theatre

Fluids: 3.75% dextrose N/4 saline, 50 mL/hr, until adequate oral intake, then TKVO (to keep vein open)

Paracetamol 360 mg every 4 hours orally, pain or fever

Warm saline mouthrinses

Encourage oral fluids, soft diet as tolerated

Watch for increase in periorbital swelling

If eye closes apply chloramphenicol 1% ointment 3 hourly

References

Behaviour management
ACS G, MOORE PA, SHUSTERMAN S, NEEDELMAN HL. The extent of trauma and postoperative pain in children. *Pediatr Dent* 1988, **10**:210.
BARON RS, SNYDERSMITH M, LOGAN H, KAO, CF, FITZPATRICK M. The effects of short-term social support from dentists on the stress experienced by parents of pediatric dental patients. *Pediatr Dent* 1991, **13**:333–338.

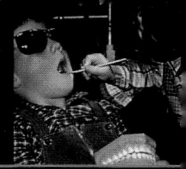

HALLONSTEN AL, KOCH G, SCHRÖDER U. Nitrous oxide-oxygen sedation in dental care. Community *Dent Oral Epidemiol* 1983, **11**:347-355.

HOLST AL, HALLONSTEN A-L, SCHRÖDER U, EK L, EDLUND K. Prediction of behaviour-management problems in 3-year-old children. *Scand J Dent Res* 1993, **101**:110-114.

HOLST A, SCHROEDER U, EK L, HALLONSTEN A-L, CROSSNER C-G. Prediction of behaviour management problems in children. *Scand J Dent Res* 1988, **96**:457-465.

NATHAN JE. Management of the difficult child: a survey of pediatric dentists' use of restraints, sedation and general anaesthesia. *J Dent Child* 1989, **56**:293-301.

RADIS FG, WILSON S, GRIFFEN AL, COURY DL. Temperament as a predictor of behavior during initial dental examination in children. *Pediatr Dent* 1994, **16**:121-127.

RANKIN JA, HARRIS MB. Dental anxiety: the patient's point of view. *J Am Dent Assoc* 1984, **109**:43-47.

ROWLAND A, LINDSAY SJE, WINCHESTER L, ZARKOWSKA E. A study of children's facial expressions of pain and fear during dental treatment and their relationship to disruptive behaviour and reports of pain and fear. *J Paed Dent* 1989, **5**:115-120.

WILLIAMS JMG, MURRAY JJ, LUND CA, Harkiss B, De FRANCO A. Anxiety in the child dental clinic. *J Child Psychol Psychiat* 1985, **26**:305-310.

WRIGHT FAC, GIEBARTOWSKI JE, MCMURRAY NE. A national survey of dentists' management of children with anxiety or behaviour problems. *Aust Dent J* 1991, **36**:378-383.

WRIGHT FAC, LANGE DE. Dental anxiety in children. *NZ Dent J* 1976, **72**:80-83.

Consent

AHAGAN PP, HAGAN JP, FIELDS HW, MACHEM JB. The legal status of informed consent for behaviour management techniques in pediatric dentistry. *Pediatr Dent* 1984, **6**:204-208.

MURPHY MG, FIELDS HW, MACHEM JB. Parental acceptance of pediatric dentistry behaviour management techniques. *Pediatr Dent* 1984, **6**:193-198.

Further reading

FOSTER MS. *Protecting our children's teeth: A guide to quality dental care from infancy through age twelve.* New York: Plenum; 1992.

INHELDER B, PIAGET J. *The growth of logical thinking from childhood to adolescence.* New York: Basic Books; 1958.

RIPA LR, BARENIE JA. *Management of dental behaviour in children.* Massachusetts: PSG Publishing Co; 1979.

THOMAS A, CHESS S. *Temperament and development.* New York: Brunner/Mazel; 1977.

WRIGHT GZ. *Behaviour management in dentistry for children.* Philadelphia: WB Saunders; 1975.

WRIGHT GZ, STARKEY PE, GARDNER DE. *Child management in dentistry.* Bristol: IOP Publishing Limited; 1987.

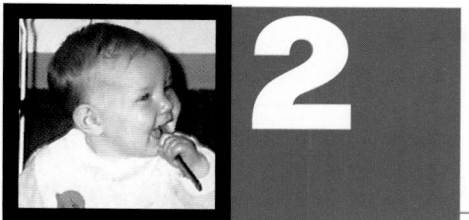

2 Fluoride modalities

Contributors

Kareen Mekertichian, Louise Brearley Messer

Introduction

Fluoride is now used widely to prevent dental caries. The caries reduction that has been achieved by the use of fluorides has been a major public health accomplishment. Community water fluoridation is safe and cost-effective and should be maintained in communities that have benefited from it and extended to low-fluoride communities wherever feasible. There is now clear evidence, on a population basis, that caries reduction is most effective when a low concentration of fluoride is maintained consistently in the oral environment. (This is in contrast to earlier concepts of the mechanism of action of fluoride which attributed the major benefit of fluoride to pre-eruptive maturation of forming enamel.) While any method of using fluoride that helps maintain this low oral concentration is desirable, community fluoridated water and fluoride toothpaste rank first as public health measures in developed countries.

Fluoride is widespread in nature, occurring in fresh water, sea water, fish, vegetables, milk and organic compounds. Physiologically, fluoride is unique in that it does not behave like the other halogens and has been termed a seeker of mineralized tissues, such as bone or forming teeth and is preferentially accumulated by the skeleton. It is absorbed into the blood from the gastrointestinal tract and is then either deposited in bones or excreted by the kidneys.

Mechanisms of action of fluoride

The concept of how fluoride prevents caries has changed considerably over the past decade and it is now recognized that the predominant effect is topical rather than systemic.

- Fluoride acts for the most part, topically, during the process of remineralization, as a posteruptive phenomenon.
- Fluoride can prevent mineral loss at crystal surfaces and enhance remineralization by calcium and phosphate groups. Because the mode of action of fluoride is predominantly posteruptive, the prevention of caries

requires lifelong exposure. When remineralization takes place in the presence of fluoride, the rebuilt enamel is more caries resistant than the original mineral and this effect is evident in even very low fluoride concentrations (less than 0.1 ppm) across the liquid phase surrounding the enamel matrix.

- Fluoride has an effect on the glycolytic pathway of oral microorganisms reducing acid production and interfering with the enzymatic regulation of carbohydrate metabolism. This reduces the accumulation of intracellular and extracellular polysaccharides (i.e. plaque).
- The continuous presence of low levels of fluoride in the plaque–enamel interface provides the most effective mode of remineralization of decalcified enamel.
- There has been a general increase in availability of fluorides from foods, beverages, dentifrices and topical agents.

This topical effect explains the efficacy of fluoridated toothpastes, dilute fluoride rinses and fluoride in drinking water. Even fluoride tablets may provide additional topical effects after eruption as well as their systemic effects during tooth formation. With concentrated topical fluoride application the formation of calcium fluoride is favoured, persisting in the pores of enamel for long periods and acting as a fluoride reservoir during remineralization.

Community water fluoridation

The naturally occurring concentration of fluoride in drinking water in Australia is typically in the range of 0.1–0.4 ppm. Fluoride is added to the reticulated water supply of most large urban populations to achieve a concentration of 1 ppm.

Caries reduction
- 20–40%

This is now considerably less than was the case when water fluoridation was first introduced into contemporary Western populations because of the general increase in fluoride availability from other sources.

- Reversal of protective benefits after removal of fluoride from water supply.
- Benefits adults as well as children.
- There is a decreased prevalence of root-surface caries in lifelong inhabitants of areas with fluoridated water.
- Preferred source of fluoride considering the cost effectiveness and population exposure.

In Western communities, the continuing existence of approximately 20% of children with a high caries experience indicates the need to maximize protection through the combined use of community water fluoridation and topical fluoride modalities.

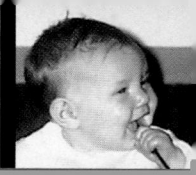

Dental fluorosis (see Chapter 7)

Recent reports in Australia, the USA and several other developed countries indicate a trend toward increasing levels of dental fluorosis. This trend is apparent in both fluoridated (a 33% increase) and non-fluoridated communities (a 10-fold increase) and is caused by the additive effects of the following:
- Fluoride supplements.
- Fluoride in the individual's diet (baby foods and beverages produced in fluoridated areas).
- Fluoride toothpastes.
- Topical applications during enamel formation.

The above levels may be sufficient to induce cosmetically noticeable fluorosis, even in areas without the addition of fluoridated water (Figure 2.1).

Definition

Dental fluorosis is a qualitative defect of enamel, resulting from an increase in concentration within the fluoride microenvironment of the ameloblasts during enamel formation. In its very severe form, however, it will also manifest as a quantitative defect.

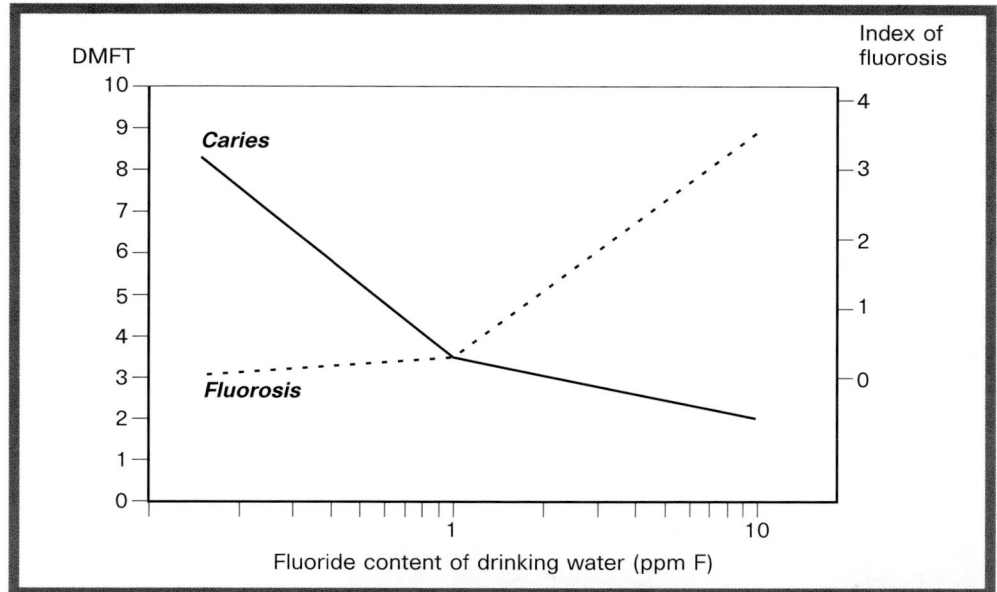

Figure 2.1 A comparison of decayed, missing and filled permanent teeth (DMFT) with Dean's index of fluorosis in relation to fluoride content of drinking water.

Threshold dose
Unknown, but suggested to be around 0.1 mg/kg body weight.

Manifestations
Dental fluorosis represents a continuum of changes in the enamel:
- Very mild—white flecks.
- Mild—fine white lines.
- Moderate—very chalky, opaque enamel which breaks apart soon after tooth eruption.
- Severe—mottling and loss of portions of the outer enamel.

As the fluoride content of water increases beyond 1 ppm (Figure 2.1) the increase in severity of fluorosis is greater than the decrease in caries.

Action of fluoride
- Production or composition of enamel matrix altered during ameloblastic secretory phase.
- Interference in initial calcification process caused by changes in ion-transport mechanisms.
- Ameloblast function may be affected and withdrawal of protein and water from calcified enamel becomes disrupted during the maturation phase.
- Fluoride toxicity itself may also affect nucleation and crystal growth in all stages of enamel formation, resulting in varying degrees of enamel porosity.

Because fluoride appears to affect the activity of the ameloblasts, excessive fluoride intake is of particular concern during the first 2–4 years of life when crowns of the maxillary incisor teeth are the most susceptible. Toothpastes have been identified as a significant source of fluoride for the young and in recent National

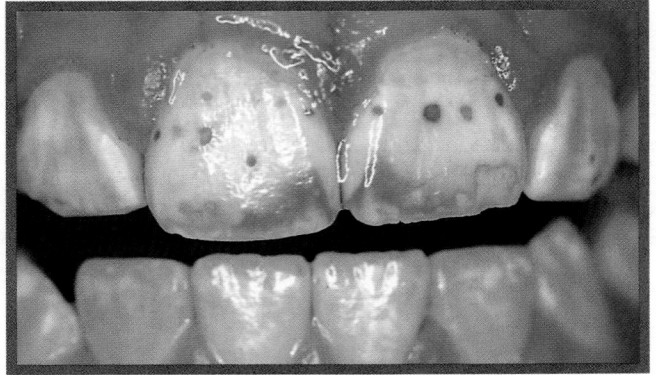

Figure 2.2 Moderate fluorosis caused by ingestion of toothpaste during infancy. Note that the brown mottling is secondary to tooth-surface wear and the acquisition of stains.

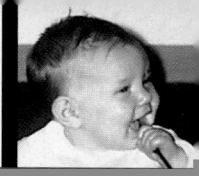

Health and Medical Research Council reviews, toothpastes account for a large percentage of ingested fluoride in young children, irrespective of the level of fluoride in the reticulated water system (see Table 2.1).

The greatest contribution, among infants, of fluoride exposure is from toothpaste ingestion. However, marked variations exist in the concentration of fluoride in infant formulas before reconstitution with water—a range of 0.9–2.8 ppm (see Table 2.2).

Table 2.1 Estimated fluoride ingestions of persons in fluoridated areas within Australia, excluding fluoride supplements and mouthrinses

	2-year-olds		Adults	
Body weight (kg)	12		75	
Daily fluoride from foods				
direct from foods (mg)	0.18–0.27		0.81–1.46	
during preparation/cooking (mg)	0.04–0.05		0.14–0.26	
Fluoride from water and beverages (mg)	0.28		1.10–1.89	
Fluoride from toothpaste (1000 ppm)				
amount of toothpaste used (g)	0.9		1.4	
% ingested 30%	30%		3–12%	
fluoride ingested per brushing (mg)	0.3		0.04–0.17	
Fluoride ingested per day (mg)	0.6		0.34	
Total fluoride (mg)	**1.10–1.20**		**2.13–3.95**	
Total fluoride (mg/kg)	0.09–0.10		0.02–0.04	
Summary of sources of ingested fluoride	**mg**	**%**	**mg**	**%**
Fluoride direct from food	0.22	19	1.13	37
Fluoride from all water sources	0.32	28	1.70	56
Fluoride from toothbrushing	0.60	53	0.21	7
Total	1.14	100	3.04	100

Source: Commonwealth Department of Health, Australia, 1985

43

Table 2.2 Mean fluoride concentration of infant formulae in Australia

	Fluoride concentration (ppm) of non-reconstituted powder/liquid	
Formula	Mean	Range
Enfamil	0.28	0.26–0.31
SMA	1.47	1.33–1.63
S 26	1.89	1.71–2.14
NAN	3.74	3.28–3.98
Digestelac	0.14	0.04–0.24
Enfalac	0.22	0.17–0.25
Lactogen	0.91	0.50–1.36
Delact	1.60	1.22–1.86
Pregestemil	2.83	2.60–3.24
Infasoy	0.32	0.14–0.45
Proso Bee (liquid)	0.68	0.66–0.70

Source: Silva and Reynolds. *Aust Dent J* 1996, **41**:37–42.

Topical fluorides

A lifetime protection against dental caries results from the continuous use of low-concentration fluoride. In addition to their use in caries prevention, topical fluorides may be used to control established carious lesions. This is effective for both adults and children.

The optimal concentration of fluoride throughout each day which, if present at both the tooth surface and in saliva, will control caries is approximately 0.1 ppm.

Factors that should be considered before committing to a fluoride regimen include:

- Caries risk—high, medium, low.
- Cariogenicity of the diet/oral clearance rate.
- Patient age and compliance.

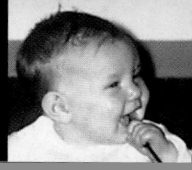

- Use of systemic and topical fluoride modalities.
- Water fluoridation levels.
- Existing medical conditions.
- Availability of fluoride modalities.

The use of fluoride toothpastes is the most feasible way of maintaining elevated fluoride concentrations at plaque–enamel interfaces.

Fluoride toothpastes

The use of fluoride toothpastes has led to a 25% reduction in the prevalence of caries in industrialized countries, with the greatest effect being observed on interproximal and smooth surfaces as well as newly erupted teeth.

Conventional toothpastes

- Contain approximately 1000–1100 ppm of fluoride (1 mg F/g paste).
- Added as sodium fluoride:
    sodium monofluorophosphate (MFP) or
    stannous fluoride.

All toothpastes have a similar effectiveness.

Fluoride mouth rinses

Studies showed that supervised fluoride-rinse programs reduce caries by 20–50%. Weekly 0.2% NaF and daily 0.05% NaF rinses were considered to be ideal public health measures.

The use of such rinses is now recommended, principally for those individuals with high caries risk or during times of increased caries susceptibility.

Daily rinses

- 0.02% acidulated phosphofluoride (APF).
- NaF (100 ppm).
- Partly acidulated solution of 0.04% NaF (200 ppm).

Weekly or fortnightly rinses

- 0.2% NaF (1000 ppm).

Indications

- Patients who are undergoing orthodontic treatment.
- Postirradiation xerostomia sufferers.
- Children unable to perform adequate toothbrushing.

Contraindications

- Not recommended for preschool-aged children.

Fluoride varnishes

Fluoride varnishes were originally developed to prolong contact times between fluoride and enamel with a view to increasing the formation of fluorapatite. Although fluoride varnishes firmly bind fluoride in enamel more than other topical fluoride preparations, the reduction of caries has been of the same order (approximately 30%).

Indications
- Hypersensitive areas.
- Newly erupted teeth.
- Arresting early caries.

Duraphat An alcoholic solution of natural varnishes containing 50 mg NaF/mL (2.5%—approximately 25 000 ppm fluoride).

This varnish remains on the teeth for up to 12 hours and there is still fixation of fluoride evident up to 48 hours after application.

Fluor Protector A silane fluoride varnish with a lower concentration of fluoride (0.8%) in a polyurethane lacquer.

With such highly concentrated fluoride products, great care must be taken to avoid overuse and ingestion. These products should not be used before the eruption of the permanent incisors.

Prophylaxis Prophylaxis is not routinely required before topical fluoride application, however, gross plaque should be removed. Fluoride uptake is not reduced by surface plaque and caries reduction can be achieved without cleaning the teeth before fluoride application. In fact, plaque can serve as a recycling reservoir for fluoride and allow access to enamel. Drying of the teeth before application facilitates adhesion and may also be beneficial for fluoride uptake.

Concentrated fluoride gels and solutions

APF gels Acidulated phosphate fluoride (APF) gels, containing 1.23% fluoride (12 300 ppm F) are used for professional applications and consist of a mixture of NaF, HF and orthophosphoric acid.
- Such highly concentrated fluoride gels should be limited to professional use and should not be dispensed for home use in children.
- The incorporation of a water-soluble polymer (i.e. sodium carboxymethyl cellulose) into aqueous APF produces a viscous solution that improves the ease of application using custom-made trays.

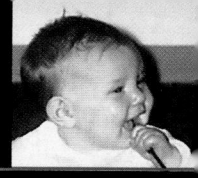

- Thixotropic gels in trays flow under pressure, so facilitating the penetration of the gel between teeth.
- APF gels are mainly used for the prevention of caries development.

Neutral 2.2% NaF
- NaF is preferred in cases of erosion, exposed dentine, carious dentine or where very porous enamel surfaces exist.
- It is chemically very stable, has an acceptable taste, is non-irritating to the gingiva and does not discolour teeth, composite resin or porcelain restorations as APF or stannous fluorides may.

Stannous fluoride SnF_2
- 10% Stannous fluoride is used to target local 'at-risk' surfaces of teeth such as deep fissures and pits.
- Rapid penetration of tin and fluoride into enamel and the formation of a highly insoluble tin–fluorophosphate complex coating on the enamel are the main mechanisms of its action. However, SnF_2 often produces discoloration of teeth and staining on margins of restorations, particularly in hypocalcified areas.
- 0.4% SnF_2 gel in a methylcellulose and glycerine base has proved effective in arresting root caries and has been incorporated into a synthetic saliva solution to reduce caries in postirradiation cancer patients.

Systemic fluorides

- Fluoride supplements (tablets and drops) have limited application as a public health measure but may be of benefit to individuals with a high risk of caries.
- Fluoride supplements are beneficial in reducing dental caries only among children in non-fluoridated communities, but this benefit is small.
- Clinical data demonstrating the caries preventive effects of prenatal fluoride supplements are limited.
- Overzealous use of supplements has been associated with dental fluorosis.
- If fluoride tablets are prescribed they should be chewed rather than swallowed whole. This will increase the topical benefit of fluoride.
- Research has identified that the period between 2 and 3 years is the time when maxillary incisor teeth are most susceptible to fluorosis. A new schedule (Table 2.3) has been proposed for supplementation of patients at high risk of developing caries who live in areas where the water supply contains less than 0.5 mg/L of fluoride. This schedule does not have an upper age limit, consistent with the view that individuals may continue to be of high caries susceptibility beyond 8 years of age.

Table 2.3 Daily fluoride supplement dosage schedule for persons considered at particularly high risk of caries

Age interval	Domestic water fluoride concentration	
	<0.3 mg/L	0.3–0.5 mg/L
6 months to <4 years	0.25	0
4 years to <8 years	0.5	0.25
8 years and above	1.0	0.50

Source: Proposed schedule from Discretionary Fluoride Committee, NH and MRC Australia (1992).
All supplements should be formulated as lozenges. Persons whose daily dose is 0.50 mg should consume one 0.25 mg tablet twice daily.

Considerations in fluoride therapy for infants and children

There is increasing recognition that young children may accumulate fluoride from a wide variety of dietary sources such as toothpastes, supplements and topicals. This can result in mild or very mild dental fluorosis. There is evidence to show that mild fluorosis will occur with ingestion of 2 mg or more of fluoride per day.

Minimizing risk
- Parents should supervise tooth brushing closely.
- Because clinical studies indicate that infants and children under 6 years of age ingest approximately 30% of toothpastes used, only use a 'pea-size' amount of toothpaste (smeared across the head of a child's toothbrush).
- Discourage swallowing of toothpaste.
- Parents should be encouraged to use low-fluoride toothpastes (400 ppm fluoride) for those infants living in optimally fluorided areas.

This level of fluoride, given that all other sources are constant and low, should result in a total fluoride intake that does not exceed the recommended upper limit of 0.07 mg/kg of body weight for a child between 2 and 7 years of age. Developing teeth are liable to experience mild fluorosis if 2 mg of fluoride or more is consumed per day, particularly in fluoridated communities.

Fluoride history
The initiation of an optimal fluoride regimen is dependent on a clear assessment of disease risk, age and the presence of other sources of fluoride.

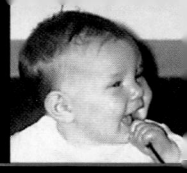

In assessing patients for additional systemic fluoride take note of such factors as:

Infants
- Breast-feeding—exclusively or partly.
- Formula use—milk or soy-based.
- Usual water source—reticulated, tank, bottled or bore.
- Baby foods used—home-made or commercial.
- Cultural feeding habits or practices.

Preschool children
- Usual water source.
- Is reticulated water fluoridated?
- Home prepared or commercial foods?
- Type of toothpaste used.
- Fluoride supplementation.
- Fluoride mouthrinses.
- Professionally applied fluoride.
- Current medications.
- Cultural feeding practices or preferences.

Water filters

Some water filters may remove fluoride, although this is mostly limited to those filters with reverse osmosis, distillation or ion exchange. Normal membrane filters will not remove a small ion such as fluoride.

To refluoridate filtered water Dissolve 1 mg of fluoride (i.e. one tablet) in 1 L of filtered water.

Recommended schedules for topical fluoridation

Low risk
Review of epidemiological data for Australia and overseas indicates that the twice-daily use of a toothpaste containing fluoride will prevent new caries development in approximately 80% of children, and an estimated 60–70% of adults.

Increased risk
Low-grade supplementation in cases of:
- Adolescent patients without access to fluoridated water.
- Patients temporarily at higher risk of caries (i.e. orthodontic patients before and during treatment).

Schedule
0.02% APF
or NaF daily mouthrinse.

Moderate caries rate
* one to two new lesions per year.

Schedule
* 0.05% neutral NaF mouthrinse daily
* or 0.2% neutral NaF mouthrinse weekly
* AND professional 1.23% APF topical applications every 3 months
* or professional 10% SnF_2 topical applications every 3 months.

High caries rate
* more than two new lesions per year.

Schedule
* Initial use of 0.2% neutral NaF mouthrinse daily and
* professional 1.23% APF topical applications every 3 months or professional 10% SnF_2 topical applications every 3 months.

Fluoride toxicity

Overwhelming evidence exists for the safety of fluorides at low concentration but high concentrations increase the possibility of toxic overdose. The first signs of fluoride overdose are enamel mottling while crippling bone fluorosis and acute toxicity occur at much higher doses. Reviews of fluoride benefits and risks, by the US Public Health Service, based on more than 50 human studies concluded that no evidence exists to show an association between fluoride and cancer. However, there is evidence of an increase in the prevalence of mild dental fluorosis.

Estimated probable toxic dose
* 5 mg F/kg of body weight.
* Gastrointestinal symptoms were noted following ingestion of 3–5 mg F/kg in young children and very frail adults.
* For a 10 kg child this corresponds to all the contents of a 45 g tube of toothpaste. Therefore, young children should not be allowed unsupervised access to fluoride toothpastes.

Certain lethal dose
* 32–60 mg F/kg of body weight.
Fatalities in children have been reported at doses of 16 mg F/kg of body weight.

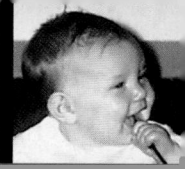

A number of concentrated topical preparations could provide such levels for young children if used in a single dose.

The inappropriate prescribing of home-fluoride treatments for very young children, particularly in nursing caries patients, is of concern. Concentrated fluoride products in excess of 1000 ppm should not be prescribed for home use.

Acute poisoning
- Cellular metabolism blocked.
- Inhibition of enolase in the glycolytic pathway.
- Interference with calcium metabolism.
- Nerve-impulse and conduction disorders.

Signs and symptoms
The clinical course in acute fluoride toxicity develops with alarming rapidity.

Generalized signs and symptoms
- Nausea and epigastric distress, often accompanied by vomiting.
- Excessive salivation, tearing, mucous discharges from the nose and mouth, and sweating.
- Headache.
- Diarrhoea.
- Generalized weakness.

Potentially lethal doses
- Myopathological signs.
- Spasm of the extremities, tetany and convulsions.
- Progressive failure of the cardiovascular system with a barely detectable pulse, hypotension and cardiac arrhythmias.
- Disturbances in electrolyte balance, particularly hypocalcaemia and hyperkalaemia.
- As respiration is depressed an accompanying respiratory acidosis progressively develops.
- Patient may become extremely disoriented before lapsing into unconsciousness.

Management
The treatment of acute fluoride toxicity is based on:
- An estimation of the amount of fluoride ingested.
- Minimizing further absorption.
- Removing fluoride from the body fluids.
- Supporting the vital signs.

If vomiting has not occurred spontaneously:
- Give as much milk as can be ingested or
- 5% calcium gluconate or calcium chloride orally.

While this immediate action is being taken, the hospital should be advised that a case of acute fluoride poisoning is in progress so that preparation for appropriate therapeutic intervention can be made.

It should be noted that while previous protocols advocated the use of an emetic such as syrup of ipecac, there has been a move away from encouraging vomiting because of the risk of aspiration of vomitus. Modern emergency room protocols advocate the use of activated charcoal in most poisonings.

Management by dosage

<5 mg/kg
- Give calcium orally (milk) and observe for a few hours.

5–15 mg/kg
- Empty stomach with emetic (ipecac syrup).
- Give calcium orally (milk, 5% calcium gluconate, calcium lactate).
- Admit to hospital and observe.

>15 mg/kg
- Admit to hospital immediately.
- Induce vomiting (syrup of ipecac or gastric lavage).
- Cardiac monitoring and life support.
- Intravenous calcium gluconate.

Calculation of fluoride ingestion
Example
- A 1000 ppm toothpaste contains 1 mg F/g toothpaste.
- A 400 ppm toothpaste contains 0.4 mg F/g toothpaste.

If a 2-year-old weighing 10 kg swallows 90 g of 0.76% MFP toothpaste (i.e. one tube of toothpaste):

1 mg/g × 90 g toothpaste/10 kg = 9 mg F/kg body weight

Treatment must be commenced.

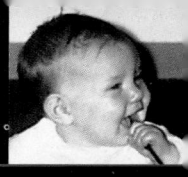

Table 2.4 Amount of toothpaste ingested to receive a probable toxic dose						
			Amount of 1000 ppm toothpaste (90 g tube = 90 mgF)		Amount of 400 ppm toothpaste (45 g tube = 18 mgF)	
Age of child	Average weight	Probable toxic dose	Weight	% tube	Weight	Tubes
2 years	12 kg	60 mg	60 g	66%	150 g	3
4 years	15 kg	75 mg	75 g	85%	188 g	4
6 years	20 kg	100 mg	100 g	over 1 tube	250 g	5

Probable toxic dose: 5 mg/kg

References

ATTWOOD D, BLINKHORN AS. Reassessment of the effect of fluoridation on cost of dental treatment among Scottish school children. *Community Dent Oral Epidemiol* 1989, **17**:79-82.
IADR Conference Report. Scientific update on fluoride and the public health. *J Dent Res* 1990, **69**:1343-1344.

Water fluoridation
NEWBRUN E. Effectiveness of water fluoridation. *J Public Health Dent* 1989, **49**:Special Issue 279-289.

Fluorosis
BELTRAN ED, SZPUNAR SM. Fluoride in toothpastes for children: suggestion for change. *Pediatr Dent* 1988, **10**:185-188.
LARSEN MJ, RICHARDS A, FEJERSKOV O. Development of dental fluorosis according to age at start of fluoride administration. *J Dent Res* 1985, **19**:519-527.
PENDRYS DG, STAMM JW. Relationship of total fluoride intake to beneficial effects and enamel fluorosis. *J Dent Res* 1990, **69**:Special Issue 529-538.
ROCK WP. Young children and fluoride toothpaste. *Br Dent J* 1994, **177**:17-20.
SZPUNAR SM, BURT BA. Trends in the prevalence of dental fluorosis in the United States: a review. *J Publ Health Dent* 1987, **47**:71-79.
World Health Organization. Report of a WHO expert committee on oral health Status and fluoride use. *Fluorides and Oral Health Technical Report Series No. 846.* Geneva: World Health Organization; 1994.

Fluoride supplementation

HOROWITZ HS. Perspectives on the use of prenatal fluorides. A symposium. *J Dent Child* 1981, **48**:100–133.

RIORDAN PJ. Fluoride supplements in caries prevention: a literature review and proposal for a new doseage schedule. *J Publ Health Dent* 1993, **53**:174–189.

Fluoride therapy

CLARKSON B FEJERSKOV O, SILVERSTONE LM, EKSTRAND J. Rational use of fluorides in caries prevention and treatment. In: Ekstand J, Fejerskov O, Silverstone LM, eds. *Fluoride in dentistry.* Copenhagen: Munksgaard; 1988: 277–288.

CRAIG GC. Towards a rational approach to topical fluoride therapy at the mixed dentition stage. *Int Dent J* 1981, **31**:121–123.

HEIFETZ SB, HOROWITZ HS. The amounts of fluoride in current fluoride therapies: safety considerations for children. *J Dent Child* 1984, **51**:257–267.

Further reading

EKSTAND J, FEJERSKOV O, SILVERSTONE LM, eds. *Fluoride in dentistry.* Copenhagen: Munksgaard; 1988.

WEI SHY, ed. *Clinical uses of fluoride.* Philadelphia: Lea and Febiger;1985.

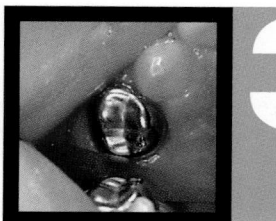
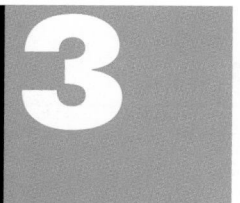

Dental caries and restorative paediatric dentistry

3

Contributors

Bernadette Drummond, Nicky Kilpatrick, Roland Bryant, James Lucas, Kerrod Hallett, Margarita Silva, Timothy Johnston, Joe Verco, Louise Brearley Messer

Dental caries

Dental caries is a multifactorial disease and the following four factors influence its progression.

Dental plaque

Plaque contains bacteria that are both acid-producing and can survive at low pH. *Mutans streptococci* are believed to be the most important bacteria in the initiation and progress of dental caries. Later, following enamel cavitation, lactobacilli become increasingly important. In the caries process, once the pH in plaque drops below a critical level (around 5.5), the acid produced begins to demineralize the enamel. This will last for 20 minutes or longer depending on the availability of substrate.

Substrates

Bacteria utilize fermentable carbohydrates for energy and the end-points of the glycolytic pathway in bacterial metabolism are acids. Sucrose is the fermentable carbohydrate most frequently implicated but it is important to remember that the bacteria can use all fermentable carbohydrates, including cooked starches. Although any carbohydrate causes the production of acid, it is the availability of glucose that drives bacterial metabolism to produce lactic acid rather than weaker by-products such as formate, acetoacetate and alcohols. Furthermore, the amount of fermentable carbohydrate is relatively unimportant, as even minute amounts of fermentable carbohydrate will be utilized immediately.

Host factors

Generally, caries is initiated in the enamel but it may also begin in dentine or cementum. Saliva plays several critical roles in the caries process. In removing substrate and buffering plaque-acid, saliva helps to slow the caries process and is critical in remineralization.

Time

When this acid challenge occurs repeatedly it may result in the collapse of enough enamel crystals to produce a visible cavity. Cavitation may take from months to years.

This means that in all mouths (and all mouths will contain some cariogenic bacteria) there is continual demineralization and remineralization of enamel. For the balance to be maintained there should be sufficient time between cariogenic challenges for the remineralization process to take place. When these challenges become too frequent, or occur when salivary flow is reduced, the rate of demineralization and subsequent tooth breakdown will increase.

Preventing dental caries

Preventing, reversing or at least slowing down dental caries generally involves altering one or more of the factors described above.

Diet modification

Although often given minimal attention by dental practitioners, diet is probably the single most important factor in determining caries risk.

Although some dietary habits have changed, the overall consumption of sugar has not altered over the last 50 years. Many foods, while not obviously cariogenic, contain hidden sugars and fermentable carbohydrates. Dietary histories may be useful in identifying those children at high risk. Achieving changes in dietary habits is extremely difficult and therefore advice must be individual, practical, and realistic.

- Frequency of intake is more important than overall quantity.
- 'Grazing' or 'snacking' between meals should be discouraged.
- The frequent consumption of soft drinks is a major problem, these being not only cariogenic but extremely erosive.
- Sweets etc. are useful rewards, but should be limited to mealtimes.
- Many foods labelled 'No added sugar' contain high levels of natural sugars.
- Dietary advice should not be all negative. Positive alternatives should be identified.

Fluorides

The principal mode of action of all fluorides (toothpastes, rinses, gels and community water fluoridation) is its topical effect on enamel. Even low concentrations of fluoride in the microenvironment around the teeth inhibit demineralization and promote remineralization of the tooth surface.

- The incorporation of systemically administered fluoride into developing enamel, however, is now thought to have a lesser role in increasing enamel resistance (see Chapter 2).

Fissure sealants

Even in communities with a low incidence of caries the pits and fissures are still susceptible. The most effective way to prevent pit and fissure caries is by fissure sealing (see 'Indications for the use of materials in paediatric dentistry' below).

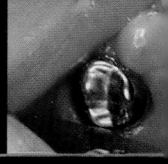

Plaque removal

Toothbrushing Toothbrushing should be regarded as topical fluoride application. In communities with water fluoridation, almost all caries occur in the pits and fissures and interproximally.

- It should be realized that the mechanical action of toothbrushing alone will not prevent caries as it does not remove plaque from the areas mentioned above. Children must be encouraged to adopt good brushing habits early and as a part of everyday hygiene.

Parents should be advised to begin cleaning their children's teeth from when they first erupt. Gauze or a face cloth on a finger, or a small very soft toothbrush may be used to remove the plaque. A smear of fluoride toothpaste should be used to give protection to the erupting teeth. It is beneficial for an adult to continue to assist with toothbrushing until the child is around 6 years old and has the dexterity to remove plaque effectively by themselves. Ideally, toothbrushing should be carried out twice a day and emphasis should be placed on brushing just before bed.

Flossing In the late preschool years, and early mixed dentition, the interproximal surfaces of the primary molars become more at risk of caries. Parents can be shown how to floss these areas when the teeth are in contact and especially if there are signs of demineralization. Older children should be taught to do this themselves and may find it easier to use one of the commercial floss holders.

Disclosing of plaque Children, their parents, and older patients find it difficult to know when they have effectively removed plaque from their teeth. Disclosing solutions and tablets are very useful for helping patients and parents to see and remove plaque more effectively (Figure 3.1).

Antimicrobials

Antibacterial mouthwashes have become part of the preventive dentistry regime in the past few years. Their role in caries prevention is limited; however, they may be useful in older children and in adolescents as an adjunct to plaque control. Their main role is in the management of high caries individuals and especially for those who are medically compromised. Systemic antimicrobials (antibiotics) cause significant alterations in oral microflora and have no use in caries prevention.

Determining patients at risk of dental caries

Before deciding what are the appropriate methods and products to use, or advise a patient to use, the patient's caries risk should be determined. This may be achieved by considering several aspects including the family background, the individuals themselves and the general oral environment.

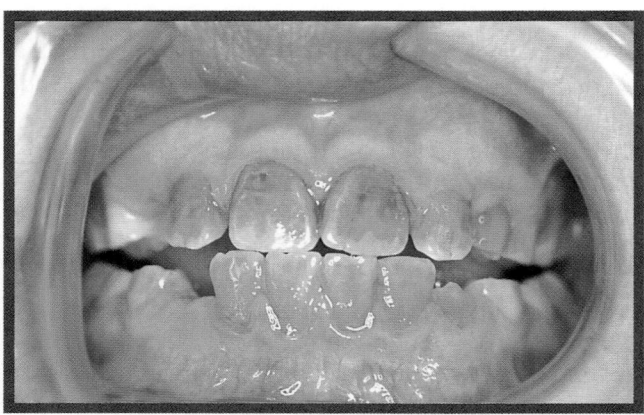

Figure 3.1 Disclosing plaque is an important part of teaching children about oral hygiene and educating parents.

Patient background
- Water fluoride levels.
- Epidemiology of caries, the caries susceptibility of the group to which the patient belongs.
- Ethnicity.
- Socioeconomic variables.

It is important to realize that these factors—especially the background factors—can only be a guide, but that they are important to consider when deciding what preventive measures to put in place for individual patients.

When the risk has been determined a preventive programme, incorporating the appropriate methods, can be used. A suggested approach is shown in Table 3.1

Individual characteristics
Age
- Different teeth sites are at risk at different ages.
- Teeth may be at particular risk in association with orthodontic treatment (Figure 3.2).

Medical history
- Frequent medication?
- Does medication alter saliva?
- Is medication sweetened with sucrose?

Diet
- Fermentable carbohydrate frequency?
- What is the patient's knowledge of foods with sugars?
- Protective foods (i.e. dairy foods)?

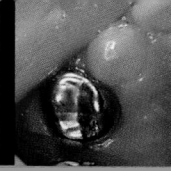

Table 3.1 Instituting preventive programs

	No caries	Early caries	Active caries
Risk	Low risk.	Medium risk: clinical/radiographic enamel demineralization.	High risk: new lesions at each recall, including risk behaviours.
Question	How to keep teeth caries-free?	How to reverse existing lesions and prevent new lesions?	How to reverse existing lesions and prevent new lesions?
Preventive plans			
Plaque	Check what the patient is doing. Either reinforce the behaviour or improve.	Disclose, have patient remove then prophy as appropriate. Advise fluoride floss or flossing with fluoride toothpaste.	Disclose, have patient remove then prophy as appropriate. Advise fluoride floss or flossing with fluoride toothpaste.
Diet	Reinforce and present good dietary habits. Check for recent changes, such as sports diets, and give advice.	Advise against frequent fermentable carbohydrate intake. Check for recent changes such as sports diets.	Check the dietary habits thoroughly with a 24-hour recording and/or a food-frequency questionnaire. Advise against frequent fermentable carbohydrate intake and check that the patient can identify these. Check for recent changes such as sports diet.
Fluoride	Check that it is being used appropriately.	Check that it is being used appropriately. Introduce daily mouthwashes if appropriate for age. Consider high-concentration fluorides for demineralized areas.	Check that it is being used appropriately. Introduce daily mouthwashes if appropriate for age. Apply concentrated fluoride treatments such as gels or varnishes.
Fissure sealants	Apply to deep retentive fissures only.	Fissure sealants to molars, especially those showing demineralization.	Ensure all open lesions are restored permanently or temporarily to reduce bacterial numbers. Fissure seal all molars and premolars.
Recall	12-monthly if there have been two 6-month periods of no caries.	6-monthly while there are signs of caries or risk remains.	6-monthly or 3-monthly with medically compromised or very high-risk children.

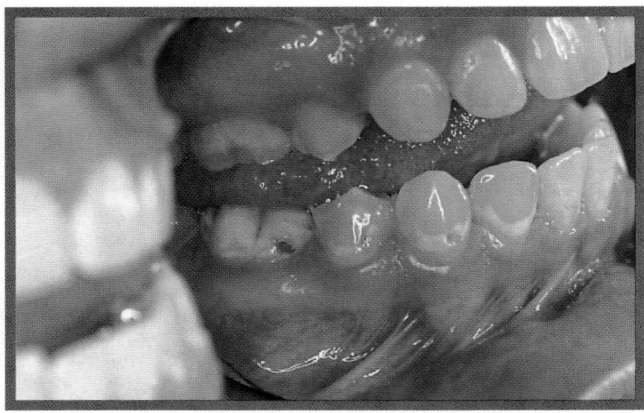

Figure 3.2 It is important to note that risk can change. A child who was previously free of caries has developed cervical lesions during orthodontic treatment.

- Are there risk habits?
- Nursing bottle in bed or at-will breast feeding?
- Frequent snacking in sports training?

Family history of caries
- Cariogenic bacteria are normally acquired from the parents and possibly other caregivers.

Intra-oral information
Caries history
- Past restorations or recurrent caries around existing restorations.
- Signs of demineralization.

Eruption of teeth
- Newly erupted teeth may be more at risk than those erupted for many years.

Oral health
- Plaque.
- How effective is the oral hygiene?
- Is plaque accumulation associated with demineralization?

Tooth morphology
- Deep fissures.
- Enamel hypoplasia or hypocalcification.
- Have the teeth been fissure sealed?

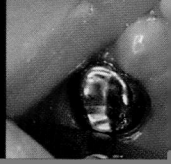

Radiographic signs
- Are lesions increasing in size?
- How fast are the lesions progressing?

Saliva
- Are the flow-rates and buffering capacity normal?

Restorative materials

Table 3.2 summarizes the main advantages and disadvantages to be considered with each material.

Amalgam
Historically, dental amalgam is the most popular restorative material. Its main advantage is that it is relatively economical and simple to use. Possibly the biggest problem associated with its use is the recent upsurge in public opinion concerning its safety. In Scandinavia, amalgam has been banned for use in children and restrictions are planned on its use in permanent teeth. The rationale for these restrictions is based upon environmental concerns rather than concerns over amalgam toxicity. Nevertheless, the dental profession may be forced into using alternatives to amalgam by a combination of public opinion and legislation.

Composite resins
The introduction of resin-based composites (along with photopolymerization) has revolutionized clinical dentistry. Although not of prime importance in the management of caries in the posterior primary dentition, the aesthetic benefits of composites have made them popular. The problems of resistance to wear, water absorption and polymerization contraction, however, have meant that the use of composite resins in posterior permanent teeth does have its limitations. Nonetheless, they may have a role to play in the restoration of the primary dentition, which is itself subject to greater wear than the permanent dentition. In addition, the bond of composite to dentine remains a problem and the actual clinical procedure is technique-sensitive.

Stainless-steel crowns
Stainless-steel crowns (SSCs) are preformed extracoronal restorations that are particularly useful in the restoration of grossly broken down teeth, primary molars that have undergone pulp therapy, and hypoplastic primary or permanent teeth. They are also indicated when restoring the dentition of children at high risk of caries, particularly those having treatment under general anaesthesia.

Glass–ionomers

One of the most significant advances in contemporary paediatric dental practice has been the development of glass–ionomers (GIs). The recent introduction of several new materials has given rise to new nomenclature.

Glass–ionomer cements (GICs) A glass–ionomer cement is one that consists of a basic glass and an acidic water-soluble powder which sets by an acid–base reaction between the two components.

Table 3.2 Advantages and disadvantages of materials used in paediatric dentistry

	Advantages	Disadvantages
Amalgam	Simple Quick Cheap Technique insensitive Durable	Not adhesive Requires mechanical retention in cavity Environmental and occupational hazards Public concerns
Composite	Adhesive Aesthetic Reasonable wear properties Command set	Technique sensitive Rubber dam required Problem of secondary caries diagnosis Expensive
Glass–ionomer cement	Adhesive Aesthetic Fluoride leaching	Long setting time Brittle Susceptible to erosion and wear Radiolucent
Resin-modified glass–ionomer cement	Adhesive Aesthetic Command set Simple to handle	Some are radiolucent Unknown durability Water absorption
Polyacid-modified composite resin	Adhesive Aesthetic Command set Simple to handle Radiopacity	Unknown durability Water absorption
Stainless-steel crowns	Very durable Protect and support remaining tooth structure Extensive tooth preparation Patient cooperation required	Extensive tooth preparation Patient cooperation required

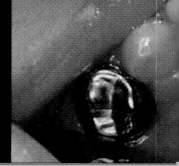

Resin-modified glass–ionomer cement A resin-modified glass–ionomer (RMGI) cement is a glass–ionomer/resin hybrid that retains significant acid–base reaction in its overall curing process and thus will set in the dark. These materials have two setting reactions:
1. The acid–base reaction between glass and polyacid.
2. A light-activated, free-radical polymerization of methacrylate groups of the polymer.

A third type of RMGI calls itself a 'tri-cured' material. It has three setting reactions:
1. The acid–base reaction between glass and polyacid.
2. A light-activated, free-radical polymerization of methacrylate groups of the polymer.
3. A dark-cure, free-radical polymerization of methacrylate groups.

The potential advantage of this material is that it will continue to cure in the depth of the cavity after the light source has been removed. Only one proprietary example of this is currently available.

Polyacid-modified composite resin (PMCR) Polyacid-modified composite resins are materials that contain either or both essential components of a GIC, but are not water-based and therefore no acid–base reaction can occur. As such, they will not set in the dark and these materials cannot strictly be described as GICs.

Restoration of the primary dentition

Choice of material

The choice of material to use in a given situation is not always simple and should not be based merely on technical considerations. Factors other than durability may be equally important in the choice of material, particularly in children.

Age The age of a child will influence their ability to cooperate with procedures such as rubber dam and local anaesthesia. The age of the child will also dictate for how long a restoration is required to remain satisfactory. A restoration in a first primary molar in a 9-year-old child does not require the same durability as one in a first permanent molar in a 6-year-old child or a second primary molar in a 4-year-old.

Caries risk Restorations placed in a child considered to be at high risk of caries may need to have slightly different objectives to those in a low-risk child. Although the use of a fluoride-releasing material has obvious preventive advantages, GIs may not be the most appropriate choice in a mouth that is at high risk of further acid attack. SSCs involve a significant amount of tooth destruction but this may be justified if it eliminates the need to re-treat in the future. Alternatively, GIs have a useful role to play in initial caries control in cases of rampant caries.

Cooperation of the child Many young children have behaviour that is not conducive to perfect, textbook, cavity preparation and restoration. In these cases highly technique-sensitive procedures are inappropriate. A more forgiving restoration such as an amalgam that can tolerate a certain amount of moisture contamination, without detriment to its longevity, may be suitable. The use of RMGIs in the management of caries in anterior primary teeth may be an excellent method of slowing the carious process and temporarily restoring aesthetics in a 2-year-old child without recourse to general anaesthesia. By the age of 3 or 4 years, the child may be able to cope with more definitive treatment with composite and strip crowns.

Restoration of primary anterior teeth

Composite resin-strip crowns
Composite is the material of choice for the restoration of primary anterior teeth. The use of anterior strip crowns with composite resins will provide a good aesthetic and durable restoration.

Method
1. Local anaesthesia and rubber-dam isolation should be used if possible. Alternatively, because of age and poor cooperation of young children, the restorative work may be completed under general anaesthesia.
2. Select the correct celluloid-crown form based upon the mesiodistal width of the teeth.
3. Remove the caries using a slow-speed round burr.
4. Reduce the incisal height by around 2 mm, prepare interproximal slices and place a labial groove at the level of gingival and middle-third of the crown (Figure 3.3). Use a high-speed tapered diamond or tungsten carbide burr.
5. Protect the exposed dentine with a GI liner (if the lesions are very deep, then a calcium hydroxide liner may be required).
6. Trim the crown-form and pierce two holes in the incisal corners with a sharp explorer.
7. Etch the enamel for 20 seconds, wash and dry.
8. Apply a thin layer of bonding resin and cure for 20 seconds and ensure all surfaces are bonded equally.
9. Fill crown-form with the appropriate shade of composite and seat with gentle, even, pressure allowing excess to exit freely. The use of small wedges may be helpful in avoiding interproximal excess.
10. Light-cure each aspect (labially, incisally and palatally) equally.
11. Remove the celluloid crown gently and adjust form and finish with either composite finishing burrs or Soflex discs.
12. Check occlusion once the rubber dam is removed.

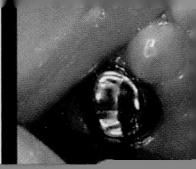

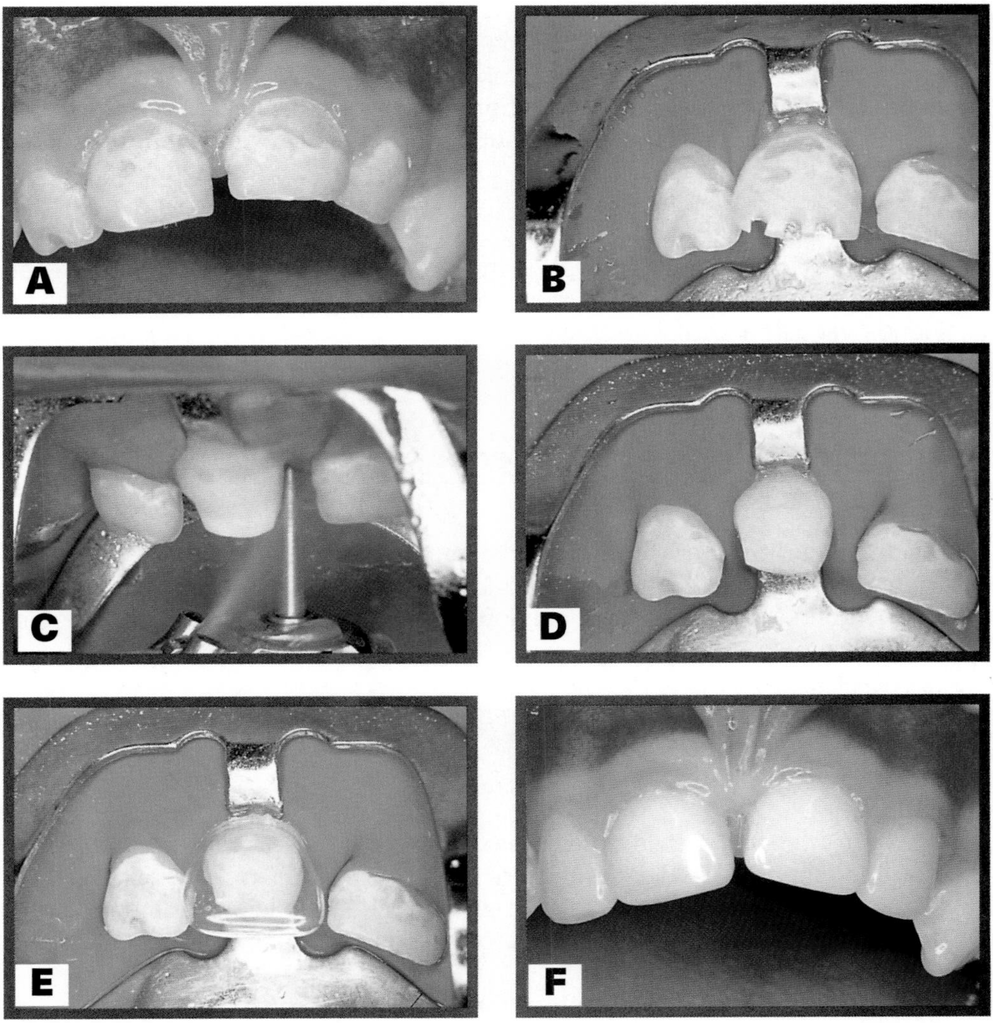

Figure 3.3 Placement of anterior-strip crowns on the primary incisors. **A** Bottle caries affecting upper anterior teeth. **B** Initial reduction of incisal edge of tooth 51 under rubber dam. Reduction guides have been used to ensure the correct amount of incisal-edge removal. **C** Proximal reduction is achieved using a high-speed tapering diamond. **D** This reduction also allows interproximal caries removal. The final preparation is shown. **E** Trial fitting of the cellulose acetate-strip crown which is then filled with composite resin. The tooth is etched, washed and dried; bonding resin applied and cured; and the strip crown placed. **F** Final restoration after polishing. (Courtesy Dr T Johnson.)

Interproximal stripping

Stripping of interproximal enamel may be used occasionally for minimal caries in anterior primary teeth. Opening of the contact points allows saliva and fluoride to arrest the carious process, even when the caries involve dentine. This is, however, an unaesthetic alternative. It goes without saying that the initiating cause, such a nursing-bottle habit, must be eliminated.

Method
- The contact points are removed with a long tapering diamond or tungsten carbide burr and a topical fluoride applied to the enamel and dentine. A fluoride varnish is useful for these cases.
- Regular follow up is required.

Restoration of primary posterior teeth

Amalgam

The use of dental amalgam to restore primary molars is common and is supported by evidence from clinical trials. Clinical studies, evaluating the durability of dental amalgam in primary molars, have laid down the benchmarks against which other restorations should be judged.

Success The success rate for class-II amalgam restorations in primary molars has been reported as between 70% and 80%.

Indications
- Amalgam is useful in children who are at moderate caries risk or who are not totally cooperative, i.e. where moisture control is a problem.
- It is appropriate for the restoration of early to moderate interproximal lesions.
- There is limited indication for the use of amalgam in class-I cavities.

Method for class-II amalgam restoration
1. Use local anaesthesia and rubber-dam isolation.
2. Complete the occlusal portion of cavity using a small pear-shaped or round diamond burr in a high-speed handpiece. The occlusal outline should not extend into all the fissures but needs to incorporate a small isthmus and a dovetail for retention (Figure 3.4).
3. Extend the cavity into the proximal area by gently proceeding gingivally until the contact point is broken. Buccolingually the cavity should extend so that a tip of an explorer can just reach the restoration margins.
4. Deeper caries should be removed using a slow-speed round burr.
5. Bevel the floor of the cavity at the junction of the axial wall and occlusal floor to increase the strength of the restoration. One of the most common sites of

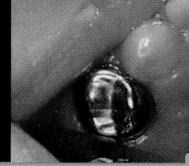

failure of the class-II amalgam is at the isthmus, which probably results from insufficient bulk of amalgam to withstand occlusal forces (Figure 3.5).

6. In deep lesions a calcium-hydroxide liner should be placed, whereas in moderate lesions a light-cured GI liner is appropriate over the whole area of dentine.
7. Adapt a matrix band to the circumference of the tooth. A narrow curved brass T band is very useful for this procedure particularly if back-to-back restorations are being placed. Both the Siqveland and Tofflemire matrix bands are adequate for single restorations. Wedging is essential for maintaining a good contact point.
8. Insert the amalgam incrementally, starting with the proximal box, using a small plugger to ensure good condensation in all the line angles.
9. Slightly overfill the cavity and carve the occlusal form using a small ball-ended burnisher and cleoid–discoid carver. An explorer is useful for creating the form of the marginal ridge.
10. Remove the matrix band carefully and pass a length of floss between the contact point to remove any debris.
11. The occlusion must be checked once the rubber dam has been removed.

Glass–ionomers

Glass–ionomer cements have an increasingly important role to play in the management of carious lesions in primary molars, because of their adhesive and fluoride-leaching properties.

Success

- The failure rate of GICs is higher than amalgam (33% over 5 years compared with 20% for amalgam).
- The average survival time for a GIC has been reported as 33 months. This may be considered satisfactory if it can be achieved with minimal destruction of sound tooth tissue and reduce the need to use local anaesthesia.

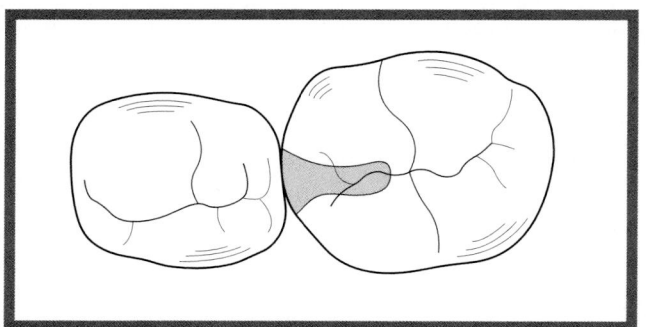

Figure 3.4 The modified outline-form of a class-II amalgam for primary molars.

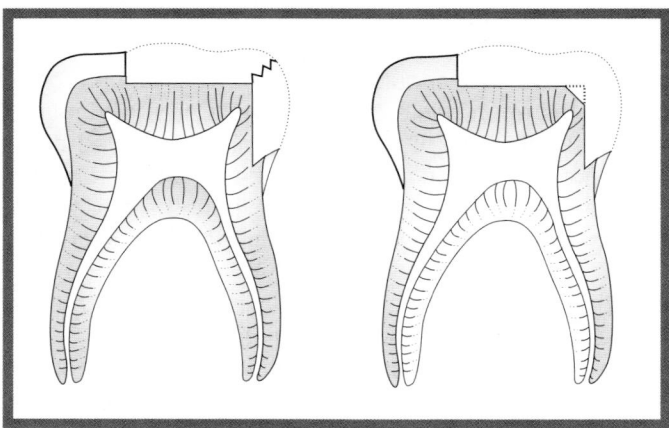

Figure 3.5 Bevelling of the axiopulpal-line angle increases the bulk of amalgam at the narrow isthmus and reduces the chance of fracture.

- The incidence of secondary caries is reduced around the fluoride-releasing materials.
- The use of PMCRs such as Dyract (Dentsply) shows considerable potential, particularly in terms of handling characteristics and radio-opacity. However, their limited fluoride-leaching ability may reduce the preventive advantage of the GICs and RMGIs. Early 2-year results would suggest that Dyract itself may be as durable as existing materials.

Indications
- Because of their lack of strength, GICs should not be used in large restorations that are to be subject to significant occlusal load.
- Class-I and limited class-II lesions.

Method for a class-I glass–ionomer restoration
1. Local anaesthesia may not always be necessary; however, rubber dam isolation should be used where possible.
2. The outline of the cavity should follow the extent of the carious lesion. There should be no extension for prevention.
3. Remove all soft caries using a slow round burr or hand instruments. Be aware of the large pulp chamber as it is easy to expose the pulp of a primary molar.
4. Pre-condition the dentine using 10% polyacrylic acid for 10 seconds, washed and dried.
5. When using encapsulated materials, ensure that the capsules are compressed for at least 3 seconds to facilitate adequate mixing of the powder and liquid components. Having mixed for 10 seconds in the amalgamator, dispense the first 3–4 mm of the mixed materials as this is often unsatisfactory. Place the remainder directly in to the cavity.

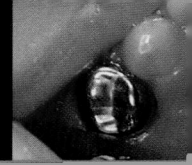

6. Once a conventional GIC has been placed in to the cavity it is compressed with a ball burnisher—the use of a small piece of 'food wrap' over the unset material prevents it from sticking to the instrument. The RMGIs should be placed and polymerized incrementally.
7. The final restoration must be protected from moisture contamination. This is best achieved by the placement of a thin layer of unfilled resin over the surface and polymerizing for 20 seconds. In young children with behaviour management problems, the use of Vaseline rather than unfilled resin may be appropriate.
8. The occlusion should be checked on removal of the rubber dam.

Modified class-II restorations using glass–ionomers Resin-modified glass-ionomers and PMCRs may be used for the restoration of interproximal carious lesions in primary molars. The method of cavity preparation is similar to that for the class-II amalgam restoration except that a small occlusal dovetail is not usually necessary but may be placed if resistance to displacement is required, particularly in the distal aspect of first primary molars. Alternatively, additional retention to minimal proximal cavities can be achieved by placing retention grooves into the dentine using very small (size 1/2) round burrs (Figure 3.6).

Composite resins
In primary molars composite is a satisfactory restorative material.

Indications Class-I or class-II cavities in children with good cooperation and low caries rates.

Success Clinical studies would suggest that class-II composite restorations in primary molars are only moderately durable, with one study reporting less than 40% success after 6 years.

Method For class-II lesions, the cavity design needs to be modified slightly from that described for amalgam in that a bevel should be prepared around the occlusal margins for additional adhesion to enamel. The biggest problem encountered with composite restorations is the integrity of the bond at the depth of the proximal box. Placement of composite is technically difficult and highly sensitive to moisture contamination. Placement of a GI liner over the dentine not only ensures a good bond at the base of the cavity, reducing microleakage, but also provides fluoride release locally. The use of rubber dam and incremental placement of composite in the proximal box may reduce handling and polymerization contraction problems.

In summary, composite is probably overly expensive and technique-sensitive without providing significant improvement in durability to make it a viable alternative to amalgam.

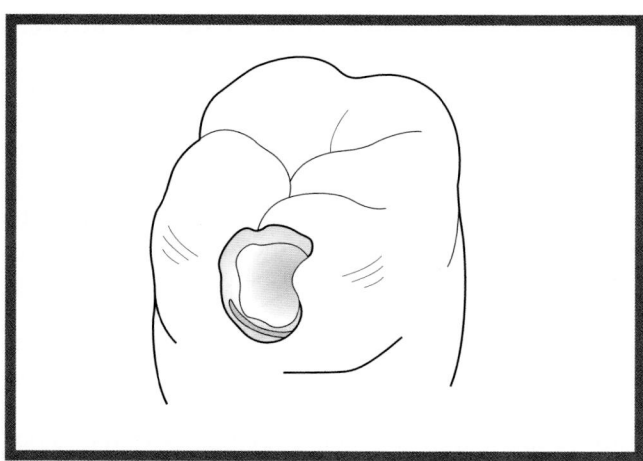

Figure 3.6 Modified class-II cavity design for the placement of RMGIs.

Stainless-steel crowns

Indications Stainless-steel crowns are preformed extracoronal restorations that are particularly useful in the restoration of:

- Grossly broken-down teeth.
- Primary molars that have undergone pulp therapy.
- Hypoplastic primary or permanent teeth.
- Dentitions of children at high risk of caries, particularly those having treatment under general anaesthesia.

Success Stainless-steel crowns undoubtedly provide the most durable restoration in the primary dentition with survival times in excess of 40 months. They are relatively expensive in relation to both time and money in the short term. However, the rate at which these restorations need to be replaced is low (3% compared with 15% replacement rate for class-II amalgam restorations). This makes them economically more attractive over the long term. They may, however, be considered unaesthetic and require a significant amount of tooth preparation and invariably local anaesthesia.

Method Irrespective of whether the tooth to be restored is vital or non-vital, local anaesthesia should be used when placing an SSC because of the soft-tissue manipulation. Rubber dam, although sometimes difficult to place in the broken-down dentition, should be used where possible.

1. Restore the tooth using a restorative type of GIC prior to preparation for the SSC (Figure 3.7A & B).
2. Reduce the occlusal surface first by about 1.5 mm using a flame-shaped or tapered diamond burr. Uniform occlusal reduction will facilitate placement of the crown without interfering with the occlusion (Figure 3.8).

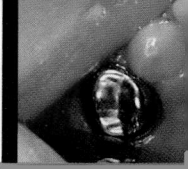

3. Using a fine, long, tapered diamond burr, held slightly convergent to the long-axis of the tooth, cut interproximal slices mesially and distally. The reduction should allow a probe to be passed through the contact area (Figure 3.8).
4. Little buccolingual reduction is needed unless there is a prominent Carabelli's cusp etc. However, such reduction should be kept to a minimum as these surfaces are important for retention (Figure 3.7C).
5. The appropriate size of precontoured crown is chosen by measuring the mesiodistal width (Ion Ni–Cro crowns are the simplest to use).
6. A trial fit is carried out before cementation. It is important that the crown should sit no more than 1 mm subgingivally. If there is excessive blanching of the gingival tissues the length of the crown should be reduced. The margins should be smoothed with a white stone.
7. Cement the crown with a GI- or polycarboxylate cement. If the crown has been built up before the placement of the crown, a GI-luting cement may be used,

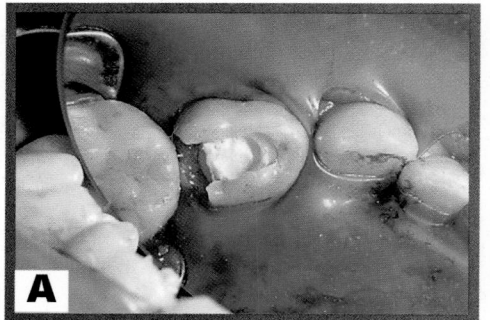
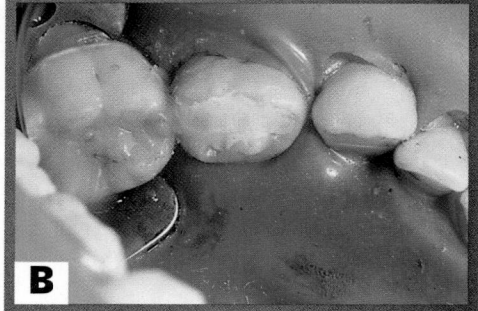
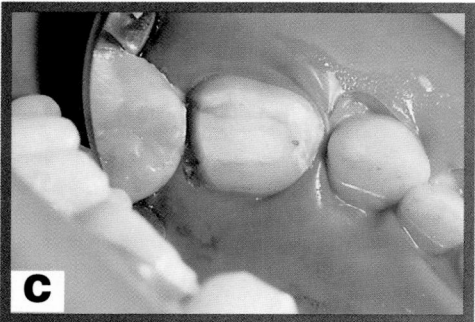
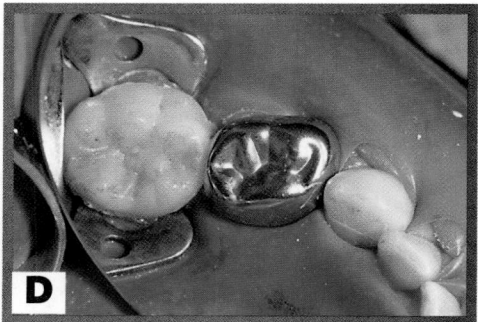

Figure 3.7 **A** Placement of a SSC after a pulpotomy. The IRM base has been covered with a GIC **B**, which has been used to rebuild the crown before crown preparation. **C** This has been cut back interproximally to remove contacts and the occlusal height reduced by 1.5 mm. **D** The completed restoration should last the lifetime of the tooth.

otherwise a restorative GIC should be used. Care should be taken to hold the crown as they are easily dropped during placement. Excess cement should be wiped away and a layer of Vaseline placed around the margins during the setting period (approximately 3 minutes, see Figure 3.7D).

Management of nursing caries

Nursing or bottle caries describes a condition of rampant caries found in young children feeding from a bottle at night. The reported prevalence ranges from 2.5% to 15%.

Characteristics
- Rampant caries affecting the maxillary anterior teeth (Figure 3.9).
- Lesions appear later on posterior teeth both maxillary and mandibular.
- Canines are affected less than first molars because of later eruption.

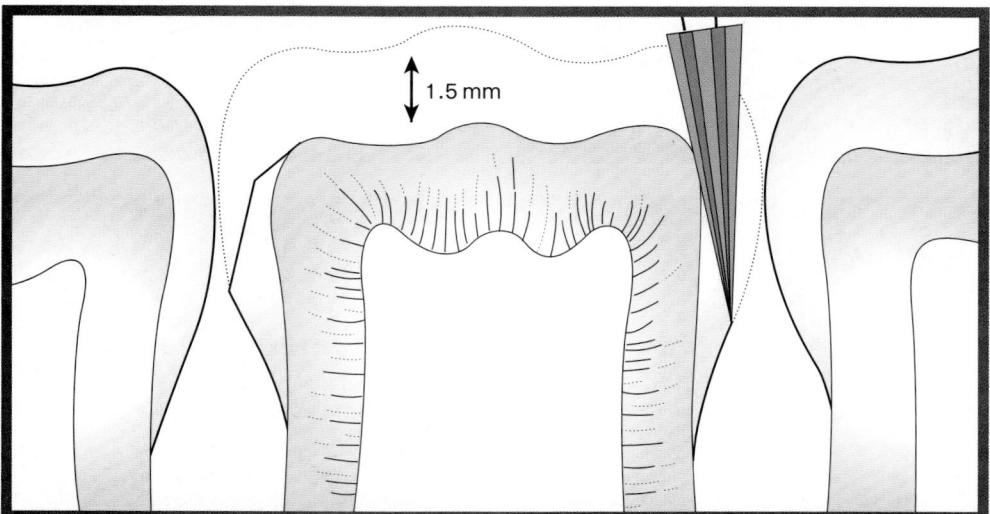

Figure 3.8 Coronal and proximal preparation required for the placement of a SSC. Note that in the proximal areas there is a smooth contour without any ledge or step. Any such step will cause great difficulty in seating the crown.

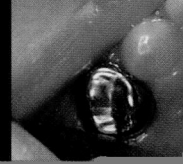

- Mandibular anterior teeth are unaffected because of salivary flow and position of tongue.
- Bottle is often used as a pacifier to get infant to sleep.
- Bottle caries occurs in all socioeconomic groups and as such often reflects the social dynamics of the family. Children who are difficult sleepers or have colic are often pacified with a bottle. The bottle can contain any liquid with fermentable carbohydrate, even milk. Commonly, vitamin-C drinks and juices are used.
- This pattern of caries may also occur with prolonged at-will breast feeding.

Aetiology
- Long periods of exposure to cariogenic substrate. The teat is held next to the palatal surfaces of the upper anterior teeth for up to 8 hours.
- Low salivary flow rate at night, and reduced buffering.

Management
- Cessation of habit.
- Fluoride application.
- Buildups of restorable teeth. This may involve GIC, composite resin-strip crowns and SSCs.
- Extractions if required. Loss of the upper anterior teeth will not result in space loss if the canines have erupted. Speech will develop normally.

It is important to give appropriate advice to the family about bottle caries. Blame should never be attributed; in many situations the condition has arisen out of ignorance, misinformation, or in frustration of coping with a sleepless infant. Elimination of the habit can be achieved by gradually reducing the amount of sugar in the bottle by diluting with water. This can be done over several weeks. Alternatively, some parents find it easier to remove the bottle immediately.

- Treatment under general anaesthesia is often required for small children.

Management of occlusal caries in permanent teeth

Of great importance is the preservation of tooth structure. Over the past decade, papers by Elderton and others have highlighted the deficiencies of the use of accepted concepts such as 'extension for prevention'. The placement of large amalgam restorations undermines the marginal ridges and weakens cusps which will eventually fracture. The tooth then requires larger restorations, with the risk of pulp disease, root-canal therapy and finally full coverage restoration. There must be a different approach to the management of permanent teeth that have not been previously restored compared with those teeth which require replacement of restorations.

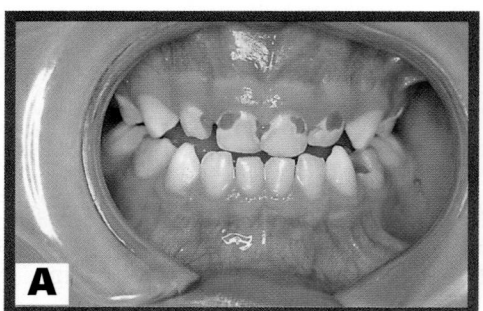

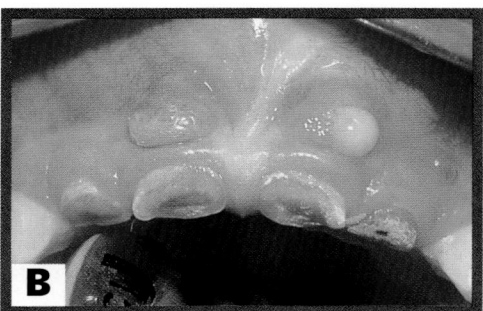

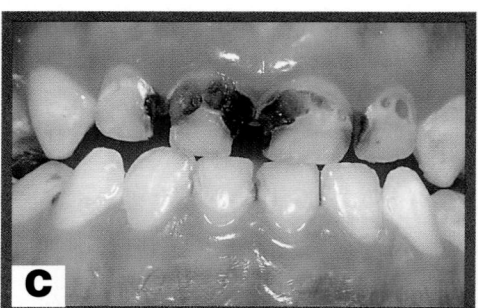

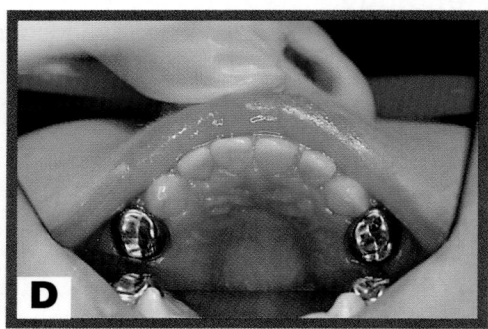

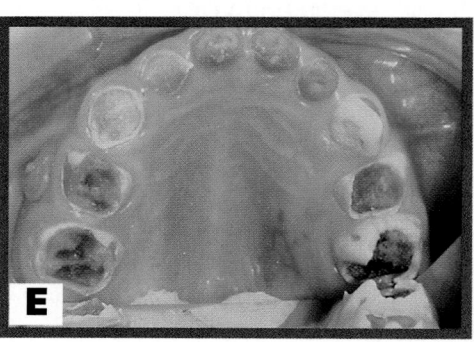

Figure 3.9 Bottle caries showing the characteristic pattern of decay. **A** The upper anterior teeth and the molars are affected but the lower anterior teeth are spared. **B** These upper anterior teeth are non-vital and require extraction. The abscesses will heal once the teeth are removed. **C** Bottle caries in an older child showing arrested caries. By removal of the cause the decay has been allowed to stop. **D** Restoration of a case of bottle caries with composite-strip crowns and SSCs on the first primary molars. **E** Gross caries in the primary dentition of a child, with a cardiac defect, living in a fluoridated community. Every tooth was carious and a full clearance was performed.

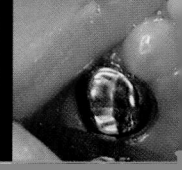

Amalgam is an inappropriate material for the restoration of early lesions on the occlusal surfaces of permanent teeth. Here, the preventive resin restoration is more desirable. Minimal tooth structure is lost in cavity preparation and has the advantage that the occlusal table is protected by a fissure sealant (Figure 3.10).

Fissure sealants

In fluoridated communities throughout Australasia, where the average DMFT (decayed, missing and filled permanent teeth) is less than 2.0, the majority of caries occur in the pits and fissures of the first permanent molar teeth. These can only be prevented by fissure sealants. Preservation of tooth structure is of vital importance. Once a cavity has been cut, a tooth will require lifelong dental care, as no restoration lasts a lifetime. It has been suggested that only those children who are at moderate risk of caries should be given sealants. Ripa (1988) believed, however, that because nearly 90% of children up to 18 years have some caries (mainly in the first permanent molars), then all teeth should be sealed. As mentioned previously, treatment should only be prescribed according to the individual needs of each patient.

Indications

- All permanent molars in children at medium or high risk of caries (see Table 3.1). Premolars should be sealed for those children at high risk.
- For those children at low risk, only those fissures that are deep and retentive need sealants.
- Primary posterior teeth for children at risk high of caries.
- The main benefit rests with those teeth which have been erupted for less than 3 years, thus a first molar in a caries-free 14-year-old child need not be fissure sealed. As mentioned previously, however, risk status can change and as the procedure is non-invasive it is prudent to seal more teeth rather than less.

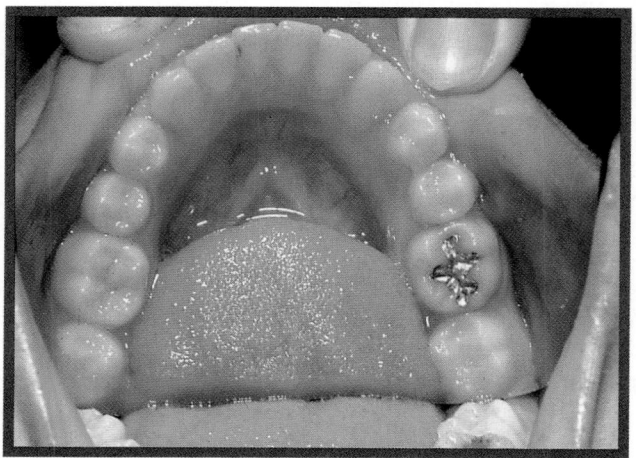

Figure 3.10 While this amalgam restoration has been well placed, it is an inappropriate restoration for a 20-year-old patient whose only caries is an incipient lesion on the occlusal surface. This amalgam will weaken the marginal ridges and supporting cusps and compromise the tooth in the long term. A preventive resin restoration is a much better alternative.

Sealant material
- Although some studies show differences, there appears to be no strong statistically significant evidence to favour light-cured over chemically cured sealants or either opaque, clear or coloured fissure sealants at this time.
- Sealants should be opaque so that they can be detected by other clinicians who might see the patient. Clear sealants show stains in the fissures that are most probably inactive caries. Other clinicians upon seeing these stains may choose to cut a cavity into a sound tooth, defeating the whole purpose of the sealant.
- Current studies support resin-based sealants over GI sealants which do not have as good retention.
- Glass–ionomer may be useful, however, in high caries-active individuals as temporary sealants until the teeth have erupted sufficiently to allow conventional fissure sealing. The main problem with the use of GICs as fissure sealants is the brittleness of the material when used in thin section over the occlusal surface. However, in one Norwegian study, despite very low retention rates, the incidence of caries under GIC sealants was significantly lower in the long term than under the resin-based sealants. It has been suggested that either the GIC is retained in the depths of the fissures at a microscopic level or that fluoride from the GIC, is taken up by the surrounding enamel so increasing the resistance of the fissure walls to demineralization.

Method
1. A recent set of bite-wing radiographs is mandatory to check for any dentinal caries. Isolate the tooth with rubber dam. If the tooth cannot be isolated then fluoride should be applied (using a fluoride varnish, for example) and one should wait 6 months until the tooth has erupted sufficiently to place a fissure sealant.
2. Clean the occlusal surface with oil-free pumice and water and run the probe through the fissures to assess their depth. If there is doubt as to the integrity of the pits or fissures they may be widened with a fine diamond burr. If this is the case then a filled resin should be used, otherwise unfilled resins are adequate.
3. Etch the tooth with gel etchant for 30 seconds and dry with copious water and air irrigation for 20 seconds.
4. If the tooth is contaminated it should be re-etched for 15 seconds.
5. Apply a thin coat of sealant to the pits and fissures making sure to include the buccal extension on lower molars and the palatal groove in upper molar teeth. Apply the white polymerization light for 20 seconds.
6. Remove the rubber dam and check the occlusion.

Preventive resin restoration
Composite is the material of choice for the treatment of early occlusal caries in permanent teeth. The development of preventive resin restoration has changed the

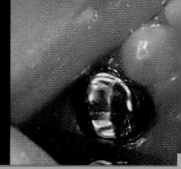

management of occlusal caries dramatically in young patients.

Indications
- Enamel-only lesions.
- Incipient lesions just into dentine.
- Small class-I lesions.

Success The durability of preventive resin restoration has been proved to be as good as occlusal-amalgam restorations and can be achieved with significantly less removal of sound tooth tissue.

Method for preventive resin restoration
1. Use local anaesthesia and rubber-dam isolation.
2. With a small high-speed diamond burr make access into the questionable fissure.
3. Remove the carious dentine. Although it is important not to remove more enamel than necessary, it is essential to have adequate access to the underlying dentine to be certain of complete caries removal. Unsupported enamel need not be removed if access and vision are clear. The cross-section outline most closely resembles a teardrop shape (Figure 3.11).
4. Deeper dentinal caries should be removed using a slow-speed round burr.
5. Place a GI liner over the dentine extending it up to the amelodentinal junction and light cure for 40 seconds.
6. Gel etchant is placed for 20 seconds on the enamel margins and occlusal surface, washed and dried. It is not necessary to etch the liner; sufficient roughening of the surface of the GIC will result from the washing process.
7. Place a thin layer of bonding resin into the cavity and cure for 20 seconds. Do not place too much resin as pooling will occur and reduce the integrity of the bond.
8. Incrementally fill and polymerize the cavity with hybrid composite resin until it is level with the occlusal surface.
9. Flow opaque unfilled fissure sealant over the restoration and the entire occlusal fissure pattern and cure for 20 seconds. There is no need to re-etch the occlusal surface before placing the fissure sealant.
10. Remove the rubber dam and check the occlusion.

Tunnel restorations
The tunnel restoration was first described in the early 1980s as a conservative method of cavity preparation. By gaining access to the proximal carious lesion from the occlusal surface it is possible to leave the marginal ridge intact (Figure 3.12). In this way the final restored tooth may be more resistant to fracture than a conventionally restored class-II lesion, although this concept has been recently questioned by Papa *et al.* (1993). In addition, preserving the marginal ridge reduces the problems often encountered when attempting to restore the contact area.

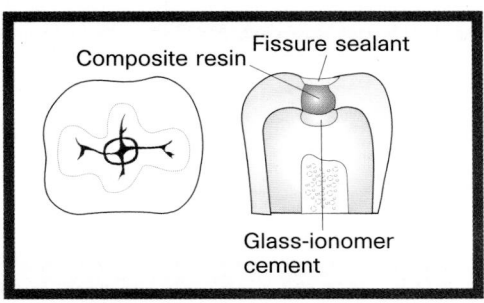

Figure 3.11 Preventive resin restoration.

Tunnel preparations would appear to offer some advantages in the permanent dentition and should be restored, with a RMGI that is radio-opaque, using composite resin to replace the occlusal enamel. In the primary dentition, however, the wider contact area, the anatomical relation of the pulp horns, the more rapid rate of progression of caries and the degree of technical difficulty involved with this type of restoration may make it inappropriate. Clinical evidence to date of its use in primary teeth is scarce.

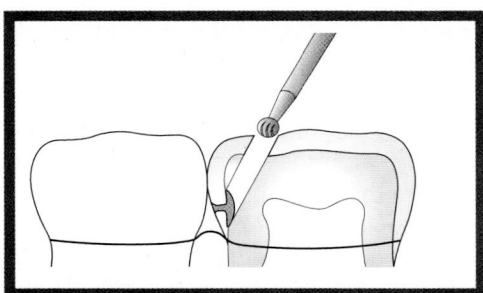

Figure 3.12 Method for preparation of a tunnel restoration. One problem is the proximity of the pulp horn to the cavity preparation. It may also be difficult to visualize the caries, especially in the roof of the tunnel.

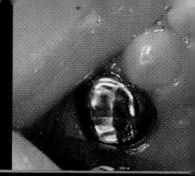

Indications for the use of materials in paediatric dentistry

These are shown in Table 3.3.

Table 3.3 Guide to the use of materials	
Primary dentition	
Class I	Glass–ionomer
	Amalgam
	Composite resin
Class II	Glass–ionomer
	Amalgam
	Composite resin
Gross carious breakdown or restoration after pulp therapy	Stainless-steel crown
Permanent dentition	
Occlusal table	Fissure sealant
Occlusal enamel caries	Fissure sealant
Occlusal caries with minimal involvement of dentine	Preventive-resin restoration
Class-I caries	Composite resin
Class II	Amalgam
Class III	Composite resin
Class V	Glass–ionomer Composite resin

References

Dental caries

AALTONEN AS, TENUOVUO J. Association between mother-infant contacts and caries resistance in children: a cohort study. *Pediatr Dent* 1994, **16**:11–16.

CARR LM. Dental health of children in Australia 1977–1985. *Aust Dent J* 1988, **33**:205–211.

ELDERTON RJ. Assessment and clinical management of early caries in young adults: invasive versus non-invasive methods. *Br Dent J* 1985, **158**:440–444.

ELDERTON RJ. Six-monthly examinations for dental caries. *Br Dent J* 1985, **158**:370–374.

GUSTAFSSON BE. The Vipeholm dental caries study. The effect of different levels of carbohydrates intakes on caries activity in 436 individuals observed for 5 years. *Acta Odontol Scand* 1954, **11**:232.

KOHLER B, ANDREEN I, JONSSON B. The effect of caries-preventive measures in mothers on dental caries and the oral presence of the bacteria *Streptococcus mutans* and Lactobacilli in their children. *Arch Oral Biol* 1984, **29**:879–883.

NAVIA JM. Caries prevention in infants and young children: which etiologic factors should we address? *J Public Health Dent* 1994, **54**:195–196.

NEWBRUN E, MATSUKUBO T, HOOVER CI, *et al.* Comparison of two screening tests for Streptococcus mutans and evaluation of their suitability for mass screenings and private practice. *Community Dent Oral Epidemiol* 1984, **12**:325–331.

POLLARD MA, CURZON MEJ. Conference report: The efficacy of caries-preventive strategies. *J Dent Res* 1992, **71**:1346.

SCHROEDER U, GRANATH L. Dietary habits and oral hygiene as predictors of caries in 3-year -old children. *Community Dent Oral Epidemiol* 1983, **11**:308–311.

TER PELKWIJK A, VAN PALENSTEIN HELDERMAN WH, VAN DIJK JWE. Caries experience in the deciduous dentition as predictor for caries in the permanent dentition. *Caries Res* 1990, **24**:65–71.

Nursing caries

BERKOWITZ RJ, TURNER J, HUGHES C. Microbial characteristics of the human dental caries associated with prolonged bottle feeding. *Arch Oral Biol* 1984, **29**:949–951.

GARDNER DE, NORWOOD JR, EISENSON JE. At-will breastfeeding and dental caries: four case reports. *J Dent Child* 1977, **43**:186–191.

JOHNSTON T, BREARLEY MESSER L. 1994, Nursing caries: literature review and report of a case managed under local anaesthesia. *Aust Dent J* **39**:373–381.

HALLONSTEN AL, WENDT LK, MEJARE I, *et al.* Dental caries and prolonge breast-feeding in 18-month-old Swedish children. *Int J Paediatr Dent* 1995, **5**:149–155.

RIPA, LW. Nursing caries: a comprehensive review. *Pediatr Dent* 1988, **10**:268–82.

Restorative materials

HATIBOVIC-KOFMAN S, KOCH, G. Fluoride release from glass ionomer cement *in vivo* and *in vitro*. *Swed Dent J* 1991, **15**:253–258.

HEYMANN HO, BAYNE SC. Current concepts in dentin bonding. *J Am Dent Assoc* 1993, **12**:27–36.

MCLEAN JW. 1988, Glass ionomer cements. *Br Dent J* **164**:293–299.

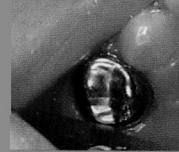
MOUNT GJ. Clinical placement of modern glass-ionomer cements. *Quint Int* 1993, **70**:99–107.

WOOLFORD M. Composite resin attached to glass polyalkenoate (ionomer) cement—the laminate technique. *J Dent* 1993, **21**:31–38.

Restoration of primary teeth

CROLL TP. Bonded composite resin crowns for primary incisors: technique update. *Quintessence* 1990, **21**:153–157.

CROLL TP, WILLIAMS RW. Six years' experience with glass-ionomer-silver cermet cement. *Quintessence* 1991, **22**:783–793.

KILPATRICK NM. Durability of restorations in primary molars. *J Dent* 1993, **21**:67–73.

MESSER LB, LEVERING NJ. The durability of primary molar restorations: I. Observations and predictions of success of stainless steel crowns. *Pediatr Dent* 1988, **10**:81–85.

LEVERING NJ, MESSER LB. The durability of primary molar restorations: I. Observations and predictions of success of amalgams. *Pediatr Dent* 1988, **10**:74–80.

OLDENBURG TR, VANN WF, DILLEY, DC. Composite restorations for primary molars: results after 4 years. *Pediatr Dent* 1987, **9**:136–143.

Restoration of permanent teeth

ELDERTON RJ. Management of early dental caries in fissures with fissure sealant. *Br Dent J* 1985, **158**:254–258.

GRAY GB, PATERSON RC. Clinical assessment of glass ionomer/composite resin sealant restorations in permanent teeth: results of a field trial after 1 year. *Int J Paed Dent* 1994, **4**:141–146.

MANTON DJ, BREARLEY MESSER L. Pit and fissure sealants: another major cornerstone in preventive dentistry. *Aust Dent J* 1995, **40**:22–29.

MITCHELL L, MURRAY JJ. Caries in fissure-sealed teeth—a retrospective evaluation. *J Paed Dent* 1990, **6**:91–96.

MJOR IA, JOKSTAD A. Five year study of class II restorations in permanent teeth using amalgam, glass polyalkenoate (ionomer) cement and resin-based composite materials. *J Dent* 1993, **21**:338–343.

PAPA J, CAIN C, MESSER HH, WILSON PR. Tunnel restorations versus Class-II restorations for small proximal lesions: a comparison of tooth strengths. *Quint Int* 1993, **70**:93–98.

VEHKALAHTI MM, SOLAVAARA L, RYTOMAA I. An eight year follow-up of the occlusal surfaces of first permanent molars. *J Dent Res* 1991, **70**:1964–1967.

WELBURY RR, WALLS AWG, MURRAY JJ MCCABE JF. The management of occlusal caries in permanent molars. A 5-year clinical trial comparing a minimal composite restoration with an amalgam restoration. *Br Dent J* 1990, **169**:361–366.

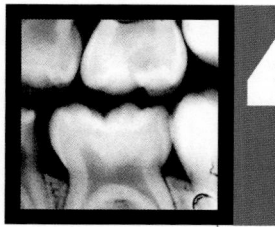
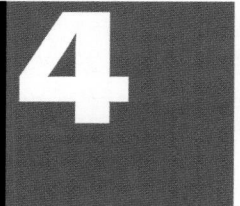

Pulp therapy for primary and young permanent teeth

Contributors

Nicky Kilpatrick, W Kim Seow, Angus Cameron, Richard Widmer

Introduction

This Chapter is concerned with the management of the pulpally involved tooth. The first decision to be made is whether the tooth should be retained. Having decided to save the tooth, some form of pulp therapy will be required.

The area of pulp therapy for primary teeth has been shrouded in controversy, mainly because of the lack of efficacious medications. Many of the procedures were developed anecdotally with few controlled longitudinal clinical trials. With this in mind it is difficult for clinicians to differentiate between case reports, 'tried and tested' remedies, and sound biological techniques.

Factors influencing the decision to retain primary teeth

Medical history

It is important that the child's medical history be taken into account before instituting any form of treatment. Medical conditions of relevance fall into a number of groupings.

Contraindications
- Congenital cardiac disease (risk of endocarditis; see Appendix E).
- Immunosuppressed patients (see Chapter 8, 'Immunodeficiency').
- Children with poor healing potential (i.e. uncontrolled diabetes).

Indications
- Bleeding disorders and coagulopathies (see Chapter 8, 'Bleeding disorders' and 'Coagulation disorders').
- Oligodontia (i.e. ectodermal dysplasia; see Chapter 7, 'Dental anomalies at different stages of tooth development').

Behaviour factors

Is the child a reasonable patient? It cannot be overstressed here how important it is to keep accurate records. The exact nature of previous treatment, the attendance history and the parental cooperation will be important considerations. Similarly, the child's ability to cooperate in the dental chair will influence the planning of treatments.

Dental factors
Is the tooth restorable? A tooth with extensive caries that has led to gross coronal breakdown or one that has caries penetrating the floor of the pulp chamber is unrestorable.

Is it necessary to keep the tooth? The amount of root remaining and the extent of surrounding bone loss will have a significant bearing on whether the tooth is extracted or maintained in the dental arch. The presence of a permanent tooth must be checked.

Contraindications
- Unrestorable tooth.
- Tooth before exfoliation.
- Acute odontogenic infection (see Chapter 6, 'Orofacial infections').

A large collection of pus cannot be drained through a primary tooth, therefore extraction is indicated. Similarly, pulp therapy is unlikely to be successful in the presence of a large periapical radiolucency.
- Excessive tooth mobility.

This may occur as a result of pathological or physiological processes.

Indications
- Well-maintained arch.
- Orthodontic considerations.

The loss of a second primary molar, before eruption of the first permanent molar, invariably leads to space loss (see Chapter 9: 'Space maintenance'). It is desirable to maintain these teeth if possible. On the other hand, space loss is minimal from the loss of the first primary molar after the eruption of the second primary molar.
- Lack of permanent successor.

The congenital absence of a premolar may influence the decision as to whether the primary molar should be preserved.

Pulpal treatment options

Indirect and direct pulp capping
Indirect and direct pulp capping, which may be indicated in permanent teeth, is not successful in the primary dentition. The size of a carious exposure in a primary tooth appears to have little effect on the clinical outcome.

Pulpotomy
Pulpotomy is the extirpation of vital inflamed pulp from the coronal chamber followed by medicament placement, over radicular pulp stumps, to fix (mummification) or stimulate repair of the remaining vital radicular pulp.

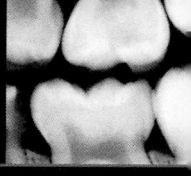

Materials   Formocresol or
             Glutaraldehyde or
             Calcium hydroxide

Pulpectomy/root canal therapy

Extirpation of soft-tissue content from the coronal pulp chamber and root canals.
The canals and the pulp chamber are then filled with a dressing.

Materials   Zinc oxide eugenol (plain) or calcium hydroxide

The controversy over pulpal medicaments

Formocresol

This medicament was introduced by Buckley at the turn of the century in the form
of 19% formaldehyde and 35% tricresol in a 15% solution of glycerin and water.
There have been extensive studies of the efficacy of this medicament over the last
20 years, with clinical success rates ranging from 70% to 100%. Concerns have
been expressed about the systemic spread of formocresol from the tooth site and
possible toxic reactions. With this in mind, it is appropriate to dilute Buckley's original formulation 1:5 in glycerine. A commercial formulation is now available.

Glutaraldehyde

This medicament has recently been advocated as a superior pulpotomy agent to
formocresol. It is a better fixative because of cross linking with low antigenic
potential. There appears to be less penetration into the tissues, because of superior fixation, and it is therefore considered to be less toxic. Although the rates of
clinical success are similar to that of formocresol, there are similar concerns over
systemic toxicity.

Calcium hydroxide

This is the only medicament that promotes biological healing and the formation of
a hard-tissue barrier over the amputated radicular pulp. Swedish authors have
advocated the use of $Ca(OH)_2$. Its use has been discounted by others, however,
because of the complications of internal resorption. Additionally, Schröder has
noted that most cases of failure resulted from inaccurate pulpal diagnosis or failure to remove the blood clot above the sectioned pulp.

Pulpotomy procedures

A final decision on whether to perform a pulpotomy, a pulpectomy or an extraction
cannot be made without an assessment of pulp status. The status of the pulp may be:
• Healthy.

- Reversible pulpitis.
- Irreversible pulpitis.
- Total pulpal necrosis.

Without histological verification, it is extremely difficult to be absolutely accurate; therefore, clinical parameters are used to differentiate between reversible and irreversible pulpitis.

Indications

- A pulpotomy is indicated when the pulp is reversibly and minimally inflamed.
- Where the marginal ridge is already destroyed in first primary molars (Figure 4.1).
- Where radiographic evidence of caries extends more than two-thirds in depth through the dentine.
- If there is any doubt as to whether or not the pulp has been exposed (mechanical or carious).

In all other situations, where there is irreversible pulpitis or there is pulpal necrosis, a pulpectomy or extraction should be performed.

Success rate

- Formocresol   90–98%
- Calcium hydroxide   60%

Pain

There may be difficulties in obtaining a meaningful pain history. The dentist should distinguish between two types of pain:

1. Provoked pain that is stimulated by heat, cold, sweets, air and chewing. When the stimulus is removed the pain is reduced or disappears. These signs often indicate minimal and reversible pulp damage.
2. The formocresol pulpotomy remains the medicament of choice.

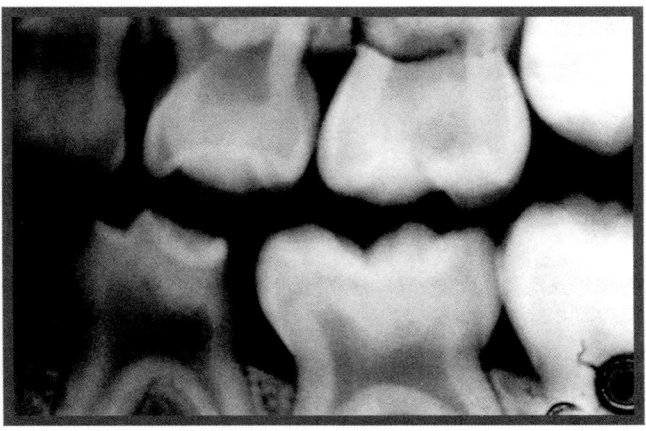

Figure 4.1 It is essential to have a good radiograph of the carious tooth. When the caries has broken through the marginal ridge, in a first primary molar, the pulp is invariably exposed.

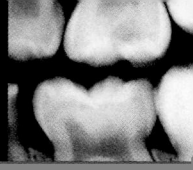

Formocresol vital pulpotomy (Figure 4.2)

1. Preoperative radiograph.
2. Local anaesthesia required and rubber dam.
3. Caries removed and endodontic access cavity.
4. Excavation of coronal pulp. Removal of coronal pulp contents with a new, slow-speed, round, 6 or 8 burr or a clean, spoon excavator.

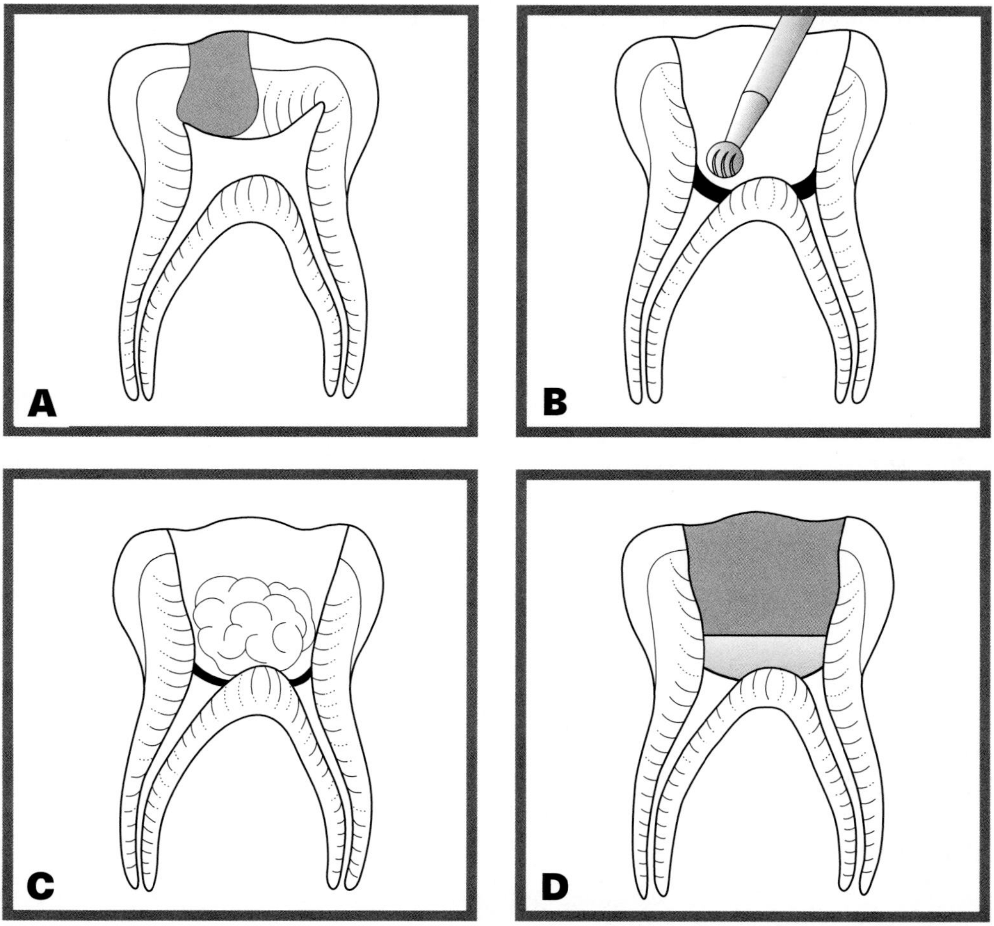

A

B

C

D

Figure 4.2 Method of performing a pulpotomy. **A** Cariously involved primary molar tooth. **B** Access cavity and removal of coronal pulp tissue with a new slow-speed round burr to the level of the canal orifices. **C** Placement of a cotton-wool pellet moistened with formocresol. **D** Capping with IRM base and crown buildup with glass–ionomer before placement of a stainless-steel crown.

5. Haemorrhage control. Place several pellets of cotton wool firmly into the excavated coronal pulp chamber. Cotton wool pellets under pressure in this manner will control the haemorrhage on the radicular pulp orifices. It is acceptable to soak the first pellet, placed in the extirpated pulp chamber, with a haemostatic agent such as local anaesthetic with adrenaline (adrenaline-impregnated gingival retraction cord should not be used because of the high concentration of adrenaline). Give the radicular pulp at least 5 minutes to stop bleeding, then remove the cotton wool and check for cessation of bleeding. Control of haemorrhage from the pulp orifices will influence success.
6. If bleeding has ceased, or if there is only a slight ooze, soak a cotton wool pellet in formocresol and blot dry. Place in the cavity over the pulp stumps and cover with an additional dry cotton wool pellet.
7. Remove after 4 minutes and, if haemostasis is achieved, fill the pulp chamber with a reinforced zinc-oxide eugenol dressing (IRM).
8. The tooth may be restored immediately with an amalgam or glass-ionomer or preferably with a stainless-steel crown (see Chapter 3).

If successful, the treated tooth should be asymptomatic. Failure is shown clinically by pain, swelling, increased mobility, fistulae and radiographic signs (radiolucency at the furcation or apex, or internal/external resorption of the root). Radiographic assessment of the tooth every 12 months is necessary. If it is noticed that the pulp therapy has failed, using the above criteria, the pulpotomy needs to be reassessed and either:

- a pulpectomy performed or
- the tooth extracted.

The success of these procedures is probably dependent more on the coronal seal and the diagnosis; these are critical. Absence or loss of a coronal seal will lead to failure. It appears that the material in contact with the pulp is of minimal importance.

Pulpectomy procedures

Where there is irreversible pulpitis, or there is pulpal necrosis, a pulpectomy or extraction should be performed.

Indications
- Evidence of pulpal necrosis.
- Hyperaemic pulp.

The most common presentation of a hyperaemic pulp is persistent bleeding during a pulpotomy procedure. In this case, the radicular pulp should be removed and a pulpectomy performed instead.

- Evidence of furcation involvement by radiographs.

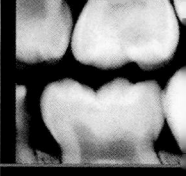

Pain Spontaneous pain that often keeps the child awake and is not relieved by analgesics. These signs usually indicate advanced, irreversible pulp damage.

Swelling Usually indicates a necrotic pulp with spread of inflammation into the soft tissues (Figure 4.3). It must be remembered, however, that not all the pulpal tissue may be necrotic and that such a tooth can still be painful when attempting to remove the remaining pulp. Considerations of the nature of the swelling include:
- The size and extent of the swelling.
- Is it only intra-oral or is there an extra-oral component?
- Has the swelling increased over the last 24 hours?

Antibiotics are usually prescribed if there are signs of systemic involvement. Drainage must be considered if the swelling is fluctuant and is best achieved by incision and extraction of the involved tooth. It is almost impossible to achieve adequate drainage through a primary tooth (see Chapter 6, 'Orofacial infections').

Pulp-sensibility (vitality) tests It should be noted that these are of little clinical benefit in young children because false positives and negatives are present too often, especially in the nervous, uncooperative child. However, percussion on a suspected tooth may be useful in accurately diagnosing the offending tooth.

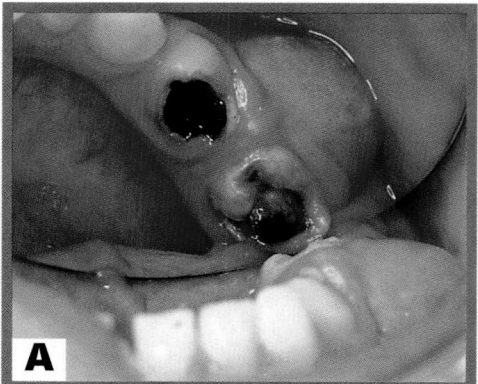
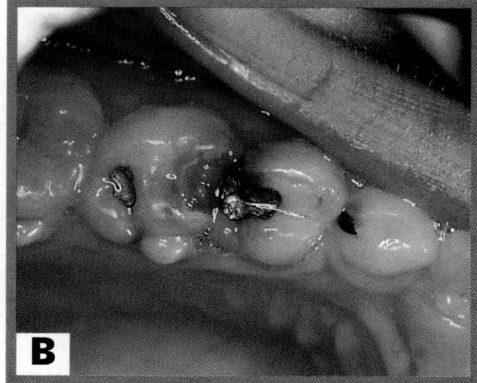

Figure 4.3 **A** Buccal swelling not only indicates pulpal necrosis and pus formation but the loss of bone and a perforation of the cortical plate. It may also be difficult to initially determine which tooth is responsible for the swelling; in this case, both teeth should be removed. **B** Much of the pain that children experience may be caused by food impaction on to gingiva that has overgrown into the cavity. Even without radiographs it is important to recognize that the pulp will always be involved when the carious lesion is of this size.

Success rate 80%.

Pulpectomy method
1. Although local anaesthesia is usually not required, as the pulp is non-vital, there may be remnants of vital, inflamed tissue in the apical 1–3 mm of the canal which may be sensitive. Furthermore, the tooth may be tender because of apical inflammation.
2. Rubber dam is required.
3. A recent periapical or bite-wing radiograph showing the root apices of the tooth is required.
4. Remove all the caries with a high-speed or slow-speed round burr. Once access has been gained into the pulp chamber, complete the endodontic access with a large round bur.
5. Debride the pulp chamber and instrument only 75% of the estimated length of the canals. Irrigate the canals with normal saline or Milton's solution and file to three sizes up from the initial file. Flush the canals with saline and dry with paper points. It is almost impossible to fully instrument the canals of primary molar teeth, but they should be debrided as much as possible.
6. Once dry, the canals should be filled with zinc-oxide eugenol (non-reinforced) or calcium hydroxide. These may be instrumented down the canals or spiralled, with care, using a spiral-filler. It may be useful to reduce the length of the spiral-filler.
7. The pulp chamber is filled with a reinforced IRM and the tooth restored, usually with a stainless-steel crown.

If the pulpectomy fails, as shown by a persistence of swelling, increased bone loss and/or resorption, then the tooth should be extracted.

Clinical problems with pulpally involved primary teeth

There are situations when it is clinically impossible or inappropriate to complete the ideal pulp therapy in one visit.

Child management difficulties
The behaviour of the child compromises the completion of the pulp treatment, such as:
- When an unexpected exposure is encountered and no local anaesthetic has been given.
- When inadequate anaesthesia has been achieved while performing a pulpotomy.
- When the child is in acute pain.

Aim
- Control and prevent pain.

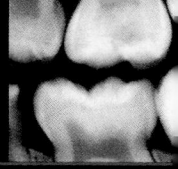

Method
- Place Ledermix paste into the pulp chamber, canals or over the site of exposure.
- Place a dry cotton-wool pellet over the dressing and restore with a temporary dressing such as IRM or glass–ionomer cement.
- Review within 7 days, at which point the tooth is re-assessed and, if asymptomatic, the appropriate pulp therapy is completed.

In the case of a tooth with persistent inflammation or infection, this therapy would be a pulpectomy or extraction. In other cases, the treatment at the second visit may involve pulpotomy, pulpectomy or extraction, depending on pulp status.

Occasionally, when clinical signs or symptoms persist, a further intermediate dressing may be desirable. Common sense will dictate how many times this treatment can be repeated before extraction is considered necessary.

Summary

Table 4.1 summarizes the options for the management of the pulpally involved primary tooth. Irrespective of the therapy employed, the long-term success is thought to be significantly influenced by the integrity of the coronal seal. The use of stainless-steel crowns in restoring the crowns of pulpally involved primary molars is strongly recommended.

Pulp therapy for young permanent molars

Similar considerations apply in the treatment-planning process for the permanent dentition as discussed earlier for the primary dentition (Figure 4.4). The treatment of choice for the cariously exposed young permanent tooth is dependent on:
- Stage of root development.
- Status of the crown.
- Orthodontic considerations for the tooth and the arch (see Chapter 9).
- Psychological and behavioural factors.

The ultimate decision in all of these cases remains the long-term advisability of retaining the tooth and the ability to adequately restore the crown. It should be remembered that the amount of crown destruction usually associated with a pulp exposure in an immature molar will mean that the tooth will require significant restorative maintenance throughout life.

Vital teeth with immature roots

Aim Preservation of vitality to ensure completion of root development.

Indirect pulp cap Indicated in vital teeth with minimal symptoms where a thin layer of carious dentine is left over the pulp, the removal of which would create an exposure. Caries control is a variation of indirect pulp capping. A child may present with multiple carious lesions, some with frank pulpal involvement and others close to the pulp. The aim of caries control is to arrest all deep active carious lesions and halt their progression. Under rubber dam, gross caries are removed followed by the placement of a glass-ionomer or a Ledermix cement dressing and the tooth restored.

Direct pulp cap Unlike primary teeth, permanent teeth respond well to direct pulp-capping procedures. Careful case selection, however, is important. Indications:
- Small carious exposures.
- Teeth with no history of swelling, spontaneous pain.
- No radiographic changes.
- Controllable bleeding at the exposure site.

Place calcium hydroxide or Ledermix cement directly on to the exposed pulp and cover with a glass-ionomer base. The tooth can be restored immediately.

Table 4.1 Treatment options for primary teeth

Clinical event	Signs or symptoms	Pulpal status	Treatment choice
Caries without exposure	No spontaneous symptoms	Healthy	Restore tooth
Caries with possible or near exposure	Occasional pain on stimulation	Minimal or reversible pulpitis	Pulpotomy
Iatrogenic/non-carious exposure	Asymptomatic	Healthy	Pulpotomy
Carious exposure	Minimal history of pain No mobility No radiographic evidence of pathology	Reversible pulpitis	Pulpotomy
Carious exposure	Spontaneous pain Swelling Mobility	Irreversible pulpitis	Pulpectomy Intermediate dressing Extraction
Carious exposure	Draining sinus Swelling Mobility Radiographic pathology (inter-radicular or periapical, root resorption)	Necrotic pulp	Pulpectomy Intermediate dressing Extraction
Gross caries	Caries through bifurcation Tooth unrestorable Extensive periapical pathology	Necrotic pulp	Extraction

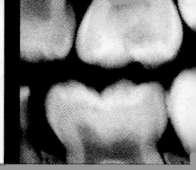

There is recent evidence to suggest that the medicament of choice in these situations is Ledermix cement. The use of calcium hydroxide is associated with calcification of the coronal and radicular pulp which may make a subsequent root-canal therapy difficult. This does not appear to be the case with Ledermix cement.

Pulpotomy

- Calcium hydroxide has been used as a pulpotomy medicament and results in rapid bridge formation over the radicular pulp stumps which may preclude root-canal therapy at a later stage.
- Formocresol pulpotomies have enjoyed equivocal success in permanent teeth. They are not recommended in teeth with mature root formation unless there are behavioural or socioeconomic constraints to performing root-canal therapy.

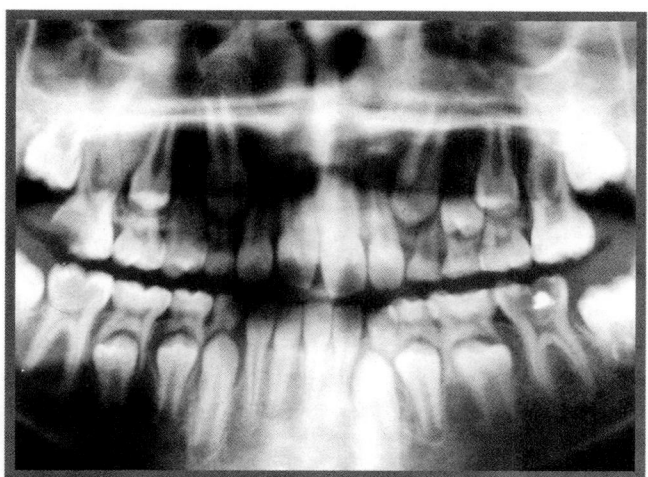

Figure 4.4 The long-term prognosis and the ability to restore a tooth are the overriding factors when assessing whether pulp therapy should be undertaken. In these cases, it is often preferable to extract the first permanent molars and allow the second molars to drift mesially.

- The use of Ledermix cement as a pulpotomy medicament would appear to be an acceptable procedure as it not only has the advantages of the obtundant effect of the corticosteroid and antibiotic but also contains both calcium hydroxide and zinc oxide eugenol. There are as yet no reports of radicular calcification with the use of Ledermix cement.

Although there are indications for partial pulp therapy in young permanent molars it must be remembered that ultimately none of these procedures enjoy the success of complete root-canal therapy. The latter should, therefore, be the treatment of choice where possible. Where partial pulp therapy has been performed, the parents and the child should be informed that problems may develop later and that periodic monitoring is essential.

Non-vital teeth with immature roots (see Chapter 9, 'Extraction of first permanent molars')

Except in exceptional circumstances these teeth should be removed, although it may be desirable to retain them in the short term for orthodontic reasons. In these cases, the canals should be cleaned and instrumented. A medicament such as non-setting calcium hydroxide or Ledermix should be placed and the crown restored with a semipermanent restoration.

References

ABBOTT PV, HEITHERSAY GS, HUME WR. Release diffusion through human tooth roots *in vitro* of corticosteroid and tetracycline trace molecules from Ledermix paste. *Endod Dent Traumatol* 1988, **4**:55–62.

FEIGAL RJ, MESSER HH. A critical look at glutaraldehyde. *Pediatr Dent* 1990, **12**:69–71.

FUKS AB, BIMSTEIN E. Clinical evaluation of diluted formocresol pulpotomies in primary teeth of school children. *Pediatr Dent* 1981, **3**:321–324.

JENG HW, FEIGAL RJ, MESSER HH. Comparison of the cytotoxicity of formocresol, formaldehyde, cresol and glutaraldehyde using human pulp fibroblast cultures. *Pediatr Dent* 1987, **9**:295–300.

RANLY DM, GARCIA-GODOY F, HORN D. Time, concentration, and pH parameters for the use of glutaraldehyde as a pulpotomy agent: an *in-vitro* study. *Pediatr Dent* 1987, **9**:199–203.

RANLY DM. Glutaraldehyde vs. formocresol. Pediatr Dent 1990, **12**:198

RANLY DM. Pulpotomy therapy in primary teeth: new modalities for old rationalies. *Pediatr Dent* 1995, **16**:403–409.

ROBERTS JF. Treatment of vital and non-vital primary molar teeth by one-stage formocresol pulpotomy: clinical success and effect upon age at exfoliation. *Int J Paediatr Dent* 1996, **6**:111–115.

SCHRÖDER U. A 2 year follow-up of primary molar pulpotomies with a gentle technique and capped with calcium hydroxide. *Scan J Dent Res* 1978, **86**:273.

SCHRÖDER U, SZPRINGER-NODZAK M, JANICHA J, WACI SKA M, BUDNY J, MLOESEK K. A one-year follow-up of partial pulpotomy and calcium hydroxide capping in primary molars. *Endod Dent Traumatol* 1987, **3**:304–306.

VERCO PJW. Microbiological effectiveness of a reduced concentration of formocresol. *Pediatr Dent* 1983, **7**:130–133

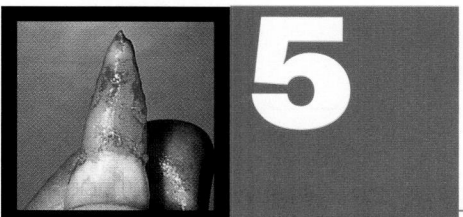

5 Trauma management

Contributors

Angus Cameron, Richard Widmer, Peter Gregory, Paul Abbott, Peter Wong, Fiona Heard, Santo Cardaci, Tony Sandler

Introduction

The management of dento-alveolar trauma in children is distressing for both child and parent (Figure 5.1) and often difficult for the dentist. However, trauma is one of the most common presentations of young children to a paediatric dentist. The patient's emergency must be the dentist's routine. The child should be carefully assessed regarding treatment needs before commenting to parents because many cases are not as bad as they first appear. Initial reassurance to both parent and child is of great value. Trauma not only compromises a previously healthy dentition but may leave a deficit that also affects the self-esteem and quality of life and commits the patient to lifelong dental maintenance.

Aetiology

Most injuries are caused by falls and play accidents. Luxation injuries to upper anterior teeth predominate in toddlers because of their frequent falls during play and attempts at walking. Injuries are generally more common in boys. Blunt trauma tends to cause greater damage to the soft tissues and supporting structures whereas high-velocity or sharp injuries cause luxations and fractures of the teeth.

Predisposing factors
- Class-II division 1.
- Overjet 3–6 mm—double the frequency of trauma to incisor teeth compared with 0–3 mm overjet.
- Overjet >6 mm—threefold increase in the risk. The study in Table 5.1 by Hall, from the Royal Children's Hospital in Melbourne, shows that falls and play accidents account for the majority of injuries. Importantly, although accounting for only 1% of all injuries, over 80% of child abuse occurs in the very young child.

Frequency
- 30% of children suffer trauma to primary dentition.
- 22% of children suffer trauma to permanent dentition by age 14 years.
- Male : female, 2 : 1.

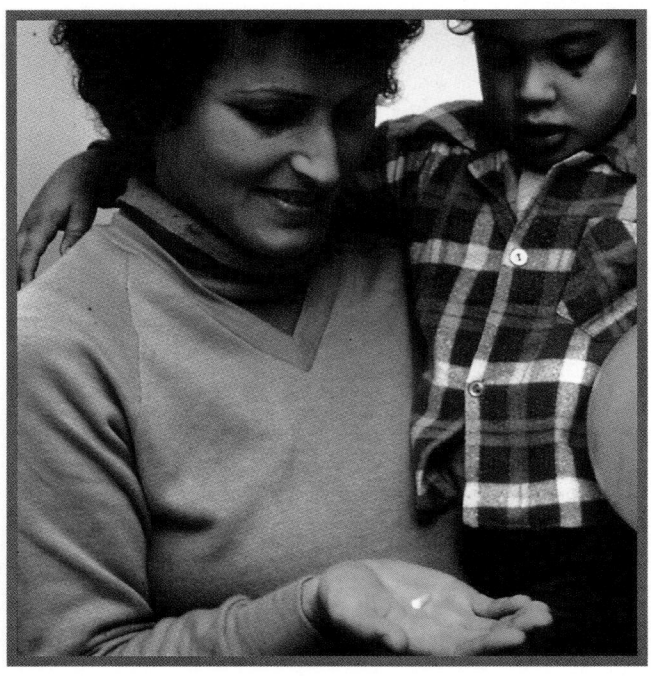

Figure 5.1 The presentation of a child with trauma is distressing for parent and child. The child in other instances may be oblivious to what has happened and is happily playing in the surgery.

Table 5.1 Aetiology of maxillofacial trauma in children

	% injuries occurring at each age group			% total injuries
	0–5 years	5–10 years	10–15 years	
Falls	50.1	32.8	17.1	43.2
Play accidents	39.5	43.5	17	17.7
Motor vehicle accidents	31.9	44.1	24	17.4
Sporting accidents	9	29.5	61.5	8.3
Dog bites	63.3	29.6	7.1	6.4
Fights and assaults	–	21.9	78.1	1.4
Child abuse	80	20	–	1
Others				4.6

Hall RK, from Royal Children's Hospital, Melbourne 1970–1979

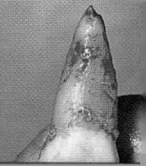

- Peak incidence at 2–4 years and rises again at 8–10 years.
- Upper anterior teeth most commonly involved.
- Usually single tooth, except with motor vehicle accidents and sporting injuries.

Child abuse

Child abuse is defined as those acts or omissions of care that deprive a child of the opportunity to fully develop his or her unique potential as a person either physically, socially or emotionally. There are four types of child abuse:
- Physical abuse.
- Sexual abuse.
- Emotional abuse.
- Neglect.

The true incidence of child abuse and neglect is unknown, and although there is increasing awareness and reporting, professionals are still reluctant to deal with it. The first step in preventing abuse is recognition and reporting. Dentists are in a strategic position to recognize and report mistreated children because they often see the child and parent/caretaker interacting during multiple visits and over a long period of time.

The orofacial region is commonly traumatized during episodes of child abuse (Figure 5.2). Injuries that do not match the given history, bruising of soft tissue not overlying bony prominences or injury that takes the shape of a recognizable object, and multiple injuries of different ages, may be the result of non-accidental trauma. Bite marks in children represent child abuse until proved otherwise. The characteristics and diagnostic findings of child abuse, and the protocol of reporting such cases, should be familiar to the dentist so that appropriate notification, treatment and prevention of further injury can be instituted.

Whenever injuries are inconsistent with the history, the patient must be investigated for abuse. There is a legal obligation in some states and countries to report the suspicion of child abuse or sexual assault. Child abuse teams are available at all paediatric hospitals or through the Departments of Family and Community Services. Dog bites, too, account for a significant number of injuries and every year several children are killed by dogs. It is common that the dog is known to the child and it cannot be stressed too highly that children must be supervised when around even the most timid of animals.

History

As dental injuries may become the subject of litigation or insurance claims, a thorough history and examination is mandatory. Where possible, injuries should

be photographed. An accurate history gives important information regarding:
- Status of the dentition at presentation.
- Prognosis of injuries.
- Other injuries sustained.
- Medical complications.
- Possible litigation.

Questions to ask:
- When did the trauma occur?
- How did the trauma occur?
- Were there any other injuries?
- What initial treatment was given?
- Have there been any other dental injuries in the past?
- Are current immunizations up to date?

Examination

Examination should be undertaken in a logical order. It is important to examine the whole body as the patient may present first to the dentist and other injuries may have occurred (Figure 5.3 and see Chapter 1).

Trauma examination and records
- Extra-oral wounds and palpation of the facial skeleton (Figure 5.4).
- Injuries to oral mucosa or gingivae.
- Palpation of alveolus.
- Displacement of teeth.
- Abnormalities in occlusion.
- Extent of tooth fractures, pulp exposure, colour changes.
- Mobility of teeth.
- Reaction to vitality tests and percussion.

Assessment of cranial nerves involved in facial trauma

I	Olfactory	Olfaction
II	Optic	Vision
III	Oculomotor	Movements of the globe
IV	Trochlear	Superior rectus
V	Trigeminal	Muscles of mastication
VI	Abducent	Lateral rectus
VII	Facial	Muscles of facial expression
VIII	Vestibulocochlear	Hearing and balance
XII	Hypoglossal	Tongue function

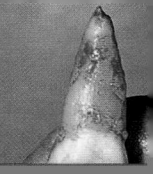

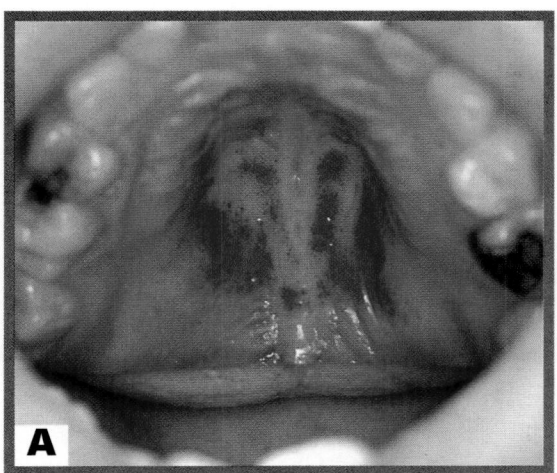
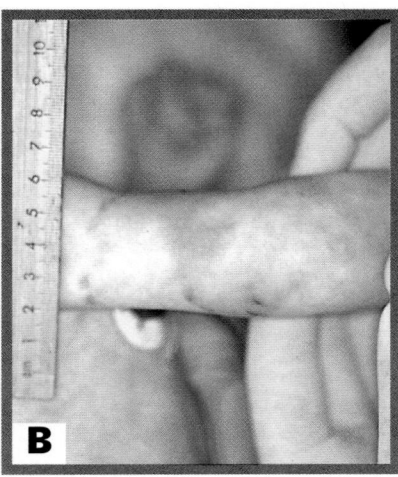

Figure 5.2 **A** Child abuse caused by sexual assault by a family member. Commonly the perpetrator is known to the child. **B** A 3-month-old infant was bitten by a 3-year-old, who was left in charge of the child. Good photographic records are required and the wounds should not be washed until specimens for DNA-testing of saliva are taken. The child-assault team will organize appropriate input from social workers, paediatricians and the police, if necessary. The dentist should also be aware of the legal requirements for recording of evidence (i.e. standardized photography with measuring scale).

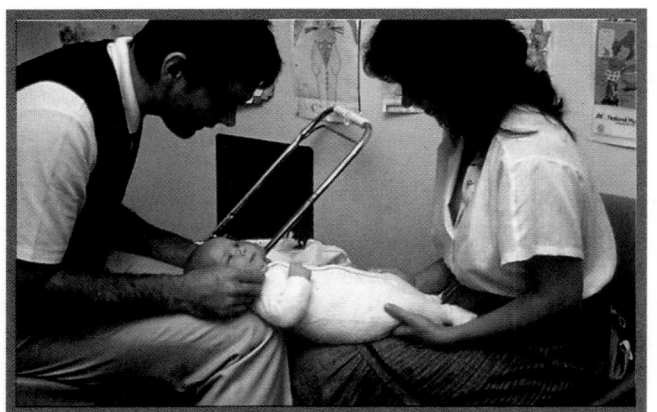

Figure 5.3 One of the easiest ways to examine young children is with the child's head in the dentist's lap. The child can see the parent, who gently restrains the arms. This gives an excellent view into the maxilla, where most trauma occurs.

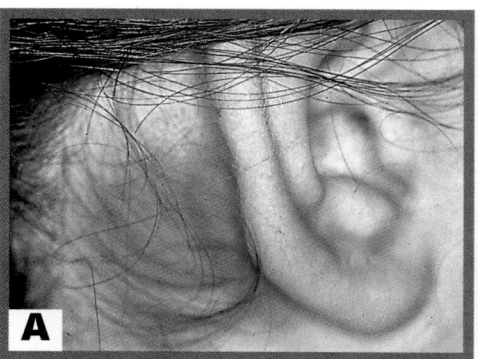
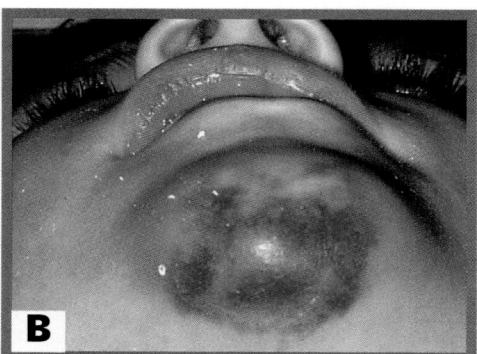

Figure 5.4 **A** The 'battle sign', or bruising of the mastoid region, is associated with a base-of-skull fracture. Examination must include all areas of the head and neck which often requires parting the hair to detect lacerations and bruising. **B** Bruising is a collection of blood which will fall to the most dependent point. The chin-point ecchymosis shown here is often associated with gingival degloving, laceration and mandibular fracture.

Head injury

Closed head injury is the most common cause of childhood mortality in accidents. Between 25% and 50% of all accidents in children up to 14 years involve the head. If there is any suggestion that a head injury has been sustained, the child should be immediately medically assessed, preferably in a paediatric casualty department.

Signs of closed head injury

- Altered or loss of consciousness.
- Bleeding from the head or ears.
- Disorientation.
- Prolonged headache.
- Nausea, vomiting, amnesia.
- Altered vision or unilateral dilated pupil.
- Seizures or convulsions.
- Speech difficulties.

Dental problems take second place if there is central nervous system involvement. If there is any loss of consciousness, hourly neurological observations should be commenced (see Appendix R). The Glasgow Coma Scale is commonly used in accident and emergency departments to assess the severity of head injury and prognosis (see Appendix L).

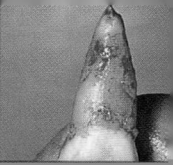

Investigations

Radiographs

The request for radiographs is obviously made after a thorough investigation. The value of extra-oral films in young children, such as panoramic radiographs, should be recognized. In the very difficult child, it may be the only way that some clinical information can be gained in the acute phase of management.

When taking periapical films, several angulations should be taken for each traumatized tooth. This is especially important to determine the presence of root fractures and tooth luxations. All traumatized teeth should be radiographed to assess:
- Stage of root development.
- Injuries to root and supporting structures.

Guide to prescription of radiographs

Dento-alveolar injuries
- Anterior maxillary occlusal or anterior mandibular occlusal.
- Panoramic radiograph.
- True lateral maxilla for intrusive luxations of primary anterior teeth.

Condylar fracture
- Panoramic radiograph, closed and open mouth.
- Lateral oblique.
- Reverse Townes.
- CT scan.

Mandibular fracture
- Panoramic radiograph.
- Posteroanterior mandible.
- True mandibular and anterior mandibular occlusal.
- Lateral oblique.

Maxillary fractures
- Panoramic radiograph.
- Occipitomental 30° (OM30 or Waters' projection).
- CT scan.

Pulp assessment tests

These are essential as a baseline measure of pulpal status. It is common that the initial responses at presentation may be inaccurate; however, it is important that results are recorded for later comparison. Young children often find it difficult to discriminate between the touch of the tester and the actual stimulus itself and so the clinician must be aware of false results. In cases that are difficult to diagnose the isolation of individual teeth under rubber dam may be required.

Pulp-sensibility testing This term relates to the assessment of pulpal health. Previously termed 'vitality testing' this new terminology stresses the fact that neural and vascular components of the pulp tissue need individual consideration. A tooth may not respond to a thermal test but may have an intact blood supply. Such discrimination of the health of pulpal elements will be important in planning treatment.

Thermal sensitivity Responses to cold stimuli give the most reliable and accurate records in children (even with immature teeth). The carbon-dioxide pencil is regarded as being the most convenient, but is also the most expensive. Ethyl-chloride spray, or ice may also be used. Cold thermal stimulation has the advantage that assessment of the pulp is possible under temporary crowns and splints.

Electrical stimulation Electrical stimulation may give a graded response to stimuli. When using these instruments the rheostat should be slowly increased so that painful aversive stimulation of the tooth is avoided. The value of electrical stimulation is equivocal in the young child.

Percussion There are two reasons to percuss teeth: (1) sensitivity in response to percussion gives information about the extent of damage to the apical tissues. Be aware that the percussion of luxated teeth will usually be painful. (2) The sound in response to percussion is also an important indicator of the likelihood of ankylosis.

Transillumination This is an extremely useful, non-invasive technique to assess the presence of cracks and/or fractures, and subtle alterations in crown colour which may indicate a change in pulpal status.

Other considerations in trauma management

Having carefully assessed the patient, the only treatment necessary may be to reassure the child and parent and discuss possible sequelae such as pulp necrosis, resorption of intruded teeth, and facial swelling.

Fasting requirements
If the patient requires extensive work under general anaesthesia it is important to check fasting details. A child over 6 years of age must be fasted for at least 6 hours without solids or liquids. Children under the age of 6 years must be fasted for 6 hours without solids and 3 hours without liquids.

Immunizations
If the patient has sustained an injury that involves contamination of the wound with soil, especially from a farm area, then a tetanus booster should be considered. If the

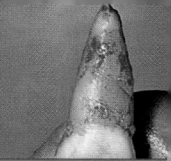

child has completed their normal immunization schedule, under normal circumstances boosters are not required (see Immunization Schedules in Appendix F).

Maxillofacial injuries

Fractures of the facial bones are uncommon in children and account for less than 5% of all maxillofacial fractures. Consequently, few surgeons have extensive experience in this area and the management of these cases must embody an understanding of the implications of such injuries for the growing child (Figures 5.5A & B)

Management principles

Management of maxillofacial trauma is complicated in a child by age, anxiety, closed head injuries and the large number of unerupted teeth. The placement of miniplates is often made difficult because of the position of unerupted permanent teeth and the potential damage that may be caused during the placement of screws. Intermaxillary fixation, however, is well tolerated in children and cap silver splints are still used. The removal of unerupted permanent teeth within lines of fracture is not indicated.

With good fixation and immobilization and antibiotics, fractures in children unite within 3 weeks. Problems such as non-union or fibrous union are almost unknown.

Fractured mandible

Most mandibular fractures involve the condylar area or the canine region of the body. The latter is often involved because it represents the area of least bone in the jaw.

Clinical signs
- Pain, swelling and stepping.
- Occlusal discrepancies.
- Limitation of jaw movement.
- Sublingual haematoma (Figure 5.6).
- Facial asymmetry.
- Mental anaesthesia or paraesthesia.

Management
- Fixation by interdental wiring, miniplate fixation or cap silver splints.
- Splints may be cemented with glass–ionomer or black copper cement, or retained with circum-mandibular wiring. Intermaxillary fixation may be achieved with elastics.

Condylar fractures

This is the most common fracture in children and results from chin-point trauma. Usually there is medial and anterior displacement of the condylar head caused by

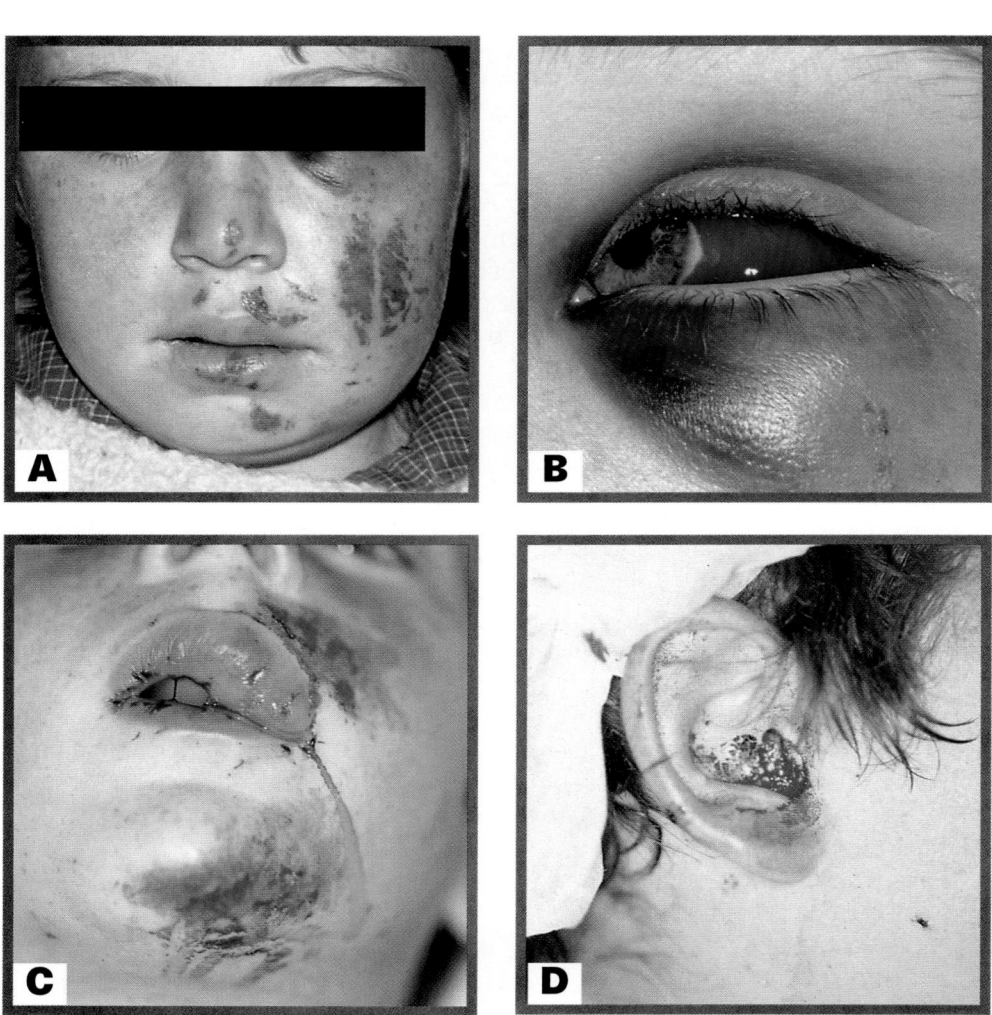

Figure 5.5 **A, B** This girl fell from a Tarzan rope on to her face. There is extensive ecchymosis around the left eye, and subconjunctival haemorrhage. The child presents with all the signs of a fractured zygoma yet, because of the immaturity of the frontozygomatic suture, which allows some displacement, there is no fracture evident. **C, D** Many children suffer chin-point trauma and it is important to check the condylar joints. This boy sustained a right subcondylar fracture. There was bleeding from the external meatus where the condylar head had perforated the anterior wall of the meatus. Under no circumstances should the ear be suctioned because the ossicles may be removed if the tympanic membrane is ruptured.

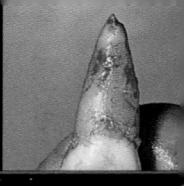

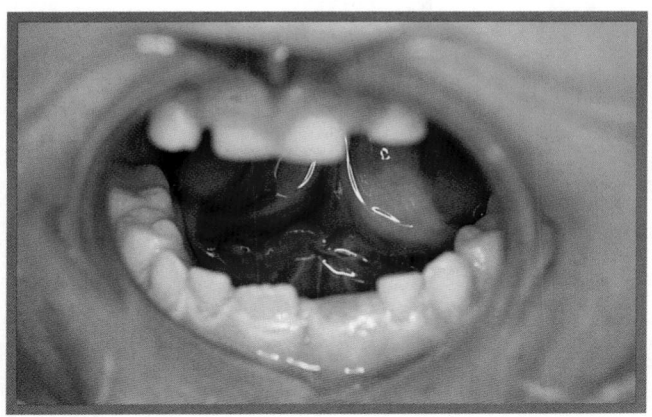

Figure 5.6 The sublingual haematoma is pathognomonic for a fractured mandible in the symphysis or in the canine region of the body.

the pull of lateral pterygoid, but there may be no occlusal disharmony. There may be cerebrospinal fluid otorrhea or bleeding from the acoustic meatus caused by perforation of the anterior wall of the meatus by the condylar head (Figure 5.5C & D). Any bleeding or discharge from the ear should be investigated by an ear, nose and throat specialist. Suctioning of the external meatus must never be performed. If the tympanic membrane is torn, the ossicles might be removed by the sucker. Rarely is there involvement of the middle cranial fossa, although these children will manifest neurological signs (see Head injury above).

Management Treatment is usually conservative with a short period of rest followed by active movement to prevent the chance of ankylosis. Bilateral cases with gross displacement may require posterior bite-blocks and a very short period of immobilization. Follow-up over many years is essential and should include a regular assessment of oral opening, study models and photographic records.

There is a greater risk of ankylosis with intracapsular fractures (Figure 5.7) and regular follow-up of growth is important to assess oral opening and asymmetry from growth-site damage. Early surgical correction of ankylosis with costochondral grafting is recommended with good success rates (Kaban, 1990).

Fractures involving telescoping or shortening of the condylar neck have been successfully treated with functional appliances for 2–3 weeks in order to distract the vertical ramus and allow better remodelling.

Fractured maxilla

Middle-third fractures are rare in children and usually present with other craniofacial trauma and head injury. The fractures do not often follow Le Fort lines, as the craniofacial sutures have not closed in young children.

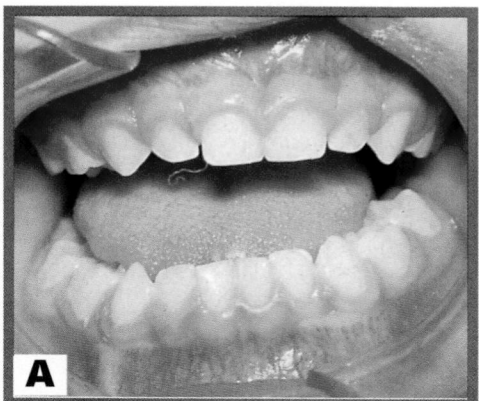 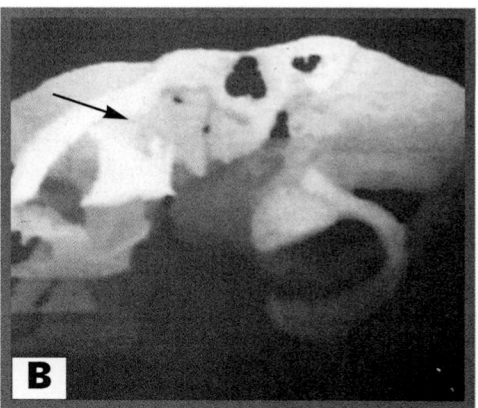

Figure 5.7 A, B Mandibular asymmetry caused by a dislocation of the left condyle after a slippery dip fell on this young girl. Imaging of these injuries can be difficult and in this case a CT scan was performed with three-dimensional reconstruction to detail the injury. The CT demonstrates the dislocation, with the condylar head (arrowed) anterior to the articular eminence and lying under the zygomatic arch. As is common with these injuries in children, an intracapsular fracture-dislocation is present, which remodelled itself without treatment. Normal function was achieved within 6 months.

Clinical signs
- Subconjunctival haemorrhage, tethering of the globe, or both.
- Strabismus and diplopia.
- Cerebrospinal fluid rhinorrhoea and epistaxis.
- Occlusal discrepancies.
- Zygomatic stepping, orbital stepping or both.
- Subcutaneous emphysema.
- Facial swelling and ecchymosis (Figure 5.8A).
- Intra-oral mucosal tears and lacerations.
- Differential movement of the maxilla.
- Anaesthesia or paraesthesia of infra-orbital nerve.

Management
- Simple maxillary fractures are managed with cap splints and intermaxillary fixation.
- Conservative management may be used when there is only minimal suture separation, without bony displacement.
- Extra-oral and miniplate fixation may be required in those cases with displacement.

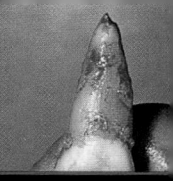

Sequelae of fractures of the jaws in children (Figure 5.8B)

Closed head injury

Children who sustain middle-third injuries usually have concomitant head injuries. A study from the Royal Children's Hospital in Melbourne found that head injury was present in 25% of cases of facial trauma. These children spend extended periods in intensive care units, undergo personality changes, suffer post-traumatic amnesia and may have episodes of neuropathological chewing.

Tooth loss

Approximately 10% of children who sustain fractures of the jaws will also suffer loss of permanent teeth.

Developmental defects of enamel

In addition to the damage caused by displacement of primary teeth into the crypts of permanent successors (see 'Sequelae after trauma to primary teeth'), unerupted teeth in the line of jaw fractures may be also be damaged. Defects may include:

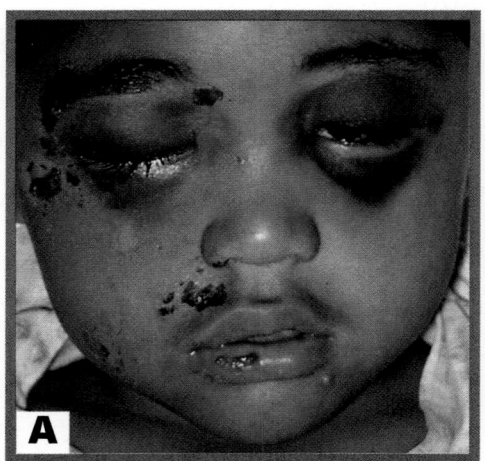

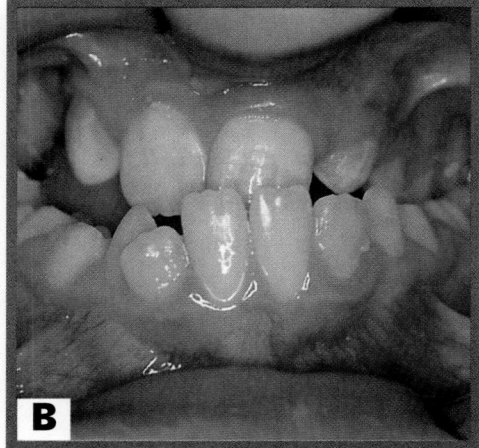

Figure 5.8 **A** Middle-third fracture in a child involved in a motor-vehicle accident. Note the bilateral periorbital ecchymosis and swelling resulting in closure of the eyes. Despite the appearance there was only minimal displacement of the maxilla, although external fixation was required to reduce the depressed nasal fracture. **B** Maxillary hypoplasia and growth retardation, in another patient with a middle-third fracture, 8 years after the trauma.

- Hypoplasia or hypomineralization of enamel.
- Dilaceration of crown and roots.
- Displacement of the developing tooth within the bone.
- Arrest of tooth development with pulp-canal obliteration.

Intra-articular damage to the temporomandibular joint

There is always a risk of ankylosis of the temporomandibular joint after significant displacement of the condylar head, intracapsular fracture or a failure to achieve early mobilization of the joint. Treatment of the ankylosis involves condylectomy and joint reconstruction with a costochondral graft.

Growth retardation

Maxillary and mandibular growth retardation may occur following major trauma. Significant scarring of soft tissues and/or tissue-loss may inhibit jaw growth. Mandibular asymmetry with antegonial notching may occur on the affected side after subcondylar fracture. The key to management is to correct asymmetries early to avoid secondary maxillary deformity.

Luxations in the primary dentition

General management considerations

Immunization If the child is not fully immunized then a tetanus booster is required:
- Tetanus toxoid 0.5 mL by immediate intramuscular injection (see Immunization Schedule, Appendix F).

Antibiotics Unless there are significant soft-tissue or dento-alveolar injuries, antibiotics are not normally required. Antibiotics are prescribed empirically as a prophylaxis against infection, but are not a substitute for proper debridement of wounds. All drugs should be prescribed according to the child's weight (see Appendix N).

Luxations

The most common injuries to the primary teeth are luxations involving a displacement of the teeth in the alveolar bone.

Concussion and subluxation (Figure 5.9A)

Concussion is an injury to the tooth and ligament without displacement or mobility of the tooth. Subluxation occurs when the tooth is mobile but is not displaced. Both involve minor damage to the periodontal ligament. All these teeth are tender to percussion, there is haemorrhage and oedema within the ligament, but gingival bleeding and mobility only occurs if the teeth have been subluxated.

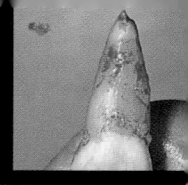

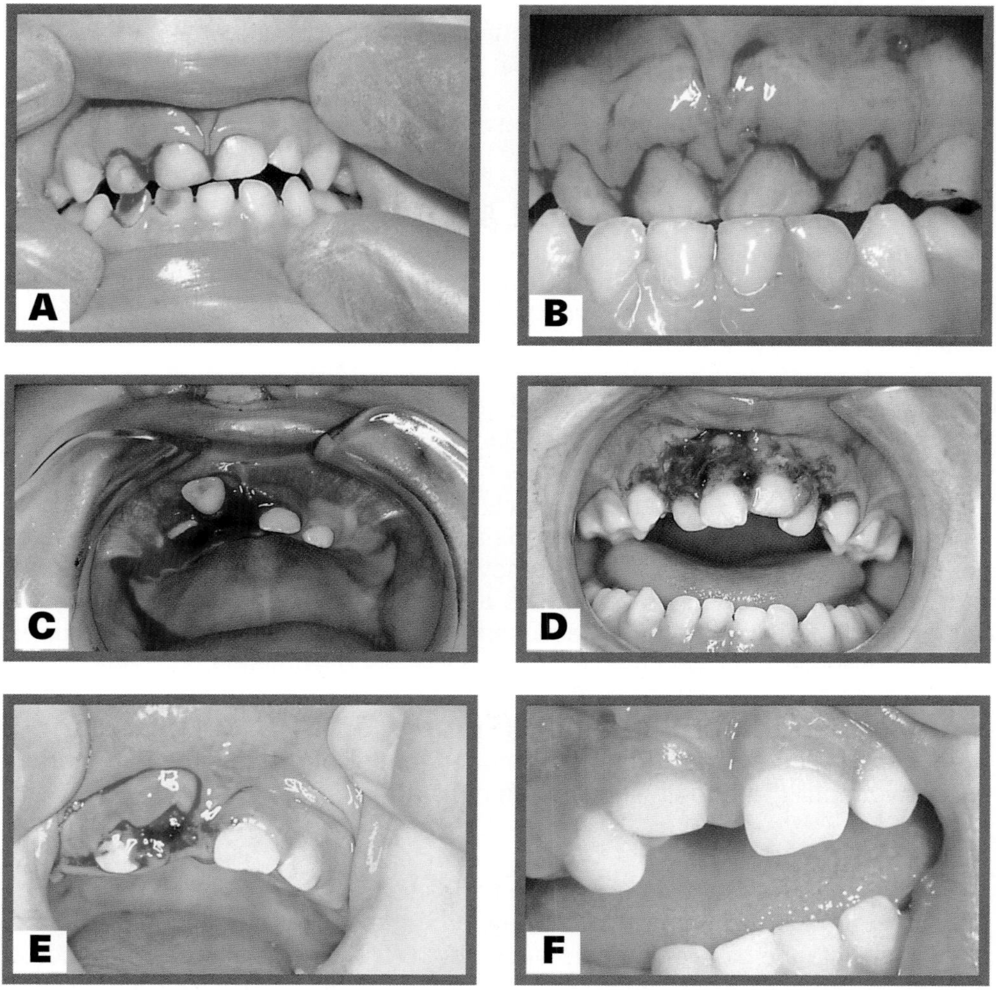

Figure 5.9 **A** Subluxation of the upper-right incisors with minimal displacement.
B Palatal luxation of the upper incisors resulting in an occlusal interference. These
teeth should be repositioned digitally, only to relieve the interference. Further anterior
movement may damage the permanent teeth. **C** Extrusive luxation of the upper-right
primary incisor teeth. These should be removed. **D** Gross displacement of all upper
anterior teeth with gingival degloving and loss of the labial plate. This child had the
displaced teeth extracted, and debridement and suturing of the gingiva performed
under general anaesthesia. **E** An intrusive luxation of the upper-right incisor tooth in
a 12-month-old child. Note the displacement of the gingiva, indicating that the tooth
has not been avulsed. The tooth partially re-erupted within a month (**F**).

Management
- Periapical radiographs as baseline.
- Soft diet for 1 week.
- Advice to the parents of possible sequelae, such as pulp necrosis.
- Individualized follow up.

Intrusive luxation (Figure 5.9E & F)

Intrusive injuries are the most common injuries to upper primary incisors. Newly erupted incisors often take the full force of any fall in a toddler. There is usually a palatal and superior displacement of the crown, which means that the apex of the tooth is forced away from the permanent follicle.

Management
- If the crown is visible and there is minor alveolar damage—leave tooth to re-erupt.
- If the whole tooth is intruded—extract.

It has been recommended that where the apex of the primary tooth has perforated the labial plate the tooth should be removed. The decision on whether to extract or to allow for re-eruption is very much a clinical one, and is based on the presentation of the injuries and the assessment of the child. More severe injuries, involving alveolar bone and gingiva, often necessitate extraction.

Extrusive and lateral luxation (Figures 5.9B, C & D; 5.11A)

Treatment is dependent on the mobility and extent of displacement. If there is excessive mobility the tooth should be removed.

Avulsion (Figure 5.10)

- Avulsed primary teeth should not be replanted.

Replacing an avulsed primary tooth may force the socket blood clot, or the root apex itself, into the developing permanent tooth. The other main reason is lack of patient cooperation. There are cases where the parent or caregiver replants the tooth and it appears to be stable and viable; in these cases the tooth could be left *in situ*.

Unless significant soft-tissue damage is present antibiotics are not required. Splinting of primary teeth may be difficult in young, traumatized children and if successfully placed must also be removed later when cooperation may not be as good.

Fractures of primary incisors

Crown fractures not involving the pulp (Fig. 5.12A)

Unlike the permanent dentition, primary teeth are more commonly displaced rather

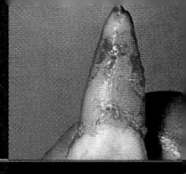

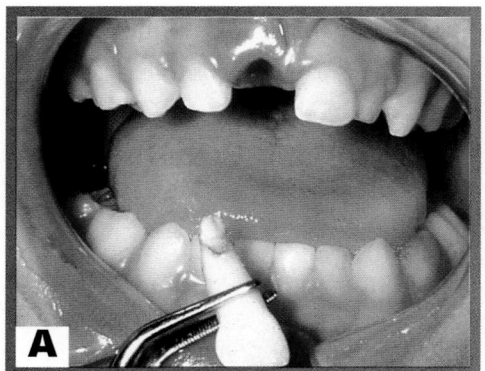
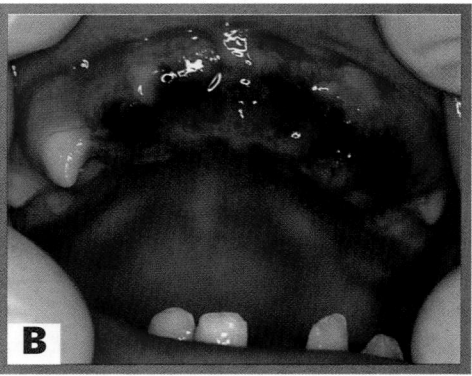

Figure 5.10 A There is almost no indication for the replantation of an avulsed primary tooth. There is more risk of damage to the permanent tooth than there is benefit gained by replacing the tooth. **B** A child involved in a motor-vehicle accident who avulsed six primary teeth. A chest radiograph was required to ensure that no teeth were swallowed or aspirated.

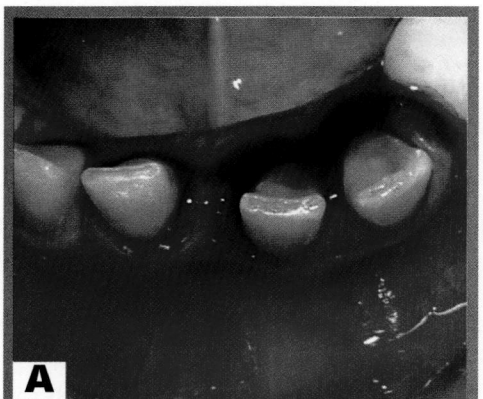
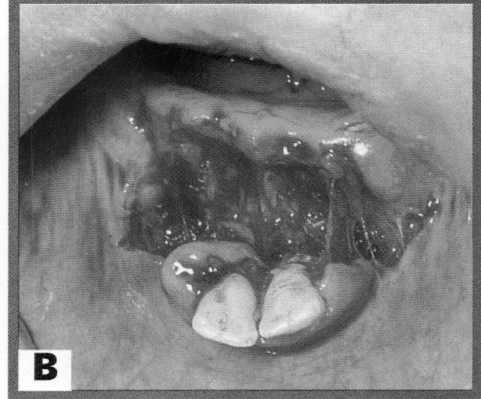

Figure 5.11 A Luxations in the mandible usually present with an anterior displacement of the incisors. This child presented 1 week after trauma with continued gingival oozing. He was subsequently diagnosed with Christmas disease (factor-IX deficiency). **B** A dento-alveolar fracture in a 6-month-old infant. In these cases it is important to reposition the bone, with or without the teeth. A thick (2-0) nylon suture passed through both labial and lingual plates can be used to provide fixation for the fragment. Teeth usually survive this trauma and there are few untoward sequelae for the permanent teeth.

than fractured. Enamel and dentine may be smoothed with a disk and if possible cover the dentine with glass–ionomer cement or composite resin. Paediatric strip crowns are often useful. A possible sequel is pulp necrosis and grey discoloration.

Complicated crown/root fractures (Figure 5.12C & D)

More commonly, fractures of primary teeth involve the pulp and extend below the gingival margin. Commonly, there are multiple fractures in individual teeth. In these cases it is not possible to adequately restore the tooth and so it should be removed. Often the fracture is not immediately evident, but the child may present several days after the trauma with a pulp polyp separating the fragments. Such a proliferative response is a protective mechanism and is not painful.

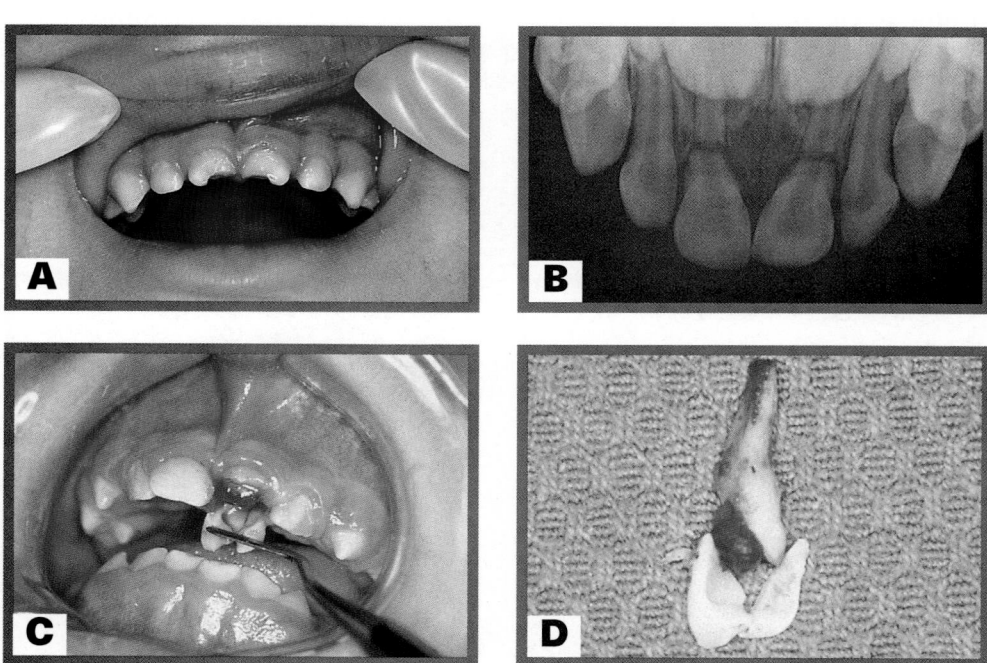

Figure 5.12 A Minor enamel/dentine fractures can be smoothed with a disk or left untreated. **B** Root fractures, again, require no treatment unless the coronal fragments are excessively mobile. The apical portions remain vital and resorb normally. **C** A complex crown/root fracture involving the upper-left primary central incisor tooth. These teeth are unrestorable and need extraction. The extent of the subgingival fracture can be seen in **D**. The pulpal polyp that forms usually causes no discomfort.

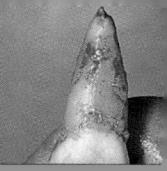

Management
- Most discomfort results from the movement of fractured pieces of enamel still held by the gingiva or periodontal ligament. In emergency management these loose tooth fragments should be removed.
- The remaining tooth can be extracted when convenient. This may necessitate the use of sedation or a short general anaesthetic.
- If a small piece of root remains in the socket after a fracture it may be safely left *in situ* where it will be resorbed as the permanent tooth erupts. It is important to keep parents adequately informed in these situations.

Root fractures (Fig. 5.12B)
As mentioned above, when children fracture primary incisors, there is usually a complex crown/root fracture that extends below the gingival margin and extraction is indicated. Isolated root fractures are uncommon. No treatment is usually necessary for primary incisors. If, at regular review, the pulp shows signs of necrosis, with excessive mobility or sinus formation, the coronal portion should be removed. Apical root fragments are always removed by resorption as the permanent tooth erupts.

Dento-alveolar fracture (Figure 5.11B)
This is more common in the mandible with the anterior teeth displaced anteriorly with the labial plate. It is often desirable to reposition the teeth with the bone to maintain the alveolar contour. This can be achieved with a thick nylon suture (2-0) passed through the labial and lingual plates of the bone. Teeth that are excessively mobile should be carefully dissected out of the sockets preserving the labial plate, which is then repositioned and sutured.

Sequelae after trauma to primary teeth (Figure 5.13)

It is important to discuss with parents the sequelae of luxated or avulsed primary incisors. Although it may be difficult to accurately predict the prognosis for permanent teeth, parents appreciate having an idea of possible outcomes.

Damage to the permanent dentition occurs more often with intrusive luxation and avulsion in very young children. It is important to warn parents of possible problems with permanent teeth but also to reassure them that, with modern restorative materials, minor defects are easily repaired. Sequelae for the permanent dentition are dependent on:
- Direction and displacement of the primary root apex (Figure 5.13B).
- Degree of alveolar damage.
- Stage of formation of the permanent tooth.

Possible damage to primary and permanent teeth
- Necrosis of the pulp of the primary tooth with grey discoloration and possible abscess formation.
- Internal resorption of the primary tooth.
- Ankylosis of the primary tooth requiring later surgical removal. This is performed just before eruption of the permanent incisor.
- Hypoplasia (Figure 5.13F) or hypomineralization (Figure 5.13D) of succedaneous teeth.
- Dilaceration of the crown, or root, varies by developmental stage (Figure 5.13E).
- Resorption of the permanent tooth germ.

Treatment options
- If the primary tooth is discolored, but asymptomatic, no treatment is usually indicated, however, masking a discoloured tooth with composite resin may be an option if aesthetics are of concern. If an abscess is present, pulpectomy or extraction is indicated.
- Hypoplasia and hypomineralization of the permanent teeth can be restored with composite resin.
- Dilaceration of the crown or root of the permanent tooth often necessitates surgical exposure and bonding of chains or brackets for orthodontic extrusion (see Figure 7.6 for details of surgical procedure). Severe cases may be untreatable and such teeth may need to be removed.

Crown and root fractures of permanent incisors

Crown infractions
An incomplete fracture (or crack) of the enamel without loss of tooth structure. Fractures do not cross the dentino-enamel junction and usually require trans-illumination or indirect light to be viewed.

Management
- Pulp-sensibility test.
- Peri-apical radiographs.

Review
- Pulp-sensibility testing after 3 and 12 months.
- Radiography after 12 months.

Uncomplicated enamel and enamel/dentine fractures
Uncomplicated fractures are confined to enamel or enamel and dentine but do not involve the pulp. The most common presentation is an oblique fracture of the mesial or distal corner of an incisor.

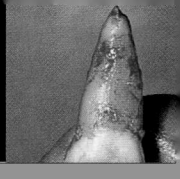

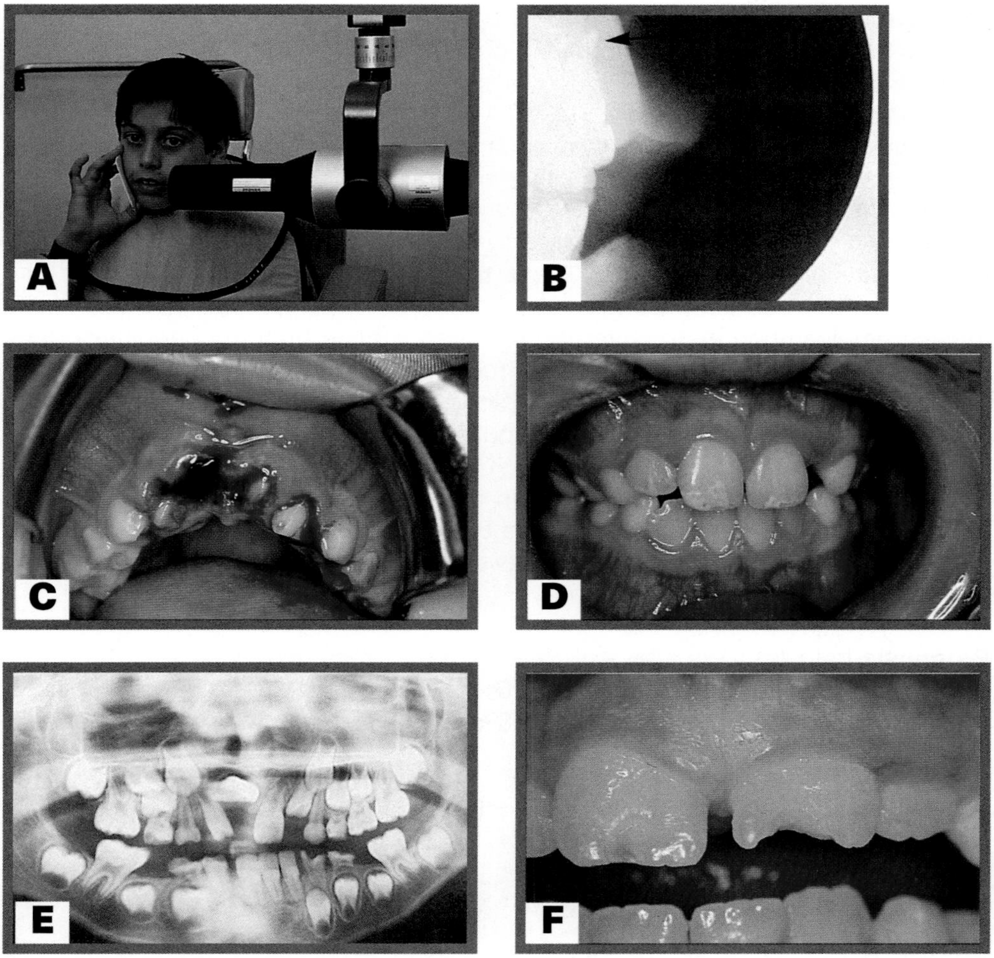

Figure 5.13 **A** Technique of taking a true lateral maxillary radiograph. This film gives a good localization of the position of the primary root apex in relation to the central incisors. **B** The root apex is clearly visible, just underneath the anterior nasal spine, having perforated the labial plate. In this situation, damage to the unerupted permanent tooth is less likely. **C** It is often difficult to predict sequelae. For example, this case of severe intrusion, and alveolar disruption, has caused little damage other than mild hypocalcification of the permanent incisors **D**. **E** Displacement and dilaceration of the upper-right permanent central incisor, following avulsion of the primary-precursor tooth, at 18 months of age. **F** Hypoplasia of the permanent central incisors resulting from trauma in the primary dentition.

Management
- Baseline periapical radiographs and pulp-sensibility tests.
- Enamel-only fractures—smooth over sharp edges with a disc or restore with composite resin if required.
- Enamel and dentine fractures—cover dentine with glass–ionomer and then restore the crown with composite resin either immediately or at review (Figure 5.14).

Review
- Pulp sensibility testing after 3, 6 and 12 months and then yearly.
- Radiographs at each review.

It is extremely important to cover the exposed dentine of permanent incisors as soon as possible. This is to prevent direct irritation of the pulp via the dentinal tubules. Parents have often saved the fractured piece of permanent incisor which can sometimes be used to restore the tooth by being bonded back onto the tooth with composite resin.

In a very immature tooth, if the pulp is very close to being exposed by the fracture, an elective Cvek pulpotomy (see below) may be indicated. This will ensure normal development of the apex and prevent the need for any possible open-apex endodontic procedure (apexification).

Prognosis Pulp necrosis after extensive proximal fracture:
- No protective coverage of dentine   54%
- With dentine coverage   8%

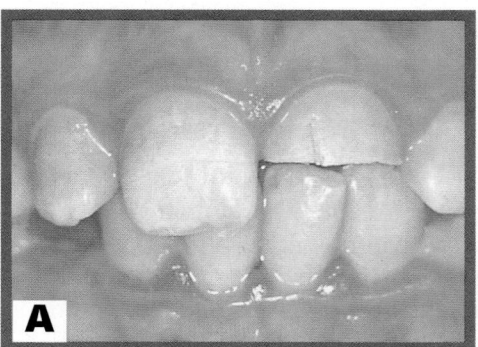 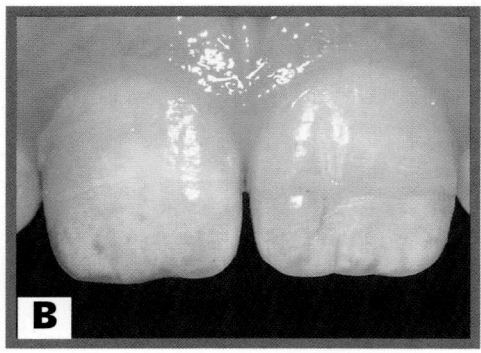

Figure 5.14 Cementation of a fractured enamel fragment. **A** A chamfer or bevel is placed around the fragment and remaining crown and the dentine covered with glass–ionomer. **B** Composite resin is then used to bind the fragment to the crown. It is often impossible to recreate the subtle hypocalcific flecks in a crown with composite resin alone; the replacement of the fractured piece is a good alternative technique if the fragments can be found.

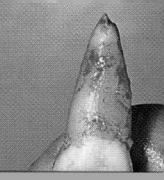

Complicated crown fractures (Figure 5.15)

Fractures involving enamel, dentine and exposure of the pulp.

- Involves laceration and exposure of the pulp to the oral environment.
- Healing does not occur spontaneously and untreated exposures will result in pulp necrosis.

The time elapsed since the injury and the stage of root development will influence treatment. If the tooth is treated within hours of the exposure conservative management is appropriate. After several days, micro-abscesses occur within the pulp, and more radical pulp amputation is required.

Aim: *To preserve vital, non-inflamed pulp tissue, biologically walled off by a hard tissue barrier* (Cvek, 1978)

In almost all situations, if vital pulp tissue can be covered with a calcium-hydroxide dressing, it is possible to form a dentine bridge over the defect. It is undoubtedly preferable to preserve tooth vitality rather than commence root-canal therapy.

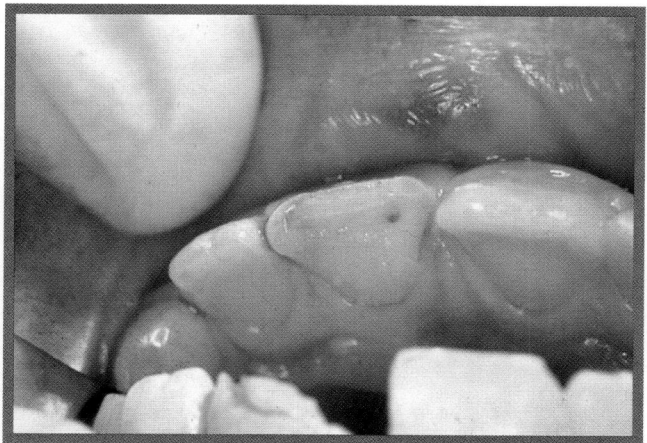

Figure 5.15
Assessment of any pulp exposure is essential, especially in cases where the tooth is immature. Immediate coverage and dressing will help to prevent pulp necrosis and the need for an open apex endodontic procedure.

Incomplete root apex with vital pulp
Cvek pulpotomy (apexogenesis) (Figure 5.16A & B)

The Cvek pulpotomy procedure involves the removal of contaminated pulp tissue with a clean round high-speed diamond burr, using saline or water irrigation. A non-setting calcium hydroxide or Ledermix cement dressing is placed directly onto uncontaminated vital tissue.

- Local anaesthesia.
- The use of rubber dam is mandatory.
- The pulp is washed with saline until the haemorrhage stops. Any clot should then be gently rinsed away.

- Non-setting calcium hydroxide is placed over the pulp remnant and this is then covered with a setting calcium hydroxide. It is essential that the calcium hydroxide is placed over vital tissue, it must not be placed over a blood clot. Alternatively, Ledermix cement may be placed directly on to the exposed pulp.
- Glass–ionomer cement base is placed over the dressings and the tooth is restored with composite resin.

This technique does not need to be limited to the coronal pulp. A 'partial pulpotomy' may be performed at any level of the root canal as there are great benefits in preserving the vitality of traumatized incisors.

Review
- 3–6 monthly with pulp vitality tests.
- Radiographs at review to check for hard-tissue barrier formation and continued root development (Figure 5.16B).

Prognosis
- Success rates 80–96%.

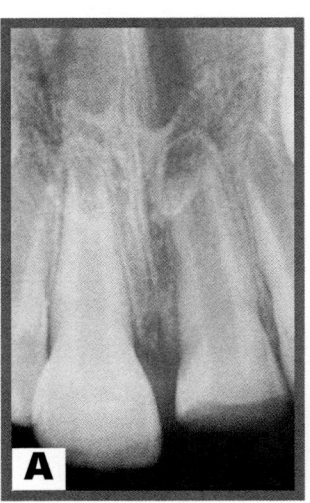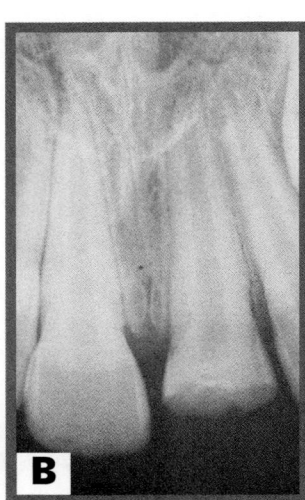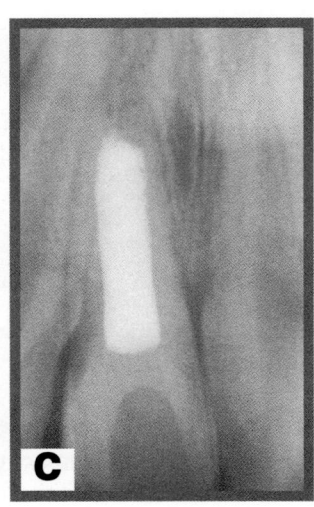

Figure 5.16 A Pulp exposure in an immature central incisor. **B** A Cvek pulpotomy (apexogenesis) has allowed normal root development with a dentine barrier in the crown. This significantly strengthens the root, especially at the cemento-enamel junction. **C** An open apex root-canal therapy is a difficult procedure, requiring apexification, and the long-term prognosis of the tooth may be questionable because of its inherent weakness.

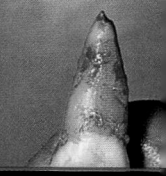

Incomplete root apex with necrotic pulp

If the pulp of a tooth with a complicated crown fracture is necrotic then extirpation and root-canal therapy is required. Although there is no difference in prognosis of the root filling in immature teeth, compared with mature teeth, long-term survival of any tooth with an open apex is reduced. This is caused by the thin cervical dentine and a short-ened root which make the tooth susceptible to fracture not only during endodontic procedures but also during function. Endodontic treatment in immature anterior teeth is difficult because of the inability to create an apical seat, the thin dentinal walls, and the difficulty in obturating the canal by the traditional method of lateral condensation.

Aim To use calcium-hydroxide therapy to create an apical hard-tissue barrier (apexification) against which the root canal filling can be placed.

Technique (apexification)
- Local anaesthesia.
- Create access cavity under rubber dam.
- Extirpate the necrotic pulp tissue.
- Mechanically prepare the canal 1 mm short of the radiographic apex.
- The canal should be carefully instrumented to completely remove necrotic debris, but preserve as much tooth structure as possible. The apical root, being very thin, is weak and may fracture if undue pressure is exerted.
- Irrigate thoroughly with sodium hypochlorite (i.e. 1% NaOCl) to dissolve pulp-tissue remnants and to disinfect the canal system.
- Ledermix should be placed as the initial dressing followed by calcium hydroxide.
- Redress a non-setting calcium hydroxide paste, after 1–2 weeks, with a paste-filler
- Compress the calcium hydroxide with a cotton-wool pellet to ensure good condensation in the canal and to allow contact with apical tissues.
- Place glass–ionomer or zinc oxide eugenol (IRM) temporary dressing

Review
- 3–6 monthly.

The formation of a calcific bridge may take up to 18 months. Once the bridge has formed the canal may be obturated. The calcium hydroxide should be changed every 2–3 months. This fresh dressing ensures an adequate concentration of calcium hydroxide and reduces the chances of infection.
- Obturation is performed with gutta-percha using either a warm vertical condensation technique or lateral condensation. An impression of the apical seat may be made with softened gutta-percha which is then cemented into the canal with an endodontic sealer. Whichever technique is used, it should be stressed that gentle pressure must be applied to avoid root splitting or pushing the calcified barrier through the apex (Figure 5.16C).

In immature teeth there is occasionally development of a small root apex, although the pulp otherwise appears necrotic. This appears to be caused by surviving remnants of Hertwig's epithelial root sheath.

Mature root apex

If the pulp of a permanent anterior tooth is exposed by trauma, and the period of exposure is short, it need not be removed, regardless of the apical development. The Cvek (partial) pulpotomy can be used to attempt to preserve the vitality of the pulp. If there are restorative considerations (i.e. the need for a post) it may be better to perform a complete extirpation and root-canal therapy immediately.

Root fractures

A fracture involving enamel, dentine and cementum which may or may not involve the pulp. Pulp necrosis occurs in 25% of cases and is related to the degree of displacement of the fragments. Progressive inflammatory or replacement root resorption is rare.

To check for horizontal root fractures, alter the vertical angulation of periapical radiographs. When looking for vertical root fractures, change the horizontal angulation.

Sometimes, a horizontal root fracture is not initially evident. This is because the fracture site opens up under the influence of an inflammatory exudate several days after the injury. Thus, for all traumatized teeth it is important to take a subsequent radiograph within 2 weeks (Figure 5.17A).

Frequency
- Primary dentition   0.5–7%
- Permanent dentition   2–4%

Healing of root fractures
- Hard-tissue union with calcified tissue (osseodentine).
- Interposition of bone.
- Interposition of fibrous connective tissue.
- Granulation tissue indicating coronal pulp necrosis.

Management
- Radiographs—several vertical angulations of periapical radiographs are usually required to adequately determine the extent of the fracture.
- Repositioning of coronal fragment.
- Rigid splinting with composite resin and wire or orthodontic appliances for at least 3 months if coronal fragment is mobile.
- High apical root fractures often require no treatment.

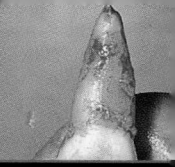

Review
- Pulp-sensibility testing every month for 6 months, then test again after a further 3 months, then test again every year for 5 years.
- Radiographs at recall appointment.

Pulp necrosis of coronal fragment
It is uncommon for the apical fragment to develop pulp necrosis. If pulp necrosis of the coronal fragment occurs, there will be radiographic signs of bone loss at the level of the fracture. Other symptoms, such as pain, excessive mobility or gingival swelling and sinus formation, may also be present.
- Extirpate the pulp from coronal fragment to 1 mm below the fracture line. Never advance an instrument through the fracture site.
- Place non-setting calcium hydroxide paste to induce hard-tissue barrier formation at the fracture site. This may take up to 18 months.
- Obturate with gutta-percha once the barrier has formed (Figure 5.17B).

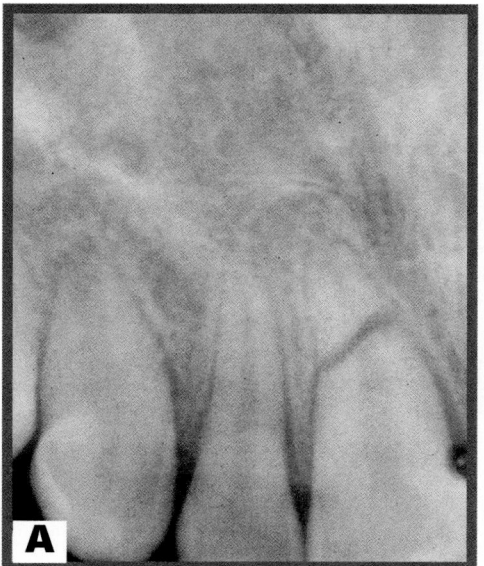
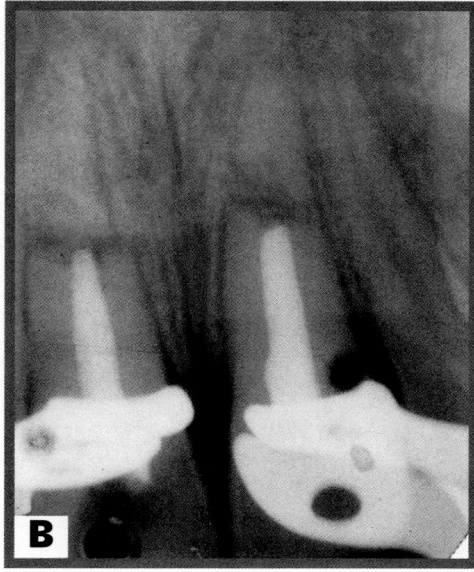

Figure 5.17 **A** High apical fractures often require no treatment. In most cases the apical fragment is not necrotic. **B** When the coronal fragments are necrotic, root-canal therapy should only be performed up to the fracture line. Long-term calcium-hydroxide therapy is required becauses the 'apex' at the fracture site will be wide open. In this case, bone is interposed between the two fragments.

Pulp necrosis of both apical and coronal fragments

When the apical fragment shows signs of necrosis the prognosis is poor. Extirpation and obturation of the coronal fragment should be performed followed by periapical surgery to remove the apical fragment. There have been reports of intraradicular splinting and endodontic implants, but both have a very poor long-term prognosis.

Crown/root fractures

The coronal fragments should always be removed to fully assess the extent of the fracture (Figure 5.18A).

Uncomplicated crown/root fracture

Where the fracture extends just below the gingival margin, cover the dentine with a glass–ionomer initially and then restore the tooth with composite resin or a crown.

Complicated crown/root fracture (pulp exposure)

- If the fracture extends below the crestal bone and the root development is complete remove the coronal fragments to assess the extent of the fracture and extirpate the pulp. Calcium hydroxide or Ledermix paste may be placed as the initial endodontic dressing.
- If the crown/root fracture does not extend below the crestal bone, and the root development is complete, a Cvek pulpotomy may be performed. This type of fracture may be restorable with composite resin whereas the more deeply extending fracture may need a cast restoration or necessitate surgical treatment.
- The prognosis for a tooth with a complicated crown/root fracture is poor.

Options for management
- Gingivectomy to expose fracture margin. If the fracture is minimal, and just below the gingival margin, then restoration of the root surface may be performed with glass–ionomer cement and a crown buildup in composite resin.
- Cast crown with extended shoulder with or without periodontal flap procedure.
- Orthodontic extrusion of the root to expose the fracture margin.
- Extraction.
- Root burial.

Orthodontic extrusion This may be a viable option in management provided there is adequate root length to support a crown. A gingivoplasty will almost always be required to reposition the gingival margin after the completion of retention. Fixed appliances are placed to extrude the root so that the margin is exposed. Retention may be difficult and a pericision is advisable. Because of the narrower emergence profile of the root compared with the crown of a normal tooth, a satisfactory aesthetic result may be difficult to achieve.

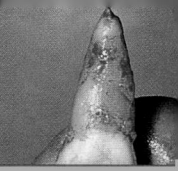

Root burial (Figure 5.19) In cases of subalveolar root fracture, root burial may be an alternative to extraction in order to preserve alveolar bone. The root is buried below the alveolar crest and a coronally repositioned flap raised to cover the defect with periosteum. In this way, it is possible for bone to grow over the root surface (Figure 5.19). The root may be vital or obturated with gutta-percha. Implants are an option in later management without the need for ridge augmentation.

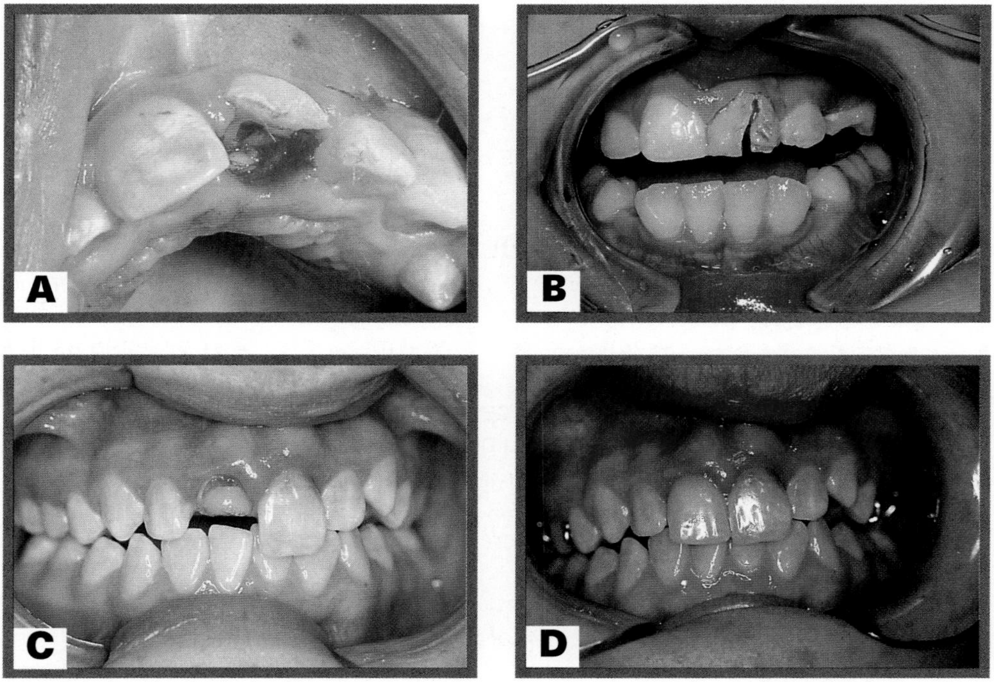

Figure 5.18 **A** The coronal fragment of a crown/root fracture should always be removed to investigate the extent of the fracture. In this case it lies just above the alveolar crest on the palate, about 4 mm below the gingival margin. Treatment will involve periodontal-flap surgery and placement of a crown with an extended shoulder. Alternatively, orthodontic extrusion may be required. **B** Vertical fractures are virtually untreatable. They may be held together with an orthodontic band or composite resin, but their prognosis is very poor. Retention in the short term may be valuable to preserve bone while planning for possible orthodontics, or implants, when growth has finished. **C** A crown/root fracture in an immature tooth with a poor prognosis. **D** A removable appliance was constructed with the pontic covering the retained root. Retention of the root will maintain alveolar bone prior to the consideration of long-term restorative needs.

Crown/root fractures in immature teeth

When complex crown/root fractures occur in teeth with incomplete apical formation, consideration should be given to maintaining the pulp vitality, where possible, to allow continuation of root development. However, if the pulp has undergone necrosis and infection, then endodontic treatment including apexification will be necessary. It is worth noting, however, that complicated crown/root fractures tend to occur in mature teeth where consideration of apical development is unnecessary. As a general comment, if the complex fracture extends below the crestal bone then the prognosis is poor.

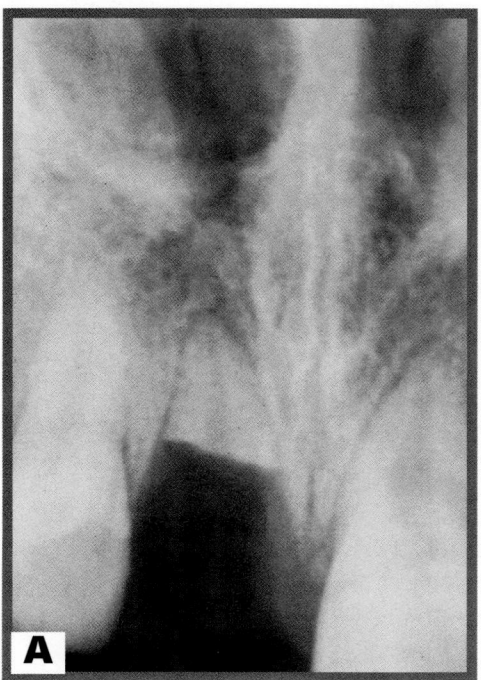 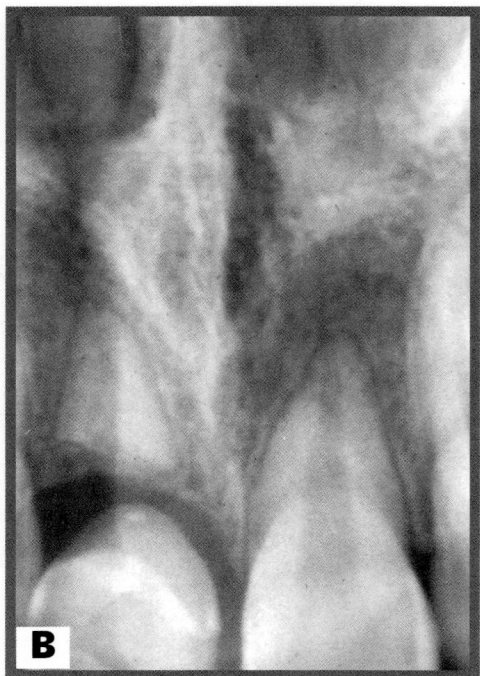

Figure 5.19 Root burial of a tooth fractured below the alveolar crest. Root burial may be an alternative to extraction in these cases. The root has been covered with a mucoperiosteal flap which has stimulated bone growth over the root. This preserves the alveolar height for later prosthodontic work. The original crown has been contoured and attached to adjacent teeth with composite resin.

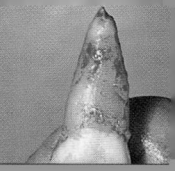

Luxations in the permanent dentition

Concussion and subluxation

These teeth are treated symptomatically. Concussed teeth will have a marked response to percussion, but the tooth will be firm in the socket. A subluxated tooth will exhibit increased mobility but will not have been displaced.

Management
- Relieve from occlusion, splinting is not required.
- Soft diet for 2 weeks.

Review
- Pulp sensibility testing at 1, 3, and 6 months then yearly.
- Radiographs at each review.

It is also important to follow these teeth for at least 4 years clinically checking pulp status, colour, mobility and radiographically assessing changes in the size of the pulp chamber and in root development.

Prognosis
- Pulp necrosis in 3–6%

Lateral and extrusive luxation

Teeth may be luxated in any direction and, depending on the extent of luxation, the teeth may need repositioning and splinting. This can be achieved with digital pressure or with forceps. If the latter are used, care must be taken to avoid damage to the root surface.

Management
- Repositioning with local anaesthesia. Early repositioning is important as it is often extremely difficult to mobilize the tooth if the patient presents after 24 hours (Figure 5.20A & B).
- Suture gingival lacerations.
- Flexible splinting with composite resin, and wire or orthodontic appliances, for up to 3 weeks for extrusive luxation, and 6–8 weeks for lateral luxation because of concomitant alveolar bone fracture, see Figure 5.20C & D).
- Antibiotics, tetanus prophylaxis, and 0.2% chlorhexidine gluconate mouthrinse if required.
- Lateral luxations always have a component of dento-alveolar fracture and it is important to mould the bone back into the correct position. Those fragments of bone attached to periosteum should be retained.

Review
- Review every 2 weeks while the splint is in place, then 1, 3, 6 and 12 monthly up to 5 years.

- Pulp-sensibility testing.
- Radiographs at each visit.

Prognosis
- Dependent on the degree of displacement and apical development, with excellent healing in immature teeth.
- Pulp necrosis occurs in 15–85% of cases and is more prevalent in teeth with closed apices.
- Pulp-canal obliteration often occurs in teeth with immature apices.
- Resorption is rare.
- Transient apical breakdown (2–12%) is an expansion of the apical periodontal ligament space. There is no indication for commencing root-canal therapy, unless there are other indicators of infection of the pulp canal.

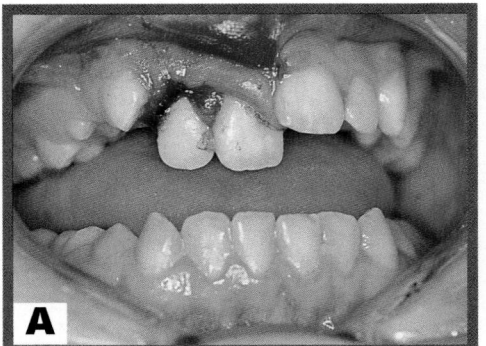
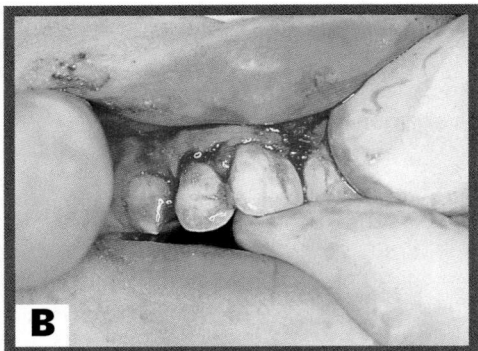
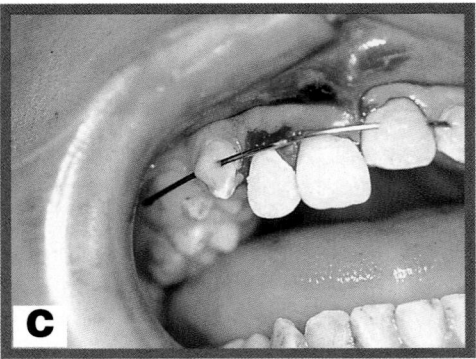
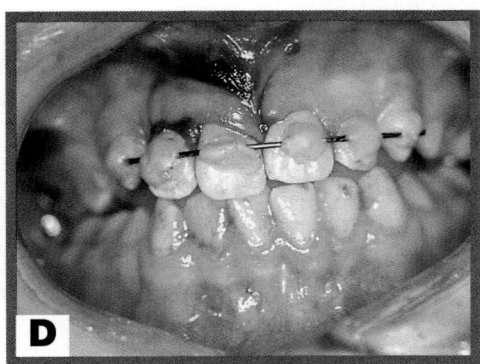

Figure 5.20 A Dento-alveolar fracture involving the upper-right central and lateral incisors. **B** The block of teeth and bone is manually replaced with finger pressure and a rigid composite resin and wire splint placed **C** and **D**. When placing a splint, attach and stabilize uninvolved teeth before splinting the displaced segment.

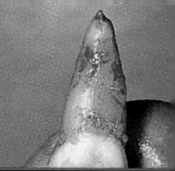

Intrusion

Intrusion (caused by the compression of the root into alveolar bone) is one of the worst injuries that can occur. There is extensive damage to the supporting structures and the neurovascular bundle. When teeth are intrusively luxated there is much discussion as to whether they should be repositioned or allowed to re-erupt on their own. Treatment may well depend on the state of apical development and, as a general rule, the partial disimpaction and flexible splinting of severely intruded teeth with incomplete root formation is preferred.

Management Current research has suggested that early repositioning of intruded permanent teeth is essential. The aims of disimpaction are to avoid ankylosis, minimize pressure necrosis of the periodontal ligament and allow access to the palatal surface of the tooth to extirpate the pulp within 14 days.

Repositioning

- If the crown remains visible and there is a very wide immature apex (>2 mm) the tooth may be allowed to re-erupt spontaneously.
- Immediate repositioning is preferred for mature teeth.
- Fixed orthodontic appliances can be used to apply traction to the intruded tooth over a 2–3-week period (Figure 5.21) OR
- Gently reposition the tooth with fingers or with forceps applied only to the crown. Avoid rotating the tooth in the socket.
- Extrusion should be rapid so that the palatal surface is exposed   and   an access cavity can be made.

Endodontics

- Extirpation of the pulp is essential in almost all cases. Ledermix paste should be placed as the initial dressing for up to 3 months, followed by calcium hydroxide for 3 months before obturation.
- If the apex is immature, then a further period of calcium-hydroxide therapy will be required for apexification before root-canal obturation.
- The only exceptions are partially-intruded extremely immature teeth which are being left to re-erupt (with regular monitoring).

Review It is essential that these teeth are regularly followed up. Progressive inflammatory resorption occurs very rapidly and an immature tooth may be lost within a number of weeks.

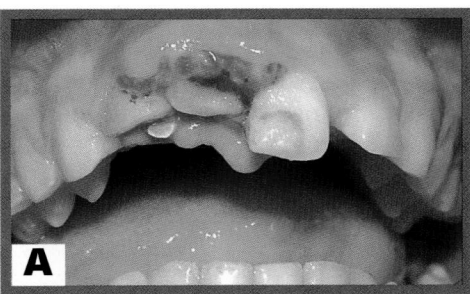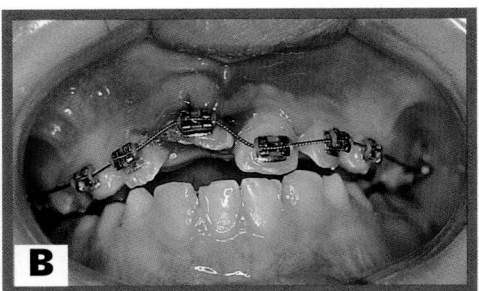

Figure 5.21 A Intrusion of the upper-right permanent incisor and canine teeth. This child was involved in a motor-vehicle accident and unfortunately no dental treatment was available. At presentation, 2 months later, the intruded teeth had become ankylosed and could not be moved orthodontically. They subsequently underwent replacement resorption and a denture was constructed. Early mobilization is essential to prevent ankylosis and allow access to the palatal surface to perform pulp extirpation. **B** An example of orthodontic appliances being used to extrude a partially intruded tooth. If the crown is completely intruded, a flap should be raised and the tooth mobilized surgically.

Prognosis
- Mature teeth undergo pulp necrosis in almost all cases (96%), and there is a high prevalence of root resorption and ankylosis.
- Immature teeth that re-erupt show pulp necrosis in 60% of cases and ankylosis in up to 50% of cases.
- Teeth treated early have a much better prognosis.

Dento-alveolar fractures
With luxation of teeth, the alveolar plate can be fractured or deformed. Use firm finger pressure on the buccal and lingual plates to reposition. It should be remembered that alveolar fractures can occur without significant dental involvement. These alveolar fractures should be splinted for 3–4 weeks in children (or 6–8 weeks in adults). Luxated or avulsed teeth usually result in alveolar bone fracture and/or displacement. Firm pressure is needed to realign bony fragments. Splinting will be required for 3–4 weeks.

Pulp vitality
Current pulp-sensibility tests only test the ability of the pulpal nerves to respond to the stimulus; they do not provide any information about the presence or absence of blood supply or the histological status of the pulp. When determining the status of the pulp in luxated permanent teeth beware of false test results. Negative results may

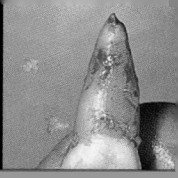

arise because of damage of sensory nerves of the pulp, even though the tooth's vascularity is maintained. It may take up to 1 year (or never) to get a positive response from such a pulp. Thus, one must be careful to judge the patient's signs and symptoms before commencing endodontics. Regular radiographs are required to assess root development and growth, evidence of external or internal root resorption, and changes in the shape of the pulp chamber. Clinically, changes in colour, excess mobility, tenderness to percussion and sinus formation are important diagnostic signs.

Radiographs
It is important to remember that when teeth have been luxated they may have suffered a crown or root fracture. The crown fractures are usually obvious but root fractures may be hidden or not yet apparent. Therefore, radiographs are always essential.

Avulsion of permanent teeth

If a permanent incisor is avulsed, the chance of successful retention is enhanced by minimizing the extra-oral time. Even if the tooth has been out of the mouth for an extended period, it is still better to replant the tooth, with the knowledge that success might be unlikely. In the mixed dentition this is important, as replantation of even questionable teeth will allow normal establishment of the arch and occlusion. Furthermore, orthodontic treatment planning is simpler if the tooth remains in the socket. These teeth are usually lost by replacement resorption, which has the benefit of preserving the alveolar bone height, making prosthodontic replacement much simpler.

First aid advice
Always check the patient's clothing for avulsed teeth that are thought to be lost. It is important that parents, caregivers and teachers have access to appropriate advice on the management of avulsed teeth. Timing is essential and this information can be given over the telephone.
- Replant the tooth immediately if clean.
- Hold the tooth in place with aluminium foil or bite gently on a handkerchief or clean cloth and seek urgent dental treatment.
- If dirty, rinse the tooth in milk and then replant.
- If unable to replant, store the tooth in isotonic media to prevent dehydration and death of the periodontal ligament cells. Use:
  Preferably milk OR
  Saline (i.e. contact lens solution)
  Wrap in plastic cling wrap.
- Do not use water as this will result in hypotonic lysis of ligament cells.
- Seek urgent dental treatment.

Management in the dental surgery

- Gently debride the root surface under copious saline, milk or tissue-culture media (Hanks balanced salt solution) irrigation. When holding teeth always do so by the crown in a wet gauze square (teeth can be very slippery, see Figure 5.22A).
- Give local anaesthesia and gently debride the tooth socket, taking care not to curette the bone or remaining ligament (Figure 5.22B).
- Replant the tooth and place a splint. The tooth usually 'clicks' back into the correct position if there has not been too much bony damage (Figure 5.22C).
- Splint for 7–10 days (Figure 5.22D).
- Reposition any degloved gingival tissues and suture if required.
- Prescribe high-dose, broad-spectrum antibiotics and check current immunization status.
- Account for any lost teeth. A chest radiograph may be required.
- Normal diet and strict oral hygiene including chlorhexidine gluconate 0.2% mouthwash

Splinting of avulsed teeth

- Composite resin and nylon fibre (0.6-mm diameter) such as fishing line (20-kg breaking strain) OR
- Orthodontic brackets with arch wire (0.014").
- Orthodontic appliances are particularly useful as the time taken to apply the brackets is half that to set composite resin.
- Splints should be flexible to allow normal physiological movement of the tooth. This helps to reduce the development of ankylosis; however, if there is a bone or root fracture present, then a rigid splint must be used so that there is no movement of the teeth and bony segments.
- Splints should generally stay in place for 7–10 days if there are no complicating factors such as alveolar or root fractures. The occlusion may need to be relieved when the degree of overbite or luxation is such that the tooth receives unwanted masticatory force. This can be achieved by minimal removal of enamel, or construction of an upper removable appliance, or placement of composite resin on the molars to open the bite. Some physiological movement is necessary.

Replanting of dry teeth

As a general rule, all teeth should be replanted whether wet or dry. Although the prognosis of the tooth may be poor, it is usually preferable to have the tooth present for 5 years during growth than not at all. Always keep options open for future treatment.

- Gently remove the dead periodontal ligament with sodium hypochlorite to chemically dissolve away the periodontal ligament. Do not scale or root plane the cementum at all.
- Create access cavity and extirpate the pulp.

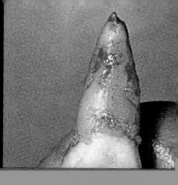

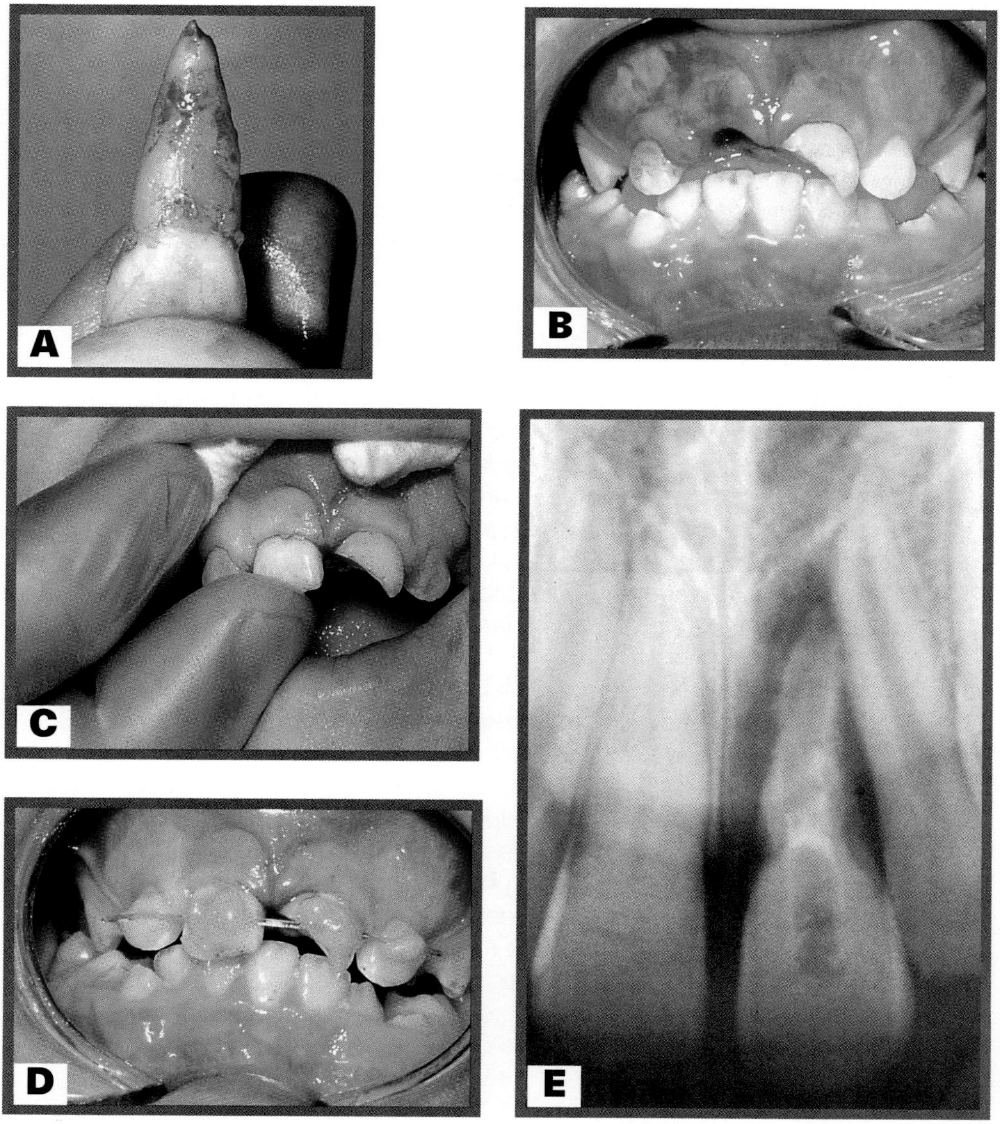

Figure 5.22 Management of avulsion. **A** Always hold the tooth by the crown and gently debride the root surface with saline. **B** The socket should be irrigated and clear of debris. **C** Replant with firm pressure. The tooth will usually click back into position. **D** Splint with a flexible splint, such as composite and nylon fishing line, to allow some physiological movement. **E** Inflammatory root resorption resulting from a failure to adequately instrument and medicate the root canal.

- Rinse the tooth in 2% NaF (pH 5.5) for 20 minutes.
- The aim is to incorporate fluoride into the dentine and cementum which may reduce ankylosis.
- Place Ledermix paste in the root canal.
- Replant and splint for 14 days.
- Replace the Ledermix with calcium hydroxide after 3 months and complete the root-canal filling after 6–12 months if there is no sign of inflammatory resorption.

Endodontics
Immature root apex
- If the tooth has been avulsed, replanted within a short period and the apex is **very** immature (>2 mm and the child is <8 years), then endodontic treatment is only needed if the symptoms and clinical signs indicate that the pulp space has become infected.
- If the canal becomes infected, then Ledermix is placed initially for 3 months and then calcium-hydroxide therapy commenced to induce apexification. The calcium hydroxide should be non-setting and placed so as to fill the radicular pulp space, and sealed with Cavit or glass–ionomer cement. This is changed 3-monthly until an apical barrier is formed and obturation is possible. There may only be a 30% survival in immature teeth even if replanted early.

Mature root apex
- In all other situations, in which the apex of the avulsed tooth is less than 2 mm open or closed, endodontics should be commenced within 10 days. Initial dressings should be Ledermix paste for 3 months followed by calcium hydroxide. The root-canal filling should be completed after 6–12 months.

Generally, it is best to always replant teeth even if they have a poor prognosis. With appropriate treatment, these teeth will be lost by progressive replacement resorption, the positive benefit is that alveolar height is maintained. The only exception are those cases with very immature roots where ankylosis will prevent alveolar bone growth and may complicate future orthodontic and prosthodontic management.

Complications in endodontic management of avulsed teeth

External inflammatory root resorption (Figure 5.22E)
- The progressive loss of tooth structure by an inflammatory process caused by the presence of infected and necrotic debris in the root canal.
- This resorption can be prevented and treated with appropriate therapy.

Factors in prevention and management include:

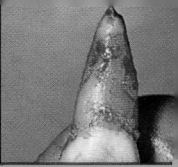

Prophylactic antibiotics
- High-dose, broad-spectrum antibiotics should be given as soon as possible after avulsion and continued for 2 weeks.

Pulp extirpation
- This should be completed as soon as possible after the replantation. It may be done at the time of trauma, but not outside the mouth. It must be done within 10 days.
- Avoid medicaments that may cause inflammation, such as calcium hydroxide, in the first 3 months after trauma. Ledermix paste is an ideal first-dressing medicament as it has been shown to prevent inflammatory root resorption and inhibit the action of clastic cells.

Management
- If inflammatory resorption is detected the canal must be thoroughly re-instrumented and dressed with Ledermix paste for 3 months, but changing the dressing every 6 weeks. Calcium hydroxide can then be placed for a further 3 months after which time, if there is no progression of the resorption, the canal can be filled.

External replacement root resorption
This is the progressive resorption of tooth structure, and replacement with bone, as part of continual bone remodelling. It results from cemental damage greater than 2 mm or from replantation of dry teeth. It cannot be treated and so the aim must be to prevent replacement resorption and subsequent ankylosis.

Factors in prevention and management include:

Extra-oral time
- Prognosis decreases dramatically after 15 minutes if tooth is dry.
- 50% of periodontal-ligament cells are dead after 30 minutes. All are dead after 60 minutes.

Storage media
- Milk is the best medium and may keep cells viable for up to 6 hours. It has the advantage that it is pasteurized, with few bacteria, is readily available and is cold. There appears to be no difference with low-fat or skimmed milks, but yoghurt and sour milk should be avoided.
- Saliva is suitable for up to 2 hours.
- Saline and plastic cling wrap will maintain cells for 1 hour.
- Water is hypotonic and causes cell lysis.
- Tissue culture media such as Hank's balanced-salt solution or RPMI is also appropriate, if available, and may give up to 24 hours' cell survival.

Mechanical damage
- Ankylosis will result if >2 mm of cementum has been removed.
Risk increases with increased handling during transport and replantation.

Splinting Flexible splinting allows physiological movement and results in less ankylosis and replacement resorption.

Management
- No treatment is possible.

Bleaching of non-vital incisors

One consequence of loss or trauma is tooth discoloration. Bleaching is a common procedure following root-canal therapy. The integrity of the root-canal seal is paramount and, above all, bleaching should not be carried out below the cemento-enamel junction because of the risk of initiating cervical resorption.

Method
1. Bleaching must be carried out under rubber dam.
2. Ensure adequate root-canal obturation and remove gutta-percha to a level 3 mm below the cemento-enamel junction.
3. Place a zinc phosphate or Cavit base just above the cemento-enamel junction.
4. Ensure that the access cavity is clean and free of all debris.
5. Acid-etch the access cavity to open dentinal tubules and place a cotton pellet, soaked in 30% H_2O_2, into the access cavity for 3 minutes.
6. Remove the cotton pellet and place a mixture of sodium perborate and hydrogen peroxide into the cavity and seal with a cotton pellet and temporary sealer such as Cavit. The perborate powder and peroxide is mixed to form a thick paste which can be packed into the chamber. This should remain in the tooth for 1 week, after which the success of the procedure is evaluated. This may be repeated several times if required.
7. The pulp chamber is then filled with a glass–ionomer base and the access cavity restored with composite resin.

Soft-tissue injuries

Alveolar mucosa and skin
Bruising (Figure 5.23C & D) The simplest and most common type of soft-tissue injury is bruising. This will often be present without any dental involvement. Treatment is symptomatic. However, be careful to check in the depths of the labial and buccal sulci for any deep soft-tissue wounds or degloving-type injuries.

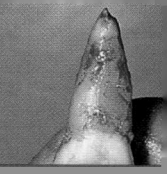

Lacerations (Figures 5.23E & F and 5.24)

- Often a full-thickness laceration of the lower lip can be undetected because of the natural contours of the soft tissues or the tentative examination of an upset child. If there has been dental injury, always look for tooth remnants in the lips.
- Careful suturing of skin wounds will be needed to avoid scarring and should be performed only by those who are competent to do so. Skin wounds must be closed within the first 24 hours and preferably within 6 hours.
- Any debris, such as gravel and dirt, must be removed by scrubbing with a brush wetted with an antiseptic surgical preparation such as povidone iodine 5% or chlorhexidine acetate 0.5%.
- Skin edges are ideally excised with a scalpel to remove necrotic tags and irregular margins.
- Muscle closure and deep suturing is achieved with a fine resorbable material such as polyglactin or polyglycoic acid.
- Final skin closure is with 6-0 monofilament nylon on a cutting needle.

Attached gingival tissues

Degloving (Figure 5.23A & B) One of the most common injuries is degloving. A full-thickness mucoperiosteal flap is stripped off the bone, the separation line usually being the mucogingival junction (Figure 5.23A). These injuries tend to occur after blunt trauma and a common presentation is a large collection of blood in the submental region (Figure 5.23C). The flap is tightly sutured and a pressure dressing placed if the lower arch is involved. This prevents the pooling of blood and prevents swelling in the submental region, which may embarrass the airway.

Interdental suturing of displaced gingival tissue is very important, especially where palatal tissue is involved.

The close re-adaptation of tissues to the tooth surface will help preserve alveolar bone especially interdentally. Suturing will also help keep the tooth in position.

Suturing (see Table 5.2)

- Suturing of torn or lacerated gingival tissues should be considered using a fine suture such as 5-0 resorbable suture (Dexon or Vicryl). Polyglactin or polyglycolic-acid sutures have good traction strength for at least 3 weeks and have less tissue reaction than catgut. As a braided material they are not as clean as monofilament sutures, but they are resorbable.
- Where strength is required, and removal of the sutures is not an issue, monofilament nylon is an excellent material.
- Suturing may prevent a periodontal defect from lack of keratinized tissue, or at least reduce the extent of periodontal work subsequently required.
- Suturing may reduce the sequestration of displaced bony fragments and may prevent bacterial contamination of the gingival sulcus. Furthermore, there is much less pain from the wound if exposed bony defects are well covered with periosteum and gingival tissues.

135

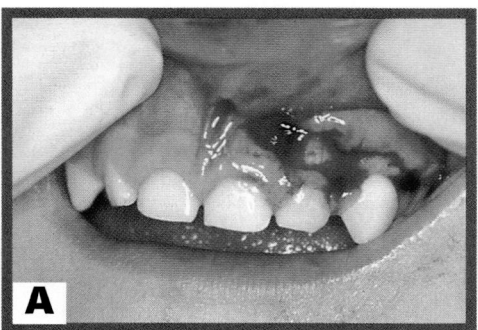
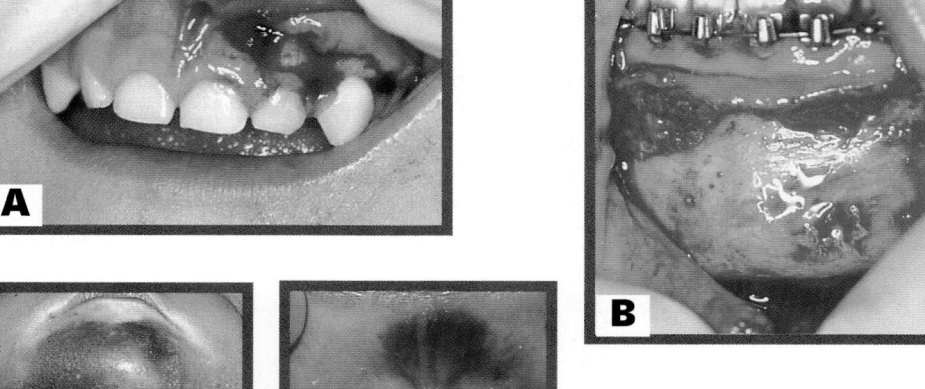
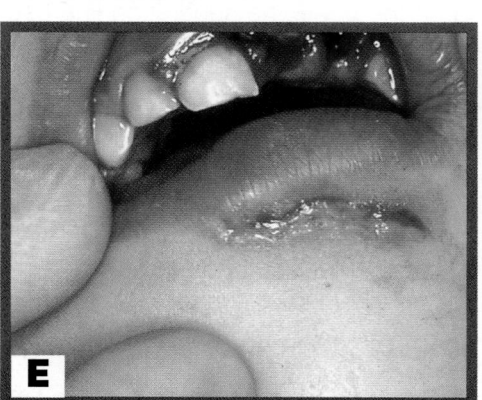
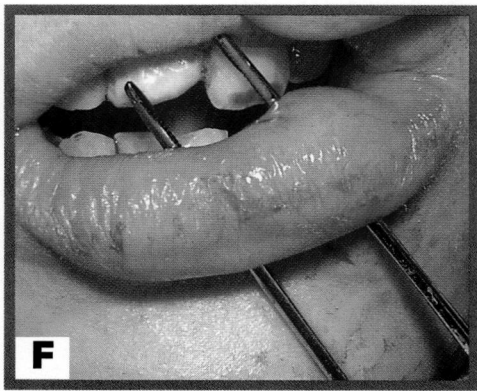

Figure 5.23 **A** Gingival degloving in a young child. Small tears such as this can be repositioned without suturing and will granulate well. **B** Severe degloving of the mandible separating at the mucogingival junction from molar to molar and to the level of the hyoid. The mental nerve on the left was severed. **C** Bruising of the chin is usually associated with severe degloving as in **B**. Bruising of the labial frenum **D** may occur from a blow across the face and child abuse should always be suspected. **E** When upper teeth are intruded, the lip is often bitten and a through-and-through laceration **F** should be identified. These lacerations must be closed in three layers, the muscle, mucosa, and skin. Always check lip lacerations for the presence of any tooth fragments if there are fractured teeth.

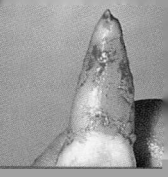

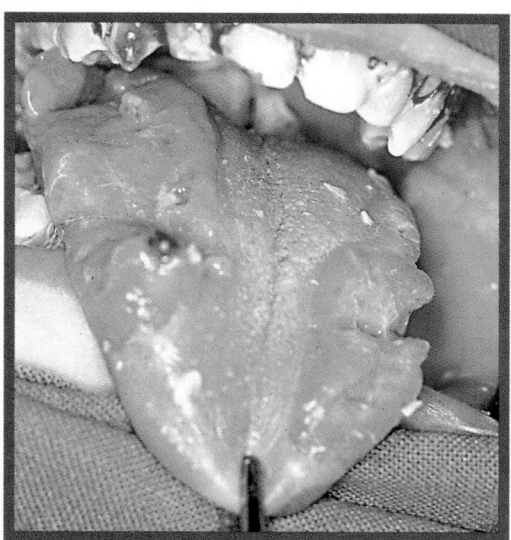

Figure 5.24 Lacerations may be caused by self-mutilation. This child has a peripheral sensory neuropathy (congenital indifference to pain). Attempts to make splints that would stop her behaviour failed and, after much agonizing, a full clearance was performed.

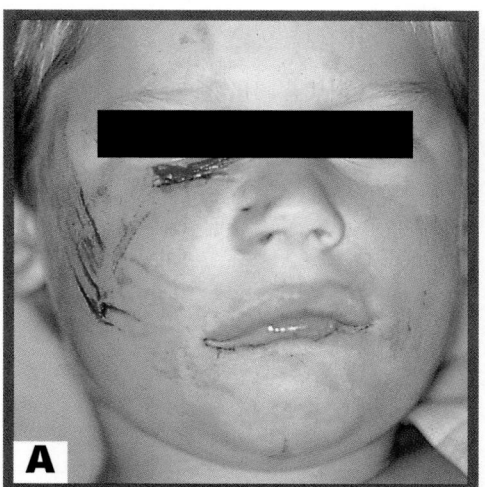

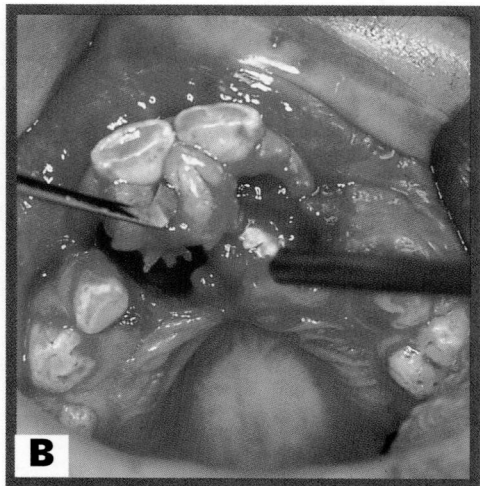

Figure 5.25 A This child was attacked by a dog. He sustained a laceration below the eye, just avoiding the nasolacrimal duct, and scratches on the side of the face. The dog's upper canine was responsible for the facial laceration; its lower canine bit into the palate causing avulsion of the unerupted upper-right permanent-central incisor and displacing a dento-alveolar fragment (**B**). This tooth was replaced in its crypt and continued to develop for a short time before undergoing necrosis. The upper-left permanent-central incisor, although exposed, erupted normally.

Table 5.2 Some indications for selection of suture material in paediatric dentistry

Suture	Indications	Size	Needle	Absorption	Tissue reaction	Notes
Surgical gut	Extraction suture	3-0	Cutting	Completely digested by 70 days. Effective strength for 2–3 days in the oral cavity.	Moderate	Used for tissue closure where strength is required for 1 or 2 days.
Chromic catgut	General closure	4-0	Taper	Completely digested by 110 days, but in the oral cavity it has effective strength for up to 5 days.	Moderate, but less than plain gut	Excellent for oral-tissue closure when longer life is required compared with plain gut.
Polyglycolic acid/ Polyglactin	Alveolar mucosa	4-0 5-0	Taper	Completely absorbed by hydrolysis after 90 days.	Mild	Polyglycolic acid has great advantages for use in the oral cavity in children It has good strength over 7 days and is resorbable.
	Attached gingiva	3-0, 4-0	Cutting			
	Large flaps where strength is required but a resorbable suture is desirable	3-0	Cutting	Faster absorption when exposed to the oral environment. Good strength for a least 2 weeks.		It is often retained for longer periods, however, and has a tendency to accumulate plaque because of its braided nature. Taper needles are useful where tissues are friable.
Monofilament nylon	Large flaps where strength is required (i.e. palate)	3-0, 4-0	Cutting	Essentially a non-resorbable material, but degrades at 15–20% per year.	Extremely low	Excellent tissue reaction and strength. Monofilament material is extremely clean and allows good wound healing but needs to be removed.
	Skin	6-0	Cutting			Skin closure must be performed with 6-0. Sutures should be removed before 7 days.
Surgical silk	General closure of most oral tissues where a non-resorbable suture is required	3-0, 4-0	Cutting	Completely degraded by 2 years.	Moderate	Traditional suture material, used where strength was required. Its use has diminished with the availability of materials such as polyglycolic acid. Is a braided material and therefore not as clean as monofilament.

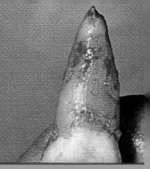

Prevention

- Education of parents and caregivers.
- Seat belts and child restraints.
- Helmets for bike riding.
- Mouthguards.
- Supervision of pets, especially dogs (Figure 5.25).

While seat belts and child restraints are covered by legislation, and more recently helmets for bike riders became mandatory in Australia, the failure of parents to observe these regulations often results in unnecessary childhood craniofacial trauma. It has been the authors' experience that there is often little trauma seen from sports, as most children are wearing mouthguards; nevertheless, there is a disproportionate amount of trauma seen from leisure activities such as skateboarding, swimming, and other 'non-contact' sports.

- Education of parents, caregivers and teachers about primary care for dental trauma is essential. The correct protocols for dealing with avulsed teeth should be available to all schools.

References

Assessment

KOPEL HM, JOHNSON R. Examination and neurological assessment of children with orofacial trauma *Endod Dent Traumatol* 1985, **18**:252–268.

STOCKWELL AJ. Incidence of dental trauma in the Western Australian School Dental Service. *Community Dent Oral Epidemiol* 1988, **16**:294–298.

SCHATZ JP, JOHO JP. A retrospective study of dento-alveolar injuries. *Endod Dent Traumatol* 1994, **10**:11–14.

Facial fractures

COSSIO PI, GALVEZ FE, *et al.* Mandibular fractures in children: a retrospective study of 99 fractures in 59 patients. *Int J Oral Maxillofac Surg* 1994, **23**:329–331.

HARDT N, GOTTSAUNER A. The treatment of mandibular fractures in children. *J Oral Maxillofac Surg* 1993, **21**:214–219.

POSNICK JC, WELLS M, *et al.* Pediatric facial fractures: evolving patterns of treatment. *J Oral Maxillofac Surg* 1993, **51**:836–844.

SILVENNOINEN U, LINDQUIST C. Dental injuries in association with mandibular condyle fractures. *Endod Dent Traumatol* 1993, **9**:254–259.

Child abuse

FONSECA MA, FEIGAL RJ, BENSEL RW. Dental aspects of 1248 cases of child maltreatment on file at a major county hospital. *Pediatr Dent* 1992, **14**:152–157.

NEEDLEMAN HL. Orofacial trauma in child abuse: types, prevalence, management, and the dental profession's involvement. *Pediatr Dent* 1986, **8**:71–79.

Primary trauma

BASSAT YB, BRIN I, FUKS A, ZILBERMAN Y. Effect of trauma to the primary incisors on permanent successors in different developmental stages. *Pediatr Dent* 1985, **7**:37–40.

BRIN I, BEN-BASSAR Y, ZILBERMAN Y, FUKS A. Effect of trauma to the primary incisors on the alignment of their permanent successors in Israelis. *Community Dent Oral Epidemiol* 1988, **16**:104–108.

HOLAN G, TOPF J. Effect of root canal infection and treatment of traumatized primary incisors on their permanent successors. *Endod Dent Traumatol* 1992, **8**:12–15.

SCHROEDER U, WENNBERG E, GRANATH LE, MOLLER H. Traumatised primary incisors—follow-up program based on frequency of periapical osteitis related to tooth colour. *Swed Dent J* 1977, **1**:95–98.

Permanent trauma

ANDREASEN FM, ANDREASEN JO. Diagnosis of luxation injuries: the importance of standardized clinical, radiographic and photographic techniques in clinical investigations. *Endod Dent Traumatol* 1985, **1**:160–169.

ANDREASEN JO, BORUM MK, *et al*. Replantation of 400 avulsed permanent incisors:1–4. *Endod Dent Traumatol* 1995, **11**:51–89.

ANDERSSON L, BODIN I, SORENSEN S. Progression of root resorption following replantation of human teeth after extended extra-oral storage. *Endod Dent Traumatol* 1988, **5**:38–47.

CVEK MJ. A clinical report on partial pulpotomy and capping with calcium hydroxide in permanent incisors with complicated crown fracture. *J Endod* 1978, **4**:232–237.

HAMMARSTROM L, BLOMLOF L, FEIGLIN B, ANDERSSON L, LINDSKOG S. Replantation of teeth and antibiotic treatment. *Endod Dent Traumatol* 1986, **2**:51–57.

HAMMARSTROM L, PIERCE A, BLOMLOF L, FEIGLAN B, LINSKOG S. Tooth avulsion and replantation–a review. *Endod Dent Traumatol* 1986, **2**:1–8.

HAMMARSTROM L, BLOMFLOF L, LINDSKOG S. Dynamics of dentoalveolar ankylosis and associated root resorption. *Endod Dent Traumatol* 1989, **5**:163–175.

HAMMARSTROM LE, BLOMLOF LB, FEIGLIN B, LINDSKOG SF. Effect of calcium hydroxide treatment on periodontal repair and root resorption. *Endod Dent Traumatol* 1986, **2**:184–189.

KRASNER P, RANKOW HJ. New philosophy for the treatment of avulsed teeth. *Oral Surg Oral Med Oral Pathol* 1995, **79**:616–623.

KLING M, CVEK M, MEJARE I. Rate and predictability of pulp revascularisation in therapeutically reimplanted permanent incisors. *Endod Dent Traumatol* 1986, **2**:83–89.

OLKARINEN K, GRUNDLACH KKH, PFEIFER G. Late complications of luxation injuries to teeth. *Endod Dent Traumatol* 1987, **3**:296–303.

Options for management

ANDREASEN FM, ANDREASEN JO, BAYER T. Prognosis of root-fractured permanent incisors—prediction of healing modalities. *Endod Dent Traumatol* 1989, **5**:11–22.

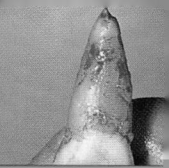

ANDREASEN JO, PAULSON HU, YU Z, SCHWARTZ O. A long-term study of 370 autotransplanted premolars. Part ii: tooth survival and pulp healing subsequent to transplantation. *Eur J Ortho* 1990, **12**:14–24.

HALL RK. Dental management of the traumatised child patient. *Ann Roy Aust Coll Dent Surg* 1986, **9**:80–99.

HEITHERSAY G. Combined endodontic-orthodontic treatment of transverse root fractures in the region of the alveolar crest. *Oral Surg Oral Med Oral Pathol* 1973, **36**:404–415.

OIKARINEN K, LAHTI J, RAUSTIA AM. Prognosis of permanent teeth in the line of mandibular fractures. *Endod Dent Traumatol* 1989, **6**:177–182.

SPALDING PM, FIELDS HW, TORNEY D, COBB HB, JOHNSON J. The changing role of endodontics and orthodontics in the management of traumatically intruded permanent incisors. *Pediatr Dent* 1985, **7**:104–110.

Self-mutilation

ALTOM RL, DI ANGELIS AJ. Multiple autoextractions: oral self mutilation reviewed. *Oral Surg Oral Med Oral Pathol* 1989, **67**:271–274.

Further reading

ANDREASEN JO, ANDREASEN FM. *Textbook and color atlas of traumatic injuries to the teeth.* 3rd ed. Copenhagen: Munksgaard; 1994.

HALL R. *Pediatric orofacial medicine and pathology.* London: Chapman and Hall Medical; 1994.

KOCH G, MODEER T, POULSEN S, RASMUSSEN P, eds. *Pedodontics—a clinical approach.* Copenhagen: Munksgaard; 1991.

ROWE NL, WILLIAMS JW. Vol I and II *Maxillofacial injuries.* Churchill Livingstone: Edinburgh; 1985.

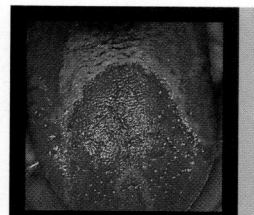

6 Paediatric oral pathology

Contributors
Michael Aldred, Roger Hall, Angus Cameron

Introduction

While some oral disease exists alone, lesions may often be a sign of a more complex medical disorder. Although much pathology is innocuous, it is essential to eliminate more serious illnesses. The presentation of pathology in children is usually different from adult pathology and these subtleties are often important in diagnosis. Additionally, many lesions change in form or extent with growth of the body. As a diagnostic aid, conditions have been grouped according to presentation.

Orofacial infections

Differential diagnosis
- Bacterial infections
    - Odontogenic
    - Scarlet fever
    - Atypical mycobacterial
    - Actinomycosis
    - Syphilis
    - Impetigo
- Viral infections
    - Primary herpetic gingivostomatitis
    - Herpes labialis
    - Herpangina
    - Hand- foot-and-mouth disease
    - Infectious mononucleosis
    - Varicella
- Fungal infections
    - Candidosis

Odontogenic infection
The basic signs and symptoms of oral infection must be familiar to all clinicians.

Acute infection Usually presents as an emergency:
- A sick, upset child.
- Raised temperature.
- Red, swollen face.
- Anxious and distressed parents.

Chronic infection Presents with none of the preceding emergencies:
- Buccal sinus may be present.
- Mobile tooth.
- Halitosis.
- Discoloured tooth.

Presentation
- Children tend to present with facial cellulitis rather than a facial abscess with pus. The patient is febrile; although, if the infection has perforated the cortical plate the child may not be in pain. The mainstay of treatment is removal of the cause. Too often, antibiotics are prescribed by medical practitioners without due regard to extraction of the tooth or extirpation of the pulp.
- Maxillary canine fossa infections (Figure 6.1A) are commonly confused by medical colleagues as a periorbital cellulitis (caused by *Haemophilus influenzae* or *Staphylococcus aureus*). Posterior spread may lead to cavernous sinus thrombosis and brain abscess.
- Mandibular infections which spread may embarrass the airway and there is the possibility of mediastinal involvement.
- Presenting problems for a young patient may include pain and dehydration. It is important to ask whether the child has urinated over the previous 12 hours and assess the fluid intake (see Appendix B, Fluid and Electrolyte Balance).

Management The treatment of infection follows two basic tenets:
- Removal of the cause and
- Local drainage and debridement.

Criteria for hospital admission
- Significant infection present or spiking temperature >39°C.
- Floor of mouth swelling.
- Dehydration.

Use of antibiotics Antibiotics should not be considered automatically as a first line of treatment unless there is systemic involvement. In a child, a temperature of 39°C or higher can be considered a significant rise (normal, 37°C).

If a child has a systemic infection resulting from a local focus of dental infection (i.e. a sick child with a high temperature, an obvious spreading infection of the face and regional lymphadenopathy), then antibiotics should be administered (see Appendix N).

Immunosuppressed patients, or those with cardiac disease, should receive antibiotics if infection is suspected.

General considerations
- Extraction of involved teeth or
- Root-canal therapy for permanent teeth if it is considered important to save particular teeth (see Chapter 4, 'Pulp therapy for young permanent molars').
- Oral antibiotics if systemic involvement.
- Amoxycillin or penicillin V are usually the drugs of first choice. The former has the advantage that it is given with food and only three times a day. Often the extraction of the abscessed tooth alone will bring about resolution without antibiotic therapy.

Severe infections
- Hospital admission.
- Extraction of involved teeth. It is impossible to drain a significant infection solely through the root canals of a primary tooth.
- Drainage of any pus present.

If the diagnosis or the correct management of an infection in the mandible has been delayed and the swelling has crossed the midline, or if there is swelling of the floor of the mouth, then extra-oral drainage with a through-and-through drain should be considered (Figure 6.1B). If a flap is raised, any granulation tissue should be removed and the area irrigated with 1% hydrogen peroxide and saline. Flaps should be apposed but not tightly sutured. Soft drains such as Penrose are better tolerated in children than corrugated drains such as Yates.

- Swabs for culture and sensitivity. It is important to take specimens for culture even though empiric antibiotic therapy needs to be commenced immediately.
- Intravenous antibiotics. Benzylpenicillin is the drug of first choice (up to 200 mg/kg/day).

First-generation cephalosporins may be used as second choice if the child is allergic to penicillin (there is some cross allergenicity in those patients allergic to penicillin and hence cephalosporins should be used with care in a child who has had a severe reaction to penicillin).

In severe infections, metronidazole can be added. Although the flora of most odontogenic infections is of a mixed type, anaerobic organisms play a significant role in pathogenesis.

Adequate doses must be used. Treat serious infections in the head and neck seriously.

- Maintenance fluids + 12% for every degree over 37.5°C until the child is drinking of their own accord.

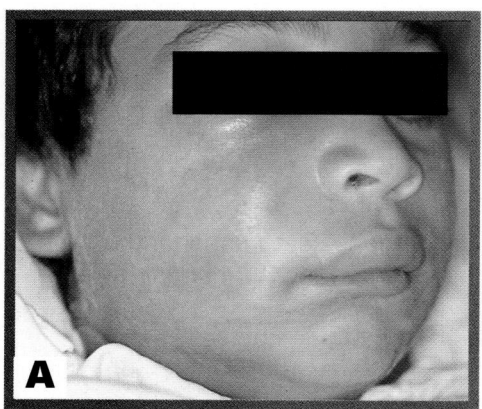
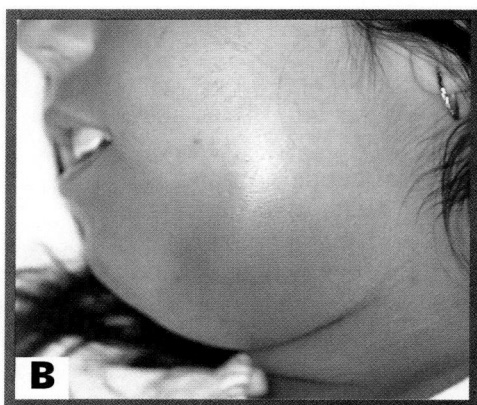

Figure 6.1 Severe facial swellings associated with odontogenic infections.
A The left eye is almost closed from the spreading infection. **B** This child
required extra-oral drainage of the facial swelling, which was caused by floor of
mouth involvement, as well as submandibular and sublingual spaces. Both
children required hospitalization and were placed on high-dose intravenous
penicillin, supplemented with metronidazole.

- Warm saline mouthrinses.
- Adequate pain control with paracetamol, 15 mg/kg, 4 hourly. Elixir (orally) or
  suppository (rectally).
- If the eye is shut, because of collateral oedema, it may be necessary to apply
  chloramphenicol eye drops, 0.5%, or ointment, 1%, to prevent conjunctivitis.

Primary herpetic gingivostomatitis (Figure 6.2)

The most common cause of severe oral ulceration in children. It is caused by herpes
simplex type-I virus. Cases of type-II (genital herpes) infection have been reported,
mainly in cases of sexual abuse; the effects of the two different strains of herpes simplex virus are, however, clinically identical. Although 60% of the population have been
infected with the virus, less than 1% manifest an acute primary infection, which occurs
after 6 months of age, often coincident with the eruption of the primary incisors. The
peak incidence occurs at 14 months. Incubation time is 3–5 days with a prodromal
48-hour history of irritability, pyrexia and malaise. Stomatitis is present with the gingival tissues becoming red and oedematous. Intra-epithelial vesicles appear after this
time and rapidly break down to form painful ulcers. Vesicles may form on any part of
the oral mucosa, including the skin around the lips. In severe cases, lesions on the
lips bleed and crusting appears with healing. Solitary ulcers are usually small (3 mm)
and painful with an erythematous margin, but larger ulcers with irregular margins can

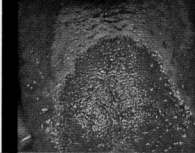

result from the coalescence of individual lesions. The disease is self-limiting and the ulcers heal spontaneously without scarring within 10–14 days.

Diagnosis
- Clinical appearance and history.
- Exfoliative cytology showing the presence of multinucleated giant cells and viral inclusion bodies.
- Indirect immunofluorescence for viral antigen.
- Viral culture.
- Blood film normal or low white-cell count.
- Lymphocytosis or monocytosis in differential count.
- Cytology and antigen detection are useful in early diagnosis.

Management
- Symptomatic care.
- Encourage oral fluids; these should be bland.
- If oral fluids cannot be taken, then intravenous fluids should be commenced.
- Analgesics—paracetamol, 20 mg/kg, 4 hourly.
- Mouthwashes for older children:
    Chlorhexidine gluconate, 0.2%, 4 hourly.
- In young children with severe ulceration, chlorhexidine can be swabbed over the affected areas with cotton wool applicators.
- Topical anaesthetics:
  Xylocaine viscous 2%.

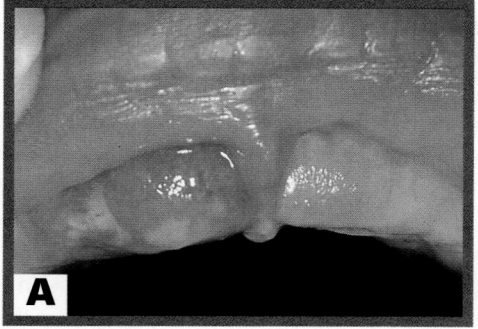
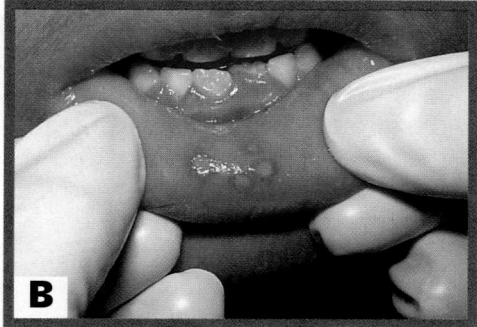

Figure 6.2 Different presentations of primary herpetic gingivostomatitis.
A Infection with primary herpes often occurs during eruption of primary teeth.
B Common presentation with multiple small ulcers on the lower lip and gingival inflammation.

- Antiviral chemotherapy:
  Acyclovir oral suspension or intravenously for severe cases and for immuno-suppressed patients.

A member of the immediate family will often have had a 'cold sore' on their lip recently. Treatment is palliative for all cases of viral ulceration.

- Severely affected young children often present dehydrated, being unable to eat or drink. Hospital admission is required for these cases with maintenance intra-venous fluids.
- Adequate pain control is also required with regular administration of paraceta-mol.
- Antibiotics are contraindicated.
- Much of the pain from oral ulceration is as a consequence of secondary bacterial infection. Chlorhexidine, 0.2%, mouthwash has been shown to be beneficial in the management of oral ulceration. In the young child this can be administered by swabbing the mouth with the solution. The authors have used Difflam (3M) (chlorhexidine 0.12%, benzydamine hydrochloride) with good results in cases of severe oral ulceration.
- Topical anaesthetics are often advocated; however, the effect of a numb mouth in a young child is often more distressing than the pain from the illness and can lead to traumatic ulceration from the decrease in sensation. Additionally, it is often difficult to initiate swallowing with a soft palate that has been anaesthetized.

The use of antiviral medications is contentious and usually reserved for children who are immunocompromised. There is some evidence to suggest, however, that the administration of aciclovir in the first 72 hours of the infection, before vesicle formation, may bring about earlier resolution of the infection. Administration after 72 hours of onset of the disease probably is of little benefit.

Herpangina and hand- foot-and-mouth disease

These infections are caused by the Coxsackie group A viruses. As with primary herpes, both of the above conditions have a prodromal phase of low-grade fever and malaise that lasts for several days before the appearance of the vesicles. In herpangina (Figure 6.3), four to five vesicles are found on the palate, pillars of the fauces and the pharynx, whereas in hand- foot-and-mouth disease up to 10 vesicles occur at these sites and elsewhere in the mouth in addition to the hands and feet (Figure 6.4A). The lesions on skin appear on the palmar surfaces of the hands and plantar surface of the feet and are surrounded by an erythematous margin. The severity of both diseases is usually milder than primary herpes and healing occurs within 10 days. Both diseases occur in epidemics, mainly affecting children.

Diagnosis
- Clinical appearance and history.
- Known epidemic.
- Viral culture.

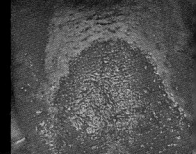

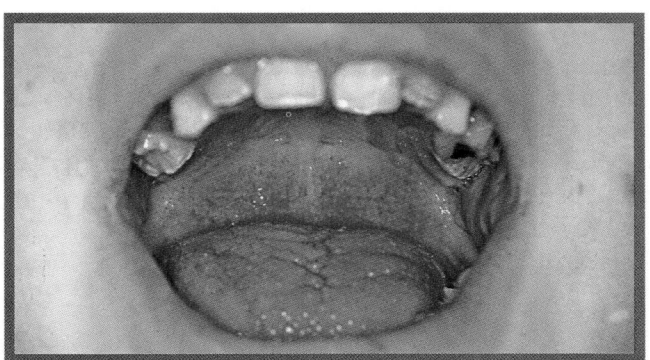

Figure 6.3
Herpangina with characteristic palatal and pharyngeal ulceration and inflammation.

Management Symptomatic care, as for other viral infections.

Infectious mononucleosis (Figure 6.4B)

This infection is caused by Epstein–Barr virus (EBV) and mainly affects late adolescent children and young adults. The disease is highly infective and is characterized by malaise, fever and acute pharyngitis. In young children, ulcers and petechiae are often found in the posterior pharynx and soft palate. The disease is self-limiting with complete recovery.

Diagnosis
- History and clinical features.
- Paul–Bunnell agglutination test.

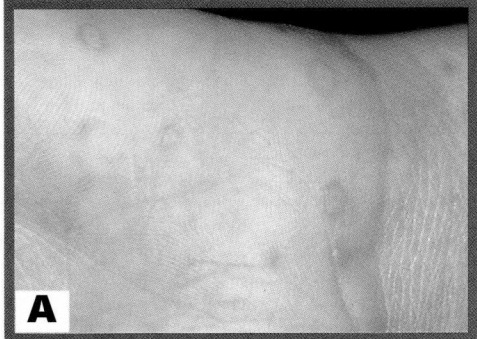

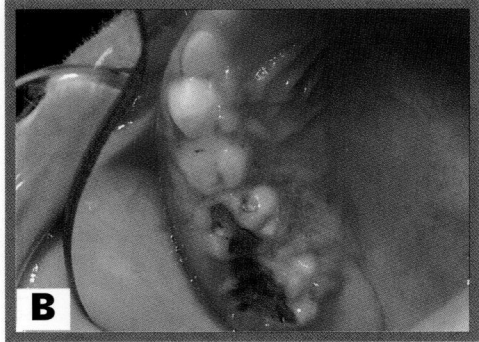

Figure 6.4 **A** Cutaneous lesions in hand- foot-and-mouth disease. **B** Gingival ulceration and stomatitis during an acute episode of infectious mononucleosis.

Varicella

This is a highly contagious infection causing both chickenpox and shingles. There is a prodromal phase of malaise and fever for 24 hours followed by macular eruptions which then form vesicles and pustules. Oral lesions occur in around 50% of cases but only a small number of vesicles occur in the mouth. These lesions may be found anywhere in the mouth in addition to other mucosal lesions such as conjunctivae, nose or anus. Healing is uneventful.

Diagnosis Clinical appearance and history.

Candidosis

Acute pseudomembranous candidiasis The most common presentation of candidal infection in infants is thrush. White plaques are present, which on removal reveal a haemorrhagic base. In older children, thrush occurs when children are immunocompromised with HIV infection or diabetes, or when prescribed broad-spectrum antibiotics, steroids, or during chemotherapy and radiotherapy for malignancies.

Diagnosis 50% of children will have *Candida albicans* as a normal commensal and culture is of little benefit. If scrapings for exfoliative cytology reveal hyphae then disease is present, but the clinical picture is usually diagnostic.

Management
- Antifungal medication for 8 weeks. Most antifungal treatment fails because of poor compliance or instruction by the clinician.
- Nystatin lozenges or ointment.
- Amphotericin B, orally or intravenously, if systemic involvement
- Ketoconazole oral (200 mg daily for 14 days) for cases of mucocutaneous candidiasis where the organism is resistant to topical treatment.
- Fluconazole oral (100 mg daily for 14 days) used for oropharyngeal candidiasis.

Ulcerative and vesiculobullous lesions

Differential diagnosis
- Traumatic
    - Postmandibular block anaesthesia
    - Riga–Fedé ulceration
- Infective
    - Primary herpetic gingivostomatitis
    - Herpangina
    - Hand- foot-and-mouth disease

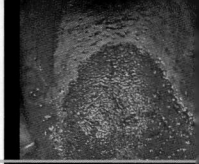

Infectious mononucleosis
Varicella
- Others
    Recurrent aphthous ulceration
    Erythema multiforme
    Stevens–Johnson syndrome
    Behçet's syndrome
    Epidermolysis bullosa
    Lupus erythematosus
    Neutropenic ulceration
    Crohn's disease
    Pemphigus
    Drug-induced (chemotherapy) lesions

Lip ulceration after mandibular block anaesthesia

This is one of the most common causes of traumatic ulceration. Always warn parents and remind children not to bite or play with their lips after mandibular block anaesthesia (Figure 6.5A).

Riga–Fedé ulceration

This is ulceration of the ventral surface of the tongue caused by trauma from continual protrusive and retrusive movements over the lower incisors (Figure 6.5B). It occurs almost exclusively in children with cerebral palsy.

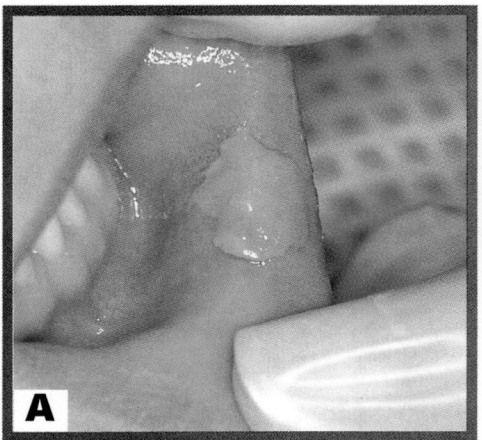
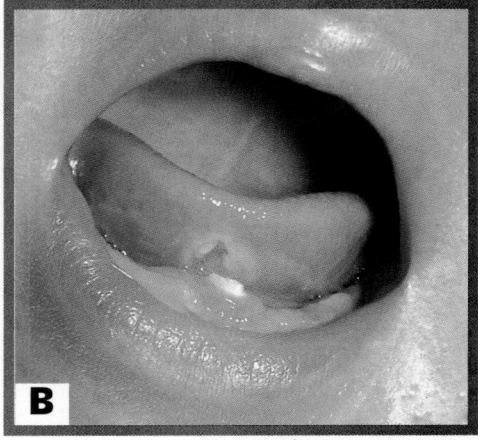

Figure 6.5 **A** Traumatic oral ulceration from biting the lip after a mandibular block injection. **B** Riga–Fedé ulcer on the ventral surface of the tongue.

Management Smooth sharp incisal edges or place domes of composite resin over the teeth. Rarely, in severe cases, extraction of the teeth may still be necessary.

Recurrent aphthous ulceration (Figure 6.6)

Recurrent aphthous ulceration (RAU) affects approximately 20% of the population. Three types are identified:

- Minor aphthae.
- Major aphthae and
- Herpetiform.

Minor aphthae account for the majority of cases with crops of shallow ulcers measuring up to 5 mm and occur on non-keratinized mucosa. There is a typical yellow pseudomembranous slough with an erythematous border. Ulcers heal within 10–14 days without scarring. The cause of RAU is contentious. Many of the British studies have suggested that RAU is associated with nutritional deficiency states and so haematological investigation is important. There is some evidence that the disease is hereditary with an increased incidence of ulceration in children where both parents suffer from RAU.

Diagnosis

- Clinical appearance and history.
- Blood tests for full blood, vitamin B_{12} folate, serum ferritin (if anaemia or latent anaemia suspected).

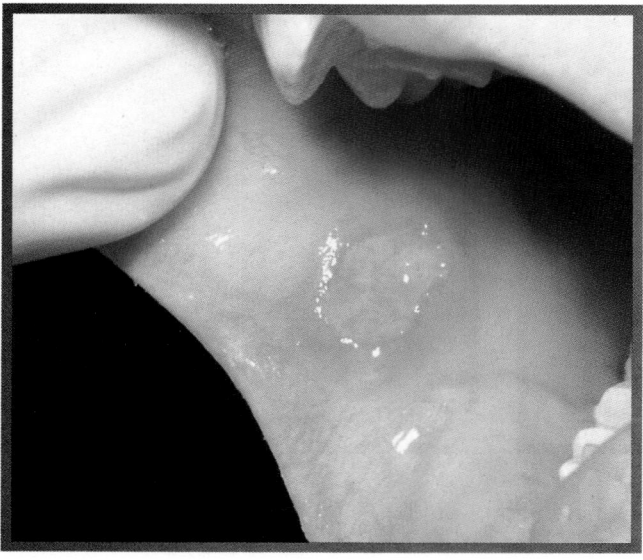

Figure 6.6 Major RAU in an adolescent girl. These lesions healed with scarring and were extremely painful. Blood chemistry revealed a low folate level, which when corrected eliminated further ulceration.

Management

- Symptomatic care with mouthrinses
    Chlorhexidine gluconate 0.2%
    Tetracycline
    Benzydamine hydrochloride 1.2% (Difflam)
    Benadryl, Mucaine, Xylocaine viscous
- Topical steroids
    Kenalog in Orabase
    Becotide spray
- Systemic corticosteroids only in most severe cases of major aphthous ulceration. Although the changes seen at biopsy are non-specific it is an important procedure to exclude other causes of oral ulceration. Blood tests should be used again to exclude deficiency states (when appropriate, replacement brings about resolution). As with all oral ulceration, symptomatic care, with appropriate analgesics and anti-septic mouthwashes, is appropriate. In those cases of severe recurrent oral ulceration, corticosteroids may be used, although their use is to be avoided in children. Tetracycline mouthwashes should not be used in children under the age of 8 years to avoid tooth discoloration. In most cases, major aphthae only occur in older children.

Behçet's syndrome

This condition is characterized by severe recurrent aphthous ulceration with both genital and ocular lesions. Behçet's syndrome is subdivided into four main types:
- Mucocutaneous form.
- Classical form with involvement of oral genital skin and conjunctiva.
- Arthritic form with arthritis in association with mucocutaneous lesions.
- Neurological form with central nervous system involvement.
- Ocular form with uveitis with signs in addition to oral and genital lesions.

Diagnosis Clinical presentation and biopsy.

Management As for recurrent aphthous ulceration, but systemic treatment is usually required.

Erythema multiforme (Figure 6.7)

This is a vesiculobullous, dermatological disease often characterized by severe oral ulceration, hypersensitivity and vasculitis. Its cause is unknown; however, there may be precipitating factors such as herpes simplex infection and sulphonamide drugs. The disease usually affects children and young adults and onset is rapid. Contiguous vesicles and bullae occur in the mouth and coalesce to form large ulcerative areas throughout the mouth. The gingival tissues are usually unaffected, the most commonly affected tissues being buccal mucosa, lips, palate and tongue.

The lesions often bleed and healing crusts form on the lips. Skin lesions are diagnostic with a 'bull's-eye' or 'target' appearance. There is a pale central macula surrounded by an erythematous margin. Healing usually takes between 3 and 4 weeks, but recurrence is common. Histopathology reveals a non-specific inflammatory infiltrate with subepithelial vesicles. Some lesions may have an intra-epithelial component.

Stevens–Johnson syndrome is a severe form of erythema multiforme with the association of conjunctival and genital ulceration.

Diagnosis
- Clinical appearance and history.
- Skin biopsy for immunofluorescence.

Management Because of the panstomatitis that presents, these children are often unable to eat and drink and so hospital admission is required. Supportive care is in the form of fluids, analgesics and regular mouthwashes with chlorhexidine and benzydamine. Systemic corticosteroids are sometimes required in severe cases. Where the condition is initiated by herpes, aciclovir may be beneficial.

Pemphigus
Pemphigus is an important bullous disease mainly affecting adults, however children can be also affected. Ulceration occurs in over 90% of these children mainly affecting the buccal mucosa, palate and lips.

Diagnosis There may be a positive Nikolsky's sign (separation of the superficial epithelium from basal layers produced by rubbing or gentle pressure) and cytological examination reveals the presence of Tzanck cells. Direct immunofluorescence using frozen sections from oral biopsy reveals intracellular immunoglobulin (IgG) deposits in the epithelium, which are diagnostic for this disease.

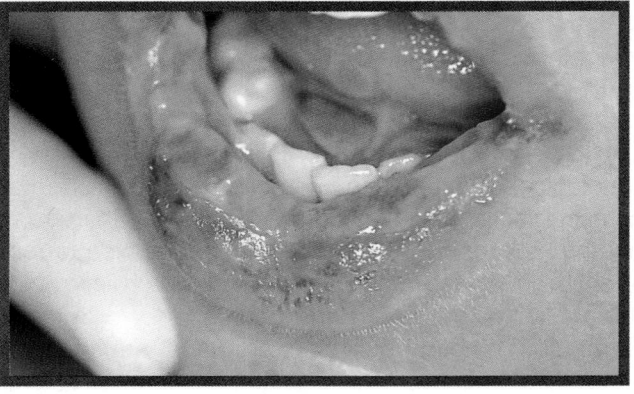

Figure 6.7 Erythema multiforme presenting with pan stomatitis and severe dehydration. This episode was initiated by exposure to sulphonamides (Bactrim). Treatment involves rehydration and symptomatic care of the ulceration. Narcotics were required to manage the pain in this patient.

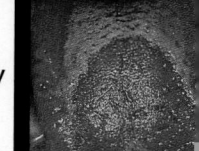

Management Systemic corticosteroid therapy.

Epidermolysis bullosa

Epidermolysis bullosa is a term used to describe several hereditary vesiculobullous diseases of the skin and mucosa. The most recent classification is based on four different types:

- Intra-epithelial, non-scarring form transmitted as an autosomal dominant or X-linked trait.
- Junctional form with hemidesmosome defect and severe scarring, transmitted as an autosomal-recessive trait.
- Dermal form with scarring and skin atrophy, and transmitted as an autosomal-dominant trait.
- Acquired form (epidermolysis bullosa acquisita)

Blisters may form from birth or appear in the first few weeks of life depending on different forms of the disease. Corneal and oral ulceration may also be present and pitting enamel hypoplasia has been reported mainly in the junctional forms of the disease.

Management Often extremely difficult because of the fragility of the skin and oral mucosa. Intensive preventive-dental care is essential to prevent dental caries and to treat early disease. Supportive care is required with the use of topical anaesthetics such as Xylocaine viscous and regular chlorhexidine mouthwashes. Fortunately children may be treated under general anaesthesia with no report of laryngeal complications. Because of stricture, however, access into the mouth is often difficult and in the older patient commissure release may be necessary. Of importance is the use of instruments covered with lubricant and the use of rubber dam.

Systemic lupus erythematosus

Systemic lupus erythematosus is a chronic inflammatory multisystem disease occurring predominantly in young women. The hallmark of Systemic lupus erythematosus is the presentation of antinuclear antibodies which form circulating immune complexes with DNA. Oral ulceration often occurs with systemic lupus erythematosus and treatment of the condition usually involves steroids which may result in immunosuppression.

Orofacial granulomatoses (Figure 6.8)

Although not primarily an ulcerative condition, oral ulceration may be the presenting sign in these conditions. Perioral and gingival swelling may be an important sign of chronic inflammatory bowel disease. The following conditions are generally classified as orofacial granulomatoses:

Crohn's disease An inflammatory condition of the gastrointestinal tract, of unknown aetiology, primarily involving the distal ileum and colon.

Presentation
- Diffuse erythematous swelling of the lips and cheeks.
- Gingival granulomatosis with diffusely swollen gingivae (Figure 6.8B).
- Linear ulceration or fissuring of the buccal and labial sulcus giving a characteristic 'cobblestone' appearance (Figure 6.8A).
- Polypoid tags of vestibular and retromolar mucosa.
- Children may also present with diarrhoea, failure to thrive, weakness, fatigue, anorexia and perianal fissuring or skin tags.
- Oral changes have been found in between 9% and 25% of patients with Crohn's disease and, importantly, their appearance may precede other systemic symptoms.

Diagnosis
- Biopsy of oral lesions.
- Endoscopy and biopsy of large and small bowel.
- Barium studies.

Management
- Prednisolone.
- Sulphasalazine.
- Strict diet and increased nutrition to manage malabsorption.

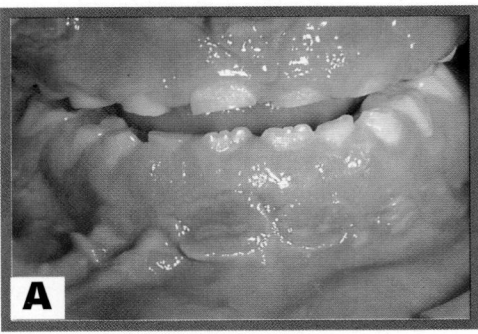 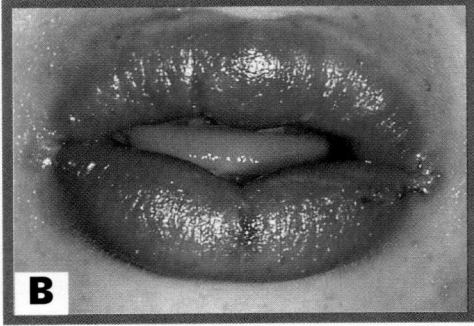

Figure 6.8 Presentations of orofacial granulomatosis and Crohn's disease. **A** The intra-oral appearance is pathognomonic with swelling of the gingivae and a 'cobblestone' ulceration of the labial and buccal sulci. **B** The patient initially presented with a painless oedematous swelling of the lips and had evidence of malabsorption, peri-anal fissuring and bowel problems. He was managed with systemic corticosteroids.

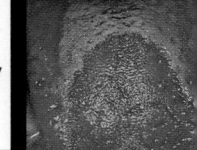

- Metronidazole for perianal disease.

Melkersson–Rosenthal syndrome
Presentation
- Persistent orofacial swelling lasting from 1 hour to several months.
- Facial nerve paralysis.
- Fissured tongue.
- Histologically indistinguishable from Crohn's disease.

Pigmented, vascular and erythematous lesions

If a lesion is red or bluish in colour there should also be the suspicion of a vascular lesion. These lesions will blanch on pressure with a glass slide (or end of a test tube if access is difficult) as the blood is removed from the vessels. True pigmented lesions are rare in children other than racial pigmentation. The only true pigmented lesion (i.e. containing melanin) in young children is the melanotic neuro-ectodermal tumour of infancy.

Differential diagnosis
Racial pigmentation (Figure 6.9)
- Vascular lesions
    Haemangioma
    Vascular malformations
    Haematoma
    Petechiae and purpura
    Hereditary haemorrhagic telangiectasia
    Sturge–Weber syndrome
- Melanin lesions
    Melanotic neuro-ectodermal tumour of infancy
    Peutz–Jeghers syndrome
    Addison's disease
- Erythematous lesions
    Peripheral giant-cell granuloma
    Eruption cyst
    Langerhans' cell histiocytosis
    Geographic tongue
    Median rhomboid glossitis
    Lingual thyroid
    Hereditary muco-epithelial dysplasia
- Other dark lesions
    Cyanosis
    Heavy-metal toxicity

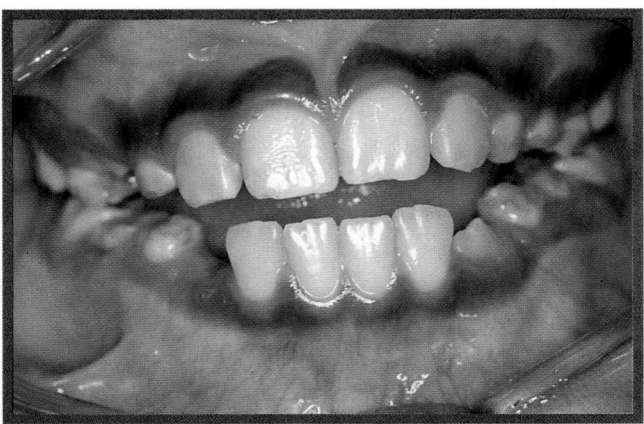

Figure 6.9 Racial pigmentation of the attached gingiva. This should not be confused with heavy-metal toxicity.

Lesions of vascular origin

Haemangioma True haemangiomas are endothelial hamartomas. Present at birth which grow rapidly in the infant, but then regress with time to disappear by adolescence. As such, they require no treatment other than observation, excepting cosmetic concerns.

Vascular malformations

Arteriovenous malformations include birthmarks, blood vessel and lymphatic anomalies. They may be life-threatening conditions which can present with profound haemorrhage. Arteriovenous malformations have been classified by Kaban and Mulliken according to their flow characteristics. They are either:

Low-flow lesions Capillary, venous, lymphatic or combined port-wine stains, Sturge–Weber syndrome.

High-flow lesions Arterial with arteriovenous fistulae (Figure 6.10).
   Present with mobile and often painful teeth, bruit and palpable pulses, bleeding from gingiva and bony involvement.

Combined lesions Extensive combined venous and arteriovenous malformations.

Diagnosis Presentation may be subtle, such as prolonged small bleeding from the gingivae after toothbrushing or alternatively a torrential haemorrhage. Vascular lesions are often warm to touch, teeth are hypermobile and may have pulsatile movements. Radiographically, there is enlargement of the periodontal ligament space and often diffuse abnormal trabeculation of the bone. As lesions expand, there may be facial asymmetry. A bruit or pulse may be felt over high-flow lesions.

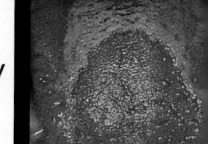

Digital subtraction angiography (Figure 6.10B) is required for definitive diagnosis of feeder vessels and the distribution of the lesion. Magnetic resonance angiography is also being used to aid diagnosis; however, digital subtraction angiography has the advantage that embolization can be performed at the same procedure.

Management Low-flow lesions can be removed by careful surgical removal and identification and ligation of feeder vessels. Others can be managed with cryotherapy, laser ablation or injection of sclerosing solutions.

Selective embolization of vessels is required for high-flow lesions, but these will generally recur after embolization due to revascularization from contralateral supply and recanalization of the embolized artery. Repeat embolization and resection of the total lesion is often necessary involving jaw reconstruction.

If a tooth is accidentally removed and a torrential haemorrhage results, the extracted tooth should be immediately replaced to control haemorrhage.

Lymphangioma

Diagnosis of developmental lymph vessel abnormalities must exclude vascular involvement. Lymphangiomas are relatively common and usually present with small raised pale or red nodules. Surgical excision is only necessary if of functional or aesthetic concern. Cystic hygroma is a term used to describe a large lymphangioma involving the floor of mouth and neck. Expansion of the lesion may cause respiratory obstruction and treatment usually involves multiple resections over time.

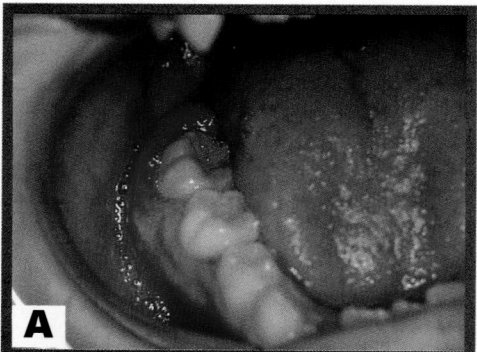
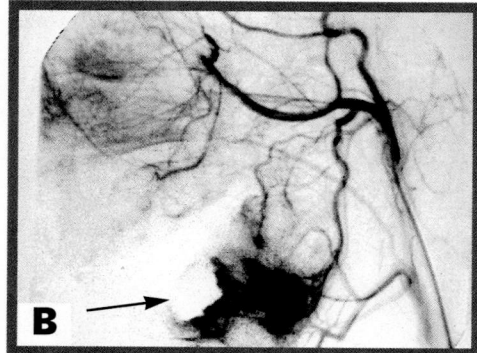

Figure 6.10 A highflow arteriovenous malformation in the mandible. This child presented with an unusual gingival erythematous enlargement around the lower right first permanent molar tooth in addition to mobile teeth **A**. During the procedure for biopsy 350 ml (20% of total volume) of blood was lost after extraction of the second primary molar. The haemorrhage was controlled with an iodoform pack (arrowed) and subsequently an angiogram **B** was ordered. The extent of the lesion posterior to the pack is seen. The lesion was embolized and later the mandible resected.

Petechiae and purpura

Petechiae are small pinpoint submucosal or subcutaneous haemorrhages. Purpura or ecchymoses present as larger collections of blood. These lesions are usually present in patients with severe bleeding disorders or coagulopathies, leukaemia and other conditions such infective endocarditis. Initially bright red in colour, they will change to a bluish-brown hue with time.

Hereditary haemorrhagic telangiectasia (Rendu–Osler–Weber disease)

An autosomal dominant disorder presenting as a developmental anomaly of capillaries. Lesions may be small raised haemorrhagic nodules or spider naevi.

Sturge–Weber syndrome (Figure 6.11)

Typically presents with encephalotrigeminal angiomatoses, epilepsy, intellectual handicap and calcification of the falx cerebri. Vascular lesions involve the leptomeninges and peripheral lesions appear along the distribution of the fifth nerve. Extraction of teeth within affected jaws should be performed with extreme caution and only after thorough investigation of the extent of the anomaly (see Vascular malformations above).

Maffucci's syndrome

Presents with multiple haemangiomas and enchondromas of the small bones in the hands and feet. Only a small number of cases will manifest with oral lesions, mainly haemangiomas.

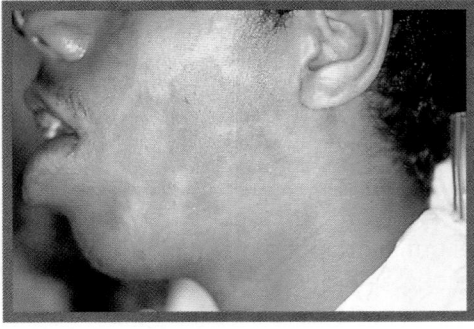 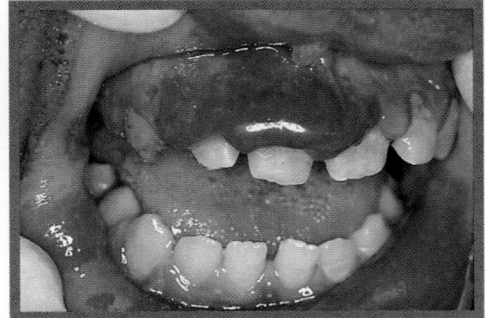

Figure 6.11 Sturge–Weber syndrome showing the extent of the capillary vascular malformation in the face which is continuous with the intra-oral involvement.

Melanin lesions

Peutz–Jeghers syndrome An autosomal dominant disorder, manifesting multiple small pigmented lesions on oral mucosa and skin appearing almost like dark freckles. Important association with intestinal polyposis coli which requires gastrointestinal investigation.

Erythematous lesions

Eruption cyst or haematoma Follicular enlargement just before eruption. These lesions may be blue–black if they contain blood and usually require no treatment unless infected. The parents and child should be reassured and the follicle allowed to burst spontaneously or it may be surgically opened if infected (Figure 6.12A).

Geographic tongue Also termed 'benign migratory glossitis', 'erythema migrans', or 'wandering rash of the tongue', it presents as an area of desquamation and erosion, with a whitish margin, on the dorsal surface of the tongue involving the filiform papillae. The lesions heal and then recur at different sites on the tongue. Sometimes symptomatic, chlorhexidine mouthwashes may be beneficial for those children in pain (Figure 6.12B).

Hereditary muco-epithelial dysplasia A rare disorder where there is a reduced number of desmosomes attaching epithelial cells. Lens cataracts, corneal lesions leading to blindness, skin keratosis and alopecia are associated with a fiery red mucosa involving both keratinized and non-keratinized mucosa.

Diagnosis Gingival and mucosal biopsy confirms the condition. Transmission electron microscopy is necessary to demonstrate reduced number of desmosomes and amorphous intracellular inclusions.

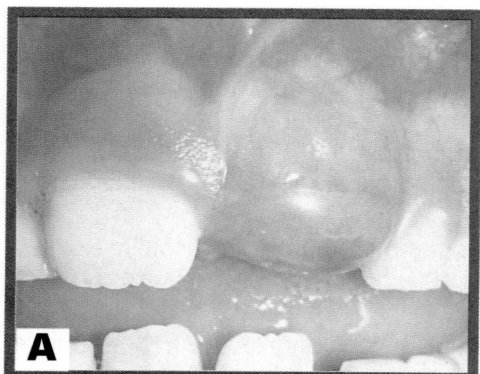 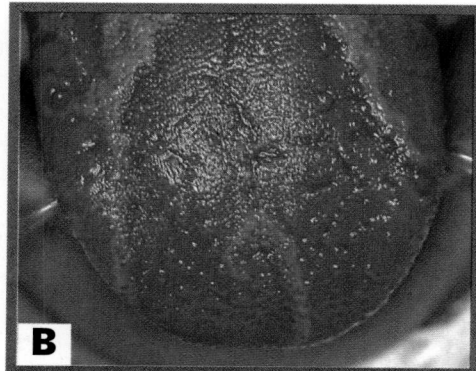

Figure 6.12 **A** Eruption cyst overlying tooth 11. **B** Geographic tongue.

Management The oral lesions are usually asymptomatic. Loss of sight is progressive due to corneal vascularization. Corneal grafts are unsuccessful as they too undergo vascularization.

Epulides and exophytic lesions

Differential diagnosis
- Inflammatory hyperplasias
  - Fibrous epulis/pyogenic granuloma
  - Peripheral giant-cell granuloma
  - Congenital epulis of the newborn
  - Papilloma/verrucous warts
- Eruption cyst/haematoma
- Melanotic neuro-ectodermal tumour of infancy
- Tuberous sclerosis
- Mucocoele
- Lymphangioma

Fibrous epulis/pyogenic granuloma (Figure 6.13A)
One of the most common epulides seen in children. A exuberant fibro-epithelial reaction to chronic inflammation or local irritation. Commonly seen behind upper incisors or in the interdental papilla, they range in colour from pink to red to bluish. The term pyogenic granuloma is confusing; however, it is often used to describe an ulcerated or highly vascular fibrous epulis that appears more erythematous in colour.

Management Surgical excision.

Peripheral giant-cell granuloma (Figure 6.13B)
These lesions usually occur in the region of the primary dentition. It is thought to represent a exuberant reaction to local irritation. The colour of these lesions tends to be dark purple and somewhat darker than the pyogenic granuloma. Bone loss of the alveolar crest is observed as 'radiographic cupping'.

Management Surgical excision, although lesions may regrow if not totally excised.

Papilloma (Figure 6.13E)
A true benign neoplasm, presenting as a cauliflower-like growth on the mucosa. The colour of the lesion depends on the degree of keratinization. The lesion is clinically indistinguishable from the verrucous wart.

Management Surgical excision with stalk and a border of normal tissue.

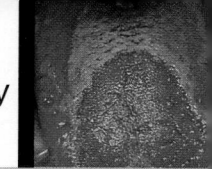

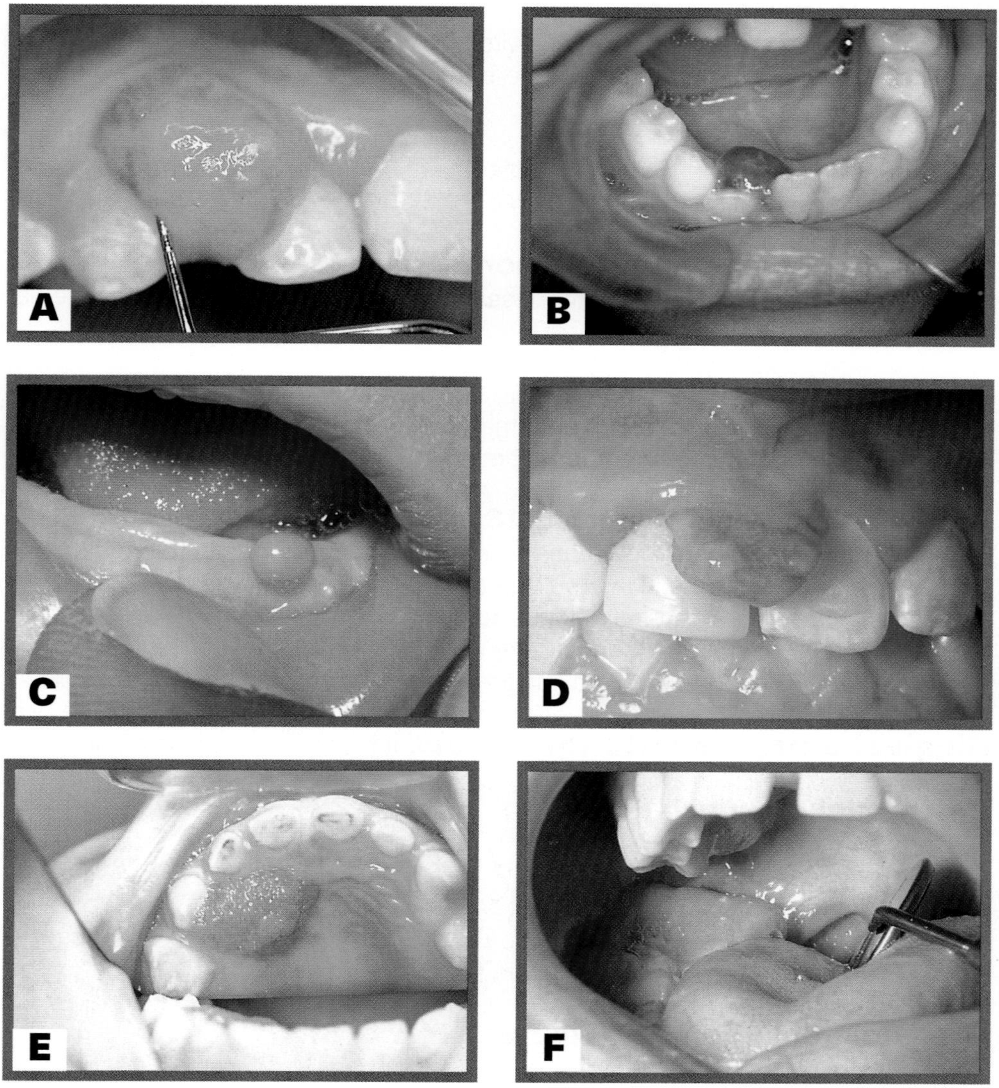

Figure 6.13 Epulides. **A** Fibrous epulis. **B** Peripheral giant-cell granuloma.
C Congenital epulis of the newborn. **D** Epulis associated with angioma in a child
with tuberous sclerosis. **E** A papilloma in the palate of a young child associated
with verrucous warts on the extremities. **F** A large gingival swelling in the
retromolar triangle associated with a metastatic fibrosarcoma. The primary lesion
occurred in the posterior abdomen and secondary lesions invaded the pelvis,
lungs and mandible.

Verrucous warts

A viral infection by the human papilloma virus. Lesions may be single or multiple and it is important to examine the rest of the body for other lesions, especially on the hands and fingers.

Management Surgical excision. If multiple lesions are present extra-orally, dermatological investigation may be required.

Congenital epulis of the newborn (Figure 6.13C)

A fibro-epithelial lesion arising from mesenchymal cells occurring on the alveolar ridges of newborns. The lesion is pedunculated.

Management Lesions often regress with time although large lesions may require surgical excision. Huge lesions sometimes occur at birth and may be life-threatening because of respiratory embarrassment.

Tuberous sclerosis (Figure 6.13D)

An autosomal dominant disorder characterized by seizures, mental retardation and adenoma sebaceum of the skin. Epulides are often present which may result from vascular malformations and may bleed profusely when excised. Hypoplasia of the enamel is often observed as surface pitting.

Gingival enlargements (overgrowth)

Differential diagnosis

- Hereditary gingival fibromatosis.
- Drug-induced hyperplasia:
    Phenytoin
    Cyclosporin A
    Nifedipine.

Phenytoin enlargement (Figure 6.14A & B)

Principally there is enlargement of the interdental papilla. There may be delayed eruption of teeth because of the bulk of fibrous tissue present and ectopic eruption. Overgrowth is because of decreased collagen degradation and phagocytosis. Withdrawal of the drug will bring about resolution in all but severe cases. Oral hygiene is most important in controlling overgrowth.

Management

- Maintenance of oral hygiene.
- Use of chlorhexidine, 0.2%, mouthwashes.
- Gingivectomy may be required to allow eruption of teeth or for aesthetics.

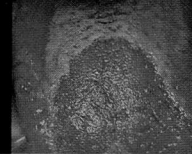

Cyclosporin-A enlargement (Figure 6.14C)

A significant number of children now undergo transplantation of kidney, liver, heart and combined heart/lung. The mainstay of immunosuppressive antirejection chemotherapy is cyclosporin. Gingival overgrowth occurs in between 30% and 70% of patients and is not dose-related. Individual patients appear to have a threshold below which gingival overgrowth will not occur.

Management
- As with phenytoin hyperplasia, maintenance of oral hygiene is mandatory.
- Gingivectomy if required.

Nifedipine enlargement

A calcium-channel blocker, used to control coronary insufficiency and hypertension in adults, its main use in children is to control cyclosporin-induced hypertension after transplantation. An increase in the extracellular compartment volume is responsible for enlargement, which is in addition to the enlargement caused by cyclosporin A.

Hereditary gingival fibromatosis (Figure 6.14D & E)

May be part of several syndromes involving mental retardation. It may occur sporadically or as an autosomal dominant transmission.

Management Gingivectomy as required to allow tooth eruption and maintain aesthetics.

Premature exfoliation of primary teeth

Premature loss of primary teeth is an important diagnostic event. Most conditions that present with early loss are serious and a child presenting with unexplained tooth loss warrants immediate investigation. Teeth may be lost because of metabolic disturbances, severe periodontal disease, loss of alveolar-bone support or self-injury.

Differential diagnosis
- Neutropenias and qualitative neutrophil defects:
    Cyclic neutropenia
    Congenital agranulocytosis
    Prepubertal periodontitis
    Juvenile periodontitis
    Leucocyte adhesion defect
    Papillon–Lefèvre syndrome
    Chediak–Higashi disease

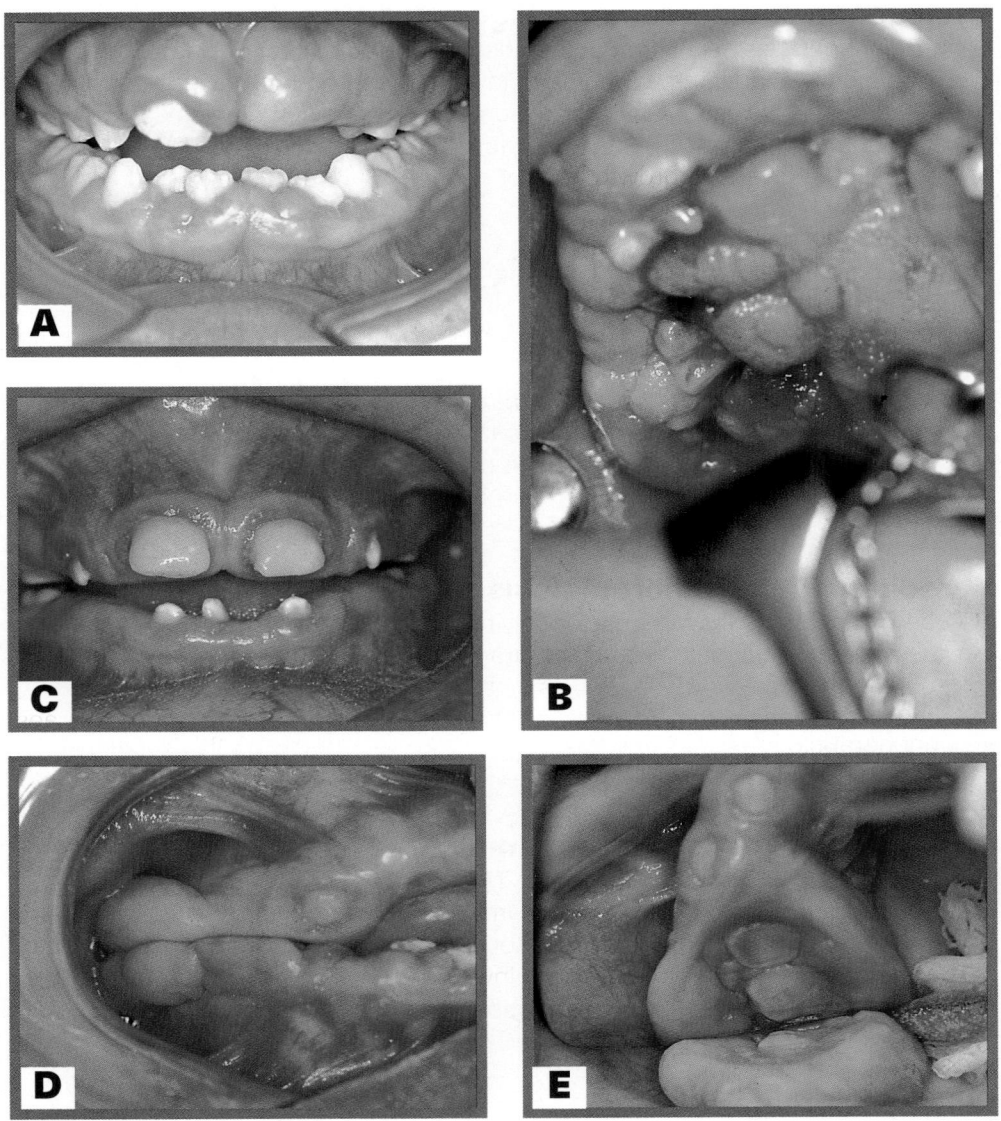

Figure 6.14 **A** Phenytoin gingival enlargement. The hyperplasia initially involves the interdental papilla and then adjacent tissues. **B** The enlargement can become extensive so as to cover the whole palate. An acute periodontal abscess was associated with this case. **C** Cyclosporin-A hyperplasia involves all gingival tissues. **D, E** Hereditary gingival fibromatosis.

- Langerhans' cell histiocytosis.
- Hypophosphatasia.
- Self-injury in congenital indifference to pain syndrome or psychotic disorder.
- Ehlers–Danlos syndrome (Type VIII).
- Acute myeloid leukaemia.
- Erythromelalgia.
- Acrodynia.
- Acatalasia.
- Scurvy.

Periodontal disease in children (Figure 6.15G)

Although gingivitis is a relatively common finding in children, periodontitis with alveolar bone loss is usually a manifestation of a serious underlying immunological deficiency. Both prepubertal periodontitis and juvenile periodontitis are associated with characteristic bacterial flora including *Actinobacillus actinomycetemcomitans, Provetella intermedia, Eikenella corrodens* and *Capnocytophagia sputigena*. The presence of these bacteria are thought to be related to decreased host resistance, specifically neutropenia or neutrophil function defects. Although B-cell defects show little oral changes, altered T-cell function will manifest with severe gingivitis, periodontitis and candidosis.

Neutropenias and qualitative neutrophil defects

Neutrophilia

- Peripheral blood levels <1500 per mL.
- Acute usually fatal.
- Chronic benign.
- Cyclic (see below).
- Intermittent as part of Shwachmann syndrome.

Cyclic neutropenia (Figure 6.15C) A condition in which there is an episodic decrease in the number of neutrophils every 3–4 weeks. Peripheral neutrophil counts usually drop to zero, and during this time the child is extremely susceptible to infection. Recurrent oral ulceration is present when cell counts are low. Gingival and periodontal involvement occurs with the appearance of teeth and is progressive.

Management

- Early preventive involvement.
- Dental care through all stages of cycle.
- Chlorhexidine 0.2% gel and mouthwashes.
- Elective extraction of primary teeth.
- In some familial cases the condition may totally regress during adolescence.

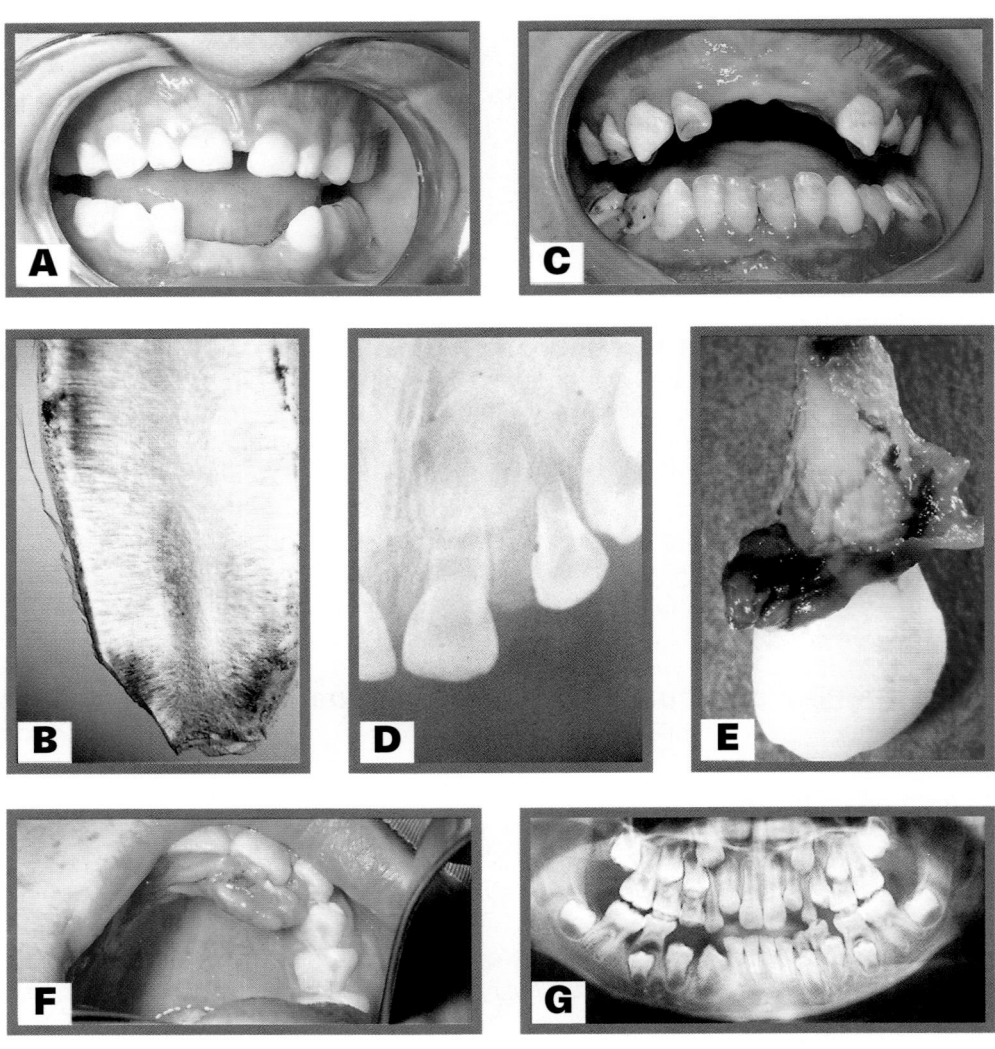

Figure 6.15 **A** Hypophosphatasia presenting with exfoliation of the upper and lower anterior teeth around 2 years of age. There is minimal gingival inflammation and hard-tissue sections (**B**) show absent cementum. **C** Gross gingival inflammation and tooth loss in a child with cyclic neutropenia. **D** Necrotic central incisor with long-standing palatal ulceration. This child had Langerhans' cell histiocytosis, the lesion is shown in **E**. **F** Severe unexplained palatal ulceration in a child with leucocyte adhesion defect. The upper left incisor exfoliated a short time later. **G** Prepubertal periodontitis also associated with leucocyte adhesion defect. It is important to assess normal eruption patterns and to be suspicious of loss of teeth in the absence of caries or other pathology.

Leucocyte adhesion defect (Figure 6.15F & G) A rare autosomal-recessive condition associated with a reduced level of adhesion molecules on peripheral leucocytes resulting in severely reduced resistance to infection. The CD11/CD18 molecules are necessary for effective phagocytosis. Children present with delayed wound healing, persistent severe oral ulceration, cellulitis without pus formation, severe gingival inflammation, periodontitis and premature loss of primary teeth. Also present is a persistently high leucocytosis and reactive marrow, without evidence of leukaemia. One important indicator of this condition is late separation of the umbilical cord after birth.

Diagnosis Diagnosis is confirmed by examining leucocytes for surface expression of CD11/CD18 markers using immunofluorescence techniques and cytofluorographic analysis.

Management
- Most children succumb to overwhelming infection.
- Granulocyte transfusion and bone marrow transplantation may be effective in some cases.

Papillon–Lefèvre syndrome An autosomal-recessive condition manifesting hyperkeratosis of the palms and feet and progressive exfoliation of all teeth from periodontal disease. *A. actinomycetemcomitans* has been implicated in the periodontal disease which is associated with a qualitative neutrophil defect. Primary teeth commence shedding from the time of eruption, with no evidence of root resorption. All primary teeth are lost before the permanent teeth erupt, when they in turn are exfoliated.

Diagnosis
- The oral changes and skin lesions are pathognomonic for this condition.
- Selective anaerobic culturing for *A. actinomycetemcomitans* is difficult and a more reliable alternative is to use an ELISA system to detect IgG against this organism.

Management
- No treatment is successful. Extraction of all remaining primary teeth before eruption of the permanent teeth. Intensive periodontal therapy with metronidazole and chlorhexidine to eliminate *A. actinomycetemcomitans* may be successful in delaying the inevitable exfoliation of teeth, although the basic neutrophil function defect remains. Treatment of other family members is also required and pets (especially dogs) if they are found to harbour the bacteria.
- Several papers have reported the use of vitamin-A derivatives in management which may improve the prognosis. All patients require planned full clearances and dentures to avoid pain and disfigurement.

Chediak–Higashi disease A rare autosomal-recessive disorder, affecting lysosomal storage, causing a qualitative neutrophil defect. There is defective neutrophil chemotaxis and abnormal degranulation which results in poor intracellular killing. There is also reported to be abnormal B-cell and T-cell function and thrombocytopenia. Most children die by 10 years of age because of overwhelming sepsis. Teeth are shed, because of severe periodontal disease with rapid alveolar bone loss.

Langerhans' cell histiocytosis (disseminated) (Figure 6.15D & E)

This condition was previously termed histiocytosis X, and described the triad of eosinophilic granuloma, Hand–Schueller–Christian disease and Letterer–Siwe disease. This is a disease of the reticulo-endothelial system with a proliferation of Langerhans' cells. Oral lesions characteristically occur in all four quadrants and characteristically arise in mucosa overlying the primary molar teeth. This lesion extends forward to the canines, but rarely involves the incisors.

Presentation
- Malaise, irritability.
- Anovulval and postauricular rash.
- Diabetes insipidus.
- Premature exposure by alveolar resorption and subsequent loss of primary teeth, especially molars.
- Radiographically, teeth appear to be 'floating in air'.
- Typically, all four quadrants are involved.

Diagnosis
- Biopsy of oral or skin lesions.
- Positive for S100 stain.
- Transmission electron microscopy of Langerhans' cells.

Management
- Conservative excision and curettage of oral lesions and extraction of involved teeth is required to control oral lesions.
- Multi-agent chemotherapy is required for disseminated disease and is effective if commenced early.

Hypophosphatasia (Figure 6.15A & B)

A decrease in serum alkaline phosphatase and an increase in the urinary excretion of phosphoenolamine (PEP) are pathognomonic for hypophosphatasia. The more usual form is transmitted as an autosomal-dominant trait, whereas the autosomal-recessive form is usually lethal. Loss of at least some of the incisor teeth usually occurs before 18 months.

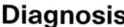

Diagnosis

- Serum alkaline phosphatase deficiency less than 90 U/litre. Normal range is 80–350 U/L, however, growing children often have levels well in excess of these values (>400 U/L).
- Urinary PEP and serum pyridoxal-5-phosphate (vitamin B$_6$) tests are required to confirm diagnosis. A skeletal survey of the long bones is necessary as rachitic changes may be present in severe cases.
- Hard-tissue sections of the exfoliated teeth show abnormal or absent cementum.

Self-mutilation (Figure 6.16)

A number of conditions exist which present with self-mutilation:

- Congenital indifference to pain syndrome.
- Lesch–Nyhan syndrome.
- Peripheral sensory neuropathies.

Because of an inability to recognize or feel pain, these children may avulse teeth and inflict extensive tears through gingiva, tongue or mucosa with their fingers or by biting and chewing.

Management

- Selective grinding of tooth cusps, or 'dome' buildups of the occlusal table, with composite resin to produce a smooth surface.
- Acrylic splints or cast silver splints to prevent gross laceration of the tongue or fingers.
- Extraction of teeth may be required as a last option in severe cases.

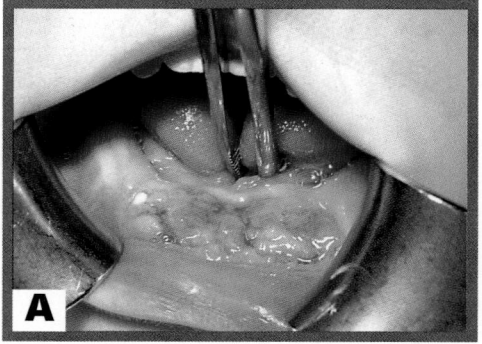

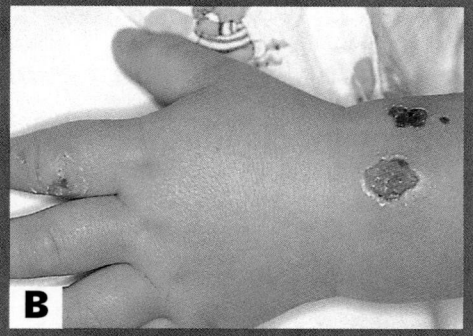

Figure 6.16 A Self-mutilation in a child with a peripheral sensory neuropathy. This child presented with exfoliation of the anterior teeth. She was investigated for many of the conditions described above until it was discovered that she herself was pulling out her teeth. Having no sensory nerve endings she could feel no pain. **B** Finger-biting is also a manifestation of neuropathies.

Ehlers–Danlos type VIII

An inborn error of metabolism presenting as a disorder of collagen formation. Typically, there is hyperextensibility of skin with capillary friability, bruising of skin, and hypermobility of the joints. Only type VIII presents with dental complications, mainly progressive periodontal disease leading to the loss of teeth.

Erythromelalgia

A very rare condition, characterized by sympathetic overactivity, causing an endarteritis and the extremities to feel hot. One case was reported with loss of primary and permanent teeth at age 4 years. The child had extreme hypermobility of joints and slept on a tiled floor in the middle of winter because of the heat in her legs. She also had an unexplained tachycardia of 200 beats per minute and presented a diagnostic dilemma for many months. The teeth exfoliated because of necrosis of alveolar bone.

Acrodynia (pink disease)

Mercury toxicity causes alveolar destruction and sequestration. Extremely rare now, although in the past seen with the use of teething powders containing mercury.

Acatalasia

Autosomal recessive catalase deficiency in neutrophils leading to periodontal destruction. Extremely rare outside Japan.

Scurvy

Almost unknown today, tooth loss results from a failure of proline hydroxylation and collagen synthesis.

Oral pathology in the newborn infant

Differential diagnosis

- Epstein's pearls.
- Bohn's nodules.
- Congenital epulis of the newborn.
- Melanotic neuro-ectodermal tumour of infancy.

Gingival (keratin) cysts in the newborn (Figure 6.17)

These hard, raised nodules are microkeratocysts and are epithelial remnants trapped along lines of fusion of embryological processes. Epstein's pearls appear in the middle of the hard palate whereas Bohn's nodules are remnants of the dental lamina and occur on the labial of the maxillary alveolar ridges. These cysts occur in all children but are normally shed *in utero*.

Management No treatment is required other than reassurance of the parents.

Melanotic neuro-ectodermal tumour of infancy (MNTI)

A rare but important paediatric tumour derived from neural-crest cells, occurs predominately in the maxilla. The condition may be present at birth and all recorded cases have been diagnosed by 4 months of age. Similar to neuroblastoma, there may be high levels of vanillymandelic acid (a catecholamine end-product) in the urine. Lesions are multicentric with close approximation to but not involving dental tissues, because of their ectomesenchymal origin. Lesions are circumscribed swellings which may be mucosal coloured or have a blue–black hue and may be associated with premature eruption of the primary incisors.

Diagnosis Computerized tomography followed by excisional biopsy because of the extremely rapid growth of the lesion.

This condition is usually so unique, at this age and at this site, that diagnosis is not difficult.

Management Enucleation of the tumour and involved primary teeth, curettage of the bony floor of the multiple cavities. Radiotherapy is contraindicated. Recurrences are extremely rare.

Diseases of salivary glands

Differential diagnosis
- Mucocoele.
- Ranula.
- Sialoliths.
- Mumps.
- Autoimmune parotitis.

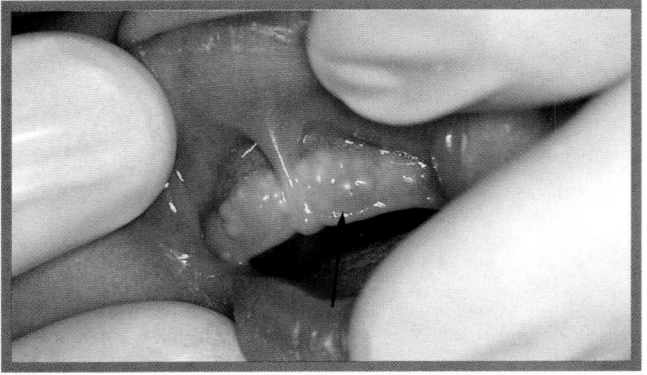

Figure 6.17 Bohn's nodules in a newborn child (arrow).

- Bilateral parotitis—bulimia.
- Congenital absence or hypoplasia of major salivary glands.

Mucocele (Figure 6.18A & B)

A mucous extravasation cyst arising from damage to one of the minor salivary glands in the lips or cheeks. Often caused from lip biting or other minor injuries, saliva builds up in connective tissue to be surrounded in a fibrous capsule. Most mucoceles are well-circumscribed bluish swellings, although long-standing lesions may have a whitish, keratinized surface.

Management
- Surgical excision together with the accessory salivary gland.
- Occasionally, cysts will burst and heal spontaneously.

Ranula

A mucous cyst of the floor of the mouth caused by damage to the duct of either the sublingual or submandibular glands. A soft, bluish swelling presents on one side of the floor of the mouth. A plunging ranula occurs when the lesion herniates through mylohyoid to involve the neck.

Management
- Complete surgical excision.
- Large lesions may require marsupialization.

Sialadenitis

Inflammation of the major salivary glands may result from:

Viral infection
- Mumps or cytomegalovirus infection. Present with bilateral non-suppurative parotitis, usually epidemic.
- HIV infection and AIDS. 10–15% of children with AIDS will manifest bilateral parotitis.

Bacterial infections
- Suppurative, usually retrograde infection.

Autoimmune
- Bilateral autoimmune parotitis, snowstorm appearance on sialogram.
- Bulimia.
- Salivary gland enlargement is a common presentation of bulimia nervosa.

Chronic sialadenitis

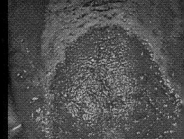

Usually caused by unilateral obstruction of a major salivary gland, either by stricture or a sialolith, and recurrent retrograde infection. Pain occurs during eating and when there is acute exacerbation of infection.

Management
- Antibiotics to control infection in the acute phase.
- Excision of calculus with sialodochoplasty to correct duct stricture.
- In long-standing cases of obstructive sialadenitis, removal of the gland may be necessary.

Salivary gland tumours
Most tumours of the salivary glands in children are vascular malformations. Pleomorphic adenomas are uncommon, whereas malignant neoplasms such as muco-epidermoid carcinoma, adenocarcinoma and sarcoma are extremely uncommon and affect mainly older children and adolescents. The parotid is the most common site.

Diagnostic imaging of the salivary glands
Radiology True mandibular occlusal film or panoramic radiographs are useful for imaging salivary calculi.

Sialography Demonstrates structure of the duct and gland architecture.

Computed tomography, magnetic resonance imaging, ultrasound If neoplasms are suspected.

Nuclear medicine Demonstrates salivary gland function.

Congenital absence of salivary glands (Figure 6.18C, D & E)
A number of cases of congenital salivary gland agenesis have been reported. Salivary gland hypoplasia is an uncommon presentation of a child with gross caries in unusual sites. Caries of the lower anterior teeth should be regarded with suspicion in a young child. It is uncommon for children to be on medication that will cause xerostomia and so congenital absence/hypoplasia should always be considered.

Diagnosis A technetium pertechnatate (^{99m}Tc) tracer seeks major protein-secreting exocrine and endocrine glands. The isotope is readily taken up by the parotid and submandibular glands, but not the sublingual gland. Lemon juice is added to assess function and clearance of the glands.

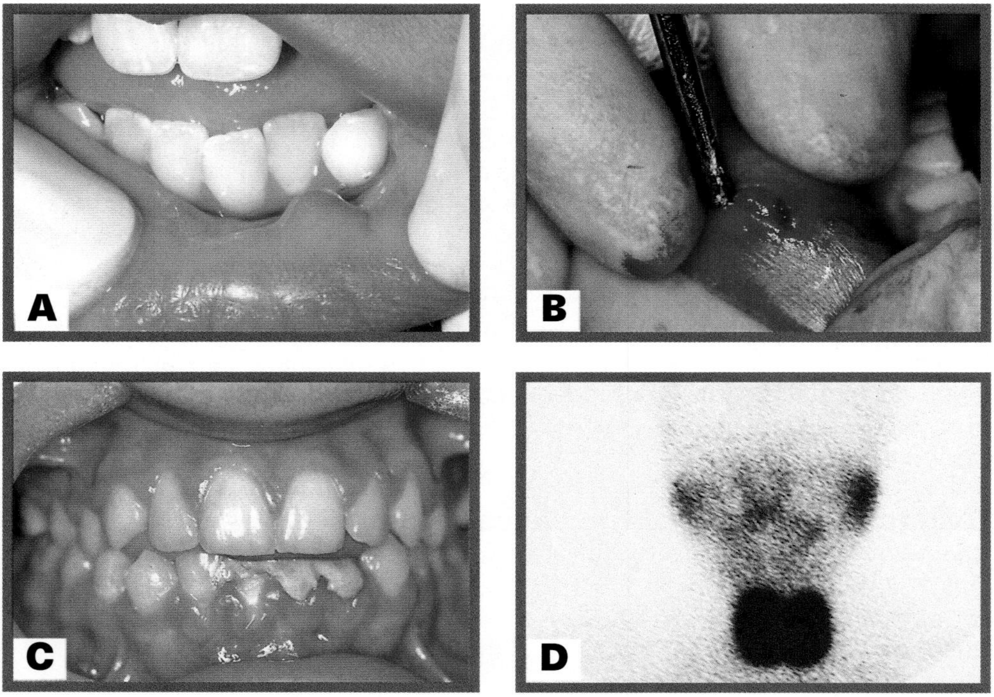

Figure 6.18 A Usual presentation of a mucocele on the lower lip. Most lesions require removal. **B** It is important to remove the lesion, and the associated minor salivary gland, in the procedure otherwise the lesion will recur. Patients must be warned that another mucocele may form from the surgery itself—causing damage to another minor salivary gland duct. **C** Gross carious destruction of the lower anterior teeth. These are the only affected teeth. The nuclear medicine scan, **D**, shows normal uptake of tracer in the parotid glands and thyroid but no function in the submandibular gland. A CT scan revealed that only small hypoplastic glands were present.

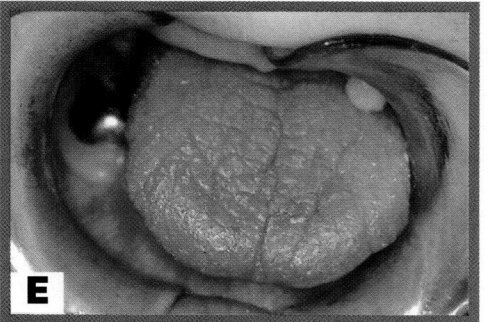

Figure 6.18 E A 4-year-old boy who, after three procedures under general anaesthesia to repair gross caries in his primary dentition, was subsequently diagnosed with complete absence of his major salivary glands.

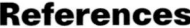

References

Infections

DOSON TB, PERROTT DH, KABAN LB. Pediatric maxillofacial infections: a retrospective study of 113 patients. *J Oral Maxillofac Surg* 1989, **47**:327–330.

KING DL, STEINHAUER W, GARCIA-GODOY F, ELKINS CJ. Herpetic gingivostomatitis and teething difficulty in infants. *Pediatr Dent* 1992, **14**:82–85.

RINDUM JL, HOLMSTRUP P, *et al.* Miconazole chewing gum for treatment of chronic oral candidosis. *Scand J Dent* Res 1993, **101**:386–390.

Oral ulceration

BORAZ RA. Oral manifestations of Crohn's disease: update of the literature and report of case. *J Dent Child* 1988, **55**:72–74.

FIELD EA, BROOKS V, TYLDESLEY WR. Recurrent aphthous ulcertion in children: a review. *Int J Paediatr Dent* 1992, **2**:1–10.

ERTURK N, DOGAN S. Distribution of *Actinobacillus actinomycetemcomitans* and *Porphyromans gingivalis* by subject age. *J Periodontol* 1991, **62**:490–494.

HARTMAN KS. Histiocytosis X: a review of 114 cases with oral involvement. *Oral Surg Oral Med Oral Pathol* 1980, **49**:38–54.

SCULLY C. Orofacial manifestations of chronic granulomatous disease of childhood. *Oral Surg Oral Med Oral Pathol* 1981, **57**:148–157.

SEDANO HO, GORLIN RJ Epidermolysis bullosa. *Oral Surg Oral Med Oral Pathol* 1989, **67**:555–563.

Gingival overgrowth

PERNU HE, PERNU LMH, HUTTUNEN KE, NIEMINEN PA, KNUUTTILA ML. Gingival overgrowth among renal transplant recipients related to immunosuppressive medication and possible local background factors. *J Periodontol* 1992, **63**:548–553.

ROSS PJ, NAZIF MM, ZULLO T, ZITELLI B, GUEVRA P. Effects of cyclosporin A on gingival status following liver transplantation. *J Dent Child* 1989, **56**:56–59.

SKRINJARIC I, BACIC M. Hereditary gingival fibromatosis; report on three families in dermatoglyphic analysis. *J Periodont Res* 1989, **24**:303–309.

Premature exfoliation of teeth

FRISKEN KW, HIGGINS T, PALMER JM. The incidence of periodontopathic micro-organisms in young children. *Oral Microbiol Immunol* 1990, **5**:43–45.

MACFAFLANE JD, SWART JGN. Dental aspects of hypophosphatasia: a case report, family study and literature review. *Oral Surg Oral Med Oral Pathol* 1989, **67**:521–526.

PREUS HR. Treatment of rapidly destructive periodontitis in Papillon–Lefevre syndrome. *J Clin Periodontol* 1988, **15**:639–643.

RASMUSSEN P. Cyclic neutropenia in an 8-year-old child. *J Pediatr Dent* 1989, **5**:121–126.

WATANABE K. Prepubertal periodontitis: a review of diagnostic criteria, pathogenesis and differential diagnosis. *J Periodontal Res* 1990, **25**:31–48.

Salivary gland agenesis

WHYTE AM, HAYWARD MWJ. Agenesis of the salivary glands: a report of two cases. *Br J Radiol* 1989, **62**:1023–1028.

Further reading

HALL RK. *Pediatric orofacial medicine and pathology*. London: Chapman and Hall Medical; 1994.

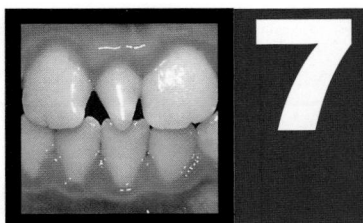

7 Dental anomalies

Contributors
Angus Cameron, Richard Widmer, Nigel King, Michael Aldred, Roger Hall, Kim Seow

Introduction

The diagnosis and management of dental anomalies constitute one of the most important areas of paediatric dentistry. Most anomalies will present in childhood and yet many are misdiagnosed or left untreated because the case is perceived to be too difficult. Genetic consultation is desirable not merely to put a name to the condition but also to give appropriate advice on the prognosis and the risk of recurrence in future offspring and for future generations. In many cases the presence of an inherited dental disorder would not stop a family from having children, but it is important to give parents and the affected children good advice. Genetic services are usually available at most paediatric hospitals.

Considerations in the management of dental anomalies

- Reassurance of child and parent.
- Genetic counselling.
- Elimination of pain.
- Restoration of aesthetics.
- Provision of adequate function.
- Maintenance of vertical dimension of occlusion.
- Delay of definitive treatment until an optimum age.
- Interdisciplinary formulation of definitive treatment plan.

Dental anomalies at different stages of tooth development

Dental lamina formation stage
Migration of neural crest cells (ectomesenchyme) into branchial arches
- Anodontia (which is usually only seen in cases of ectodermal dysplasia).
- Duplication of dental arches.

Initiation and proliferation
Induction of oral ectoderm by ectomesenchyme
- Oligodontia (isolated and in syndromes such as ectodermal dysplasia).
- Supernumerary teeth.
- Geminated or fused teeth.
- Ameloblastic fibroma/fibro-odontoma (dependent on differentiation and the presence of calcification within the lesion).
- Odontogenic keratocysts (primordial cysts).
- Ameloblastoma.
- Odontoma (compound).

Histodifferentiation
Developmental defects of multiple dental tissues
- Odontome (complex).
- Regional odontodysplasia.

Morphodifferentiaton
Abnormalities of size and shape
- Macrodontia.
- Microdontia (isolated or as part of a syndrome).
- Dens invaginatus.
- Dens evaginatus.
- Hutchinson's incisors, mulberry molars in congenital syphilis.
- Carabelli cusp.
- Talon cusp.
- Taurodontism.

Apposition
Organic matrix apposition and primary mineralization stage
- Dentine:
    Dentinogenesis imperfecta.
    Dentinal dysplasia.
    Dentinal cysts.
- Enamel:
    Amelogenesis imperfecta (hypoplastic).
    Enamel hypoplasia.

Calcification
Secondary enamel and dentine mineralization stage
- Enamel defects:
    Amelogenesis imperfecta (hypomineralized forms).
    Enamel opacities.
    Severe fluorosis.

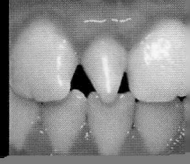

Maturation
Removal of water and enamel proteins
- Enamel defects:
    Amelogenesis imperfecta (hypomineralized forms).
    Milder forms of fluorosis.

Eruption stage and root development
- Premature eruption.
- Natal and neonatal teeth.
- Delayed eruption.
- Ectopic eruption.
- Eruption cysts.
- Transposition of teeth.
- Impactions.
- Arrested root development from systemic illness.

Oligodontia

Congenital absence of teeth is common, occurring sporadically or with a hereditary component. The most common teeth to be absent are the last teeth in each series (i.e. the lateral incisor, the second premolar and the third molar). The presence of conical teeth is frequently associated with the absence of the same teeth on the opposite side of the arch. An example of this is the peg lateral incisor. Further, that lateral incisor itself may be congenitally absent in subsequent generations. There are over 120 syndromes of the head and neck that manifest missing teeth. It is not so important how many teeth are missing but which types of teeth are absent. It is particularly rare to be missing a central incisor, a canine or a first permanent molar.

Alternative terminology
Hypodontia.

Frequency

Primary teeth	0.1–0.7%	male : female	unknown
Permanent teeth	2–9%	male : female	1 : 1.4

Major conditions manifesting oligodontia
- Ectodermal dysplasia.
- Clefting.
- Down syndrome.
- Chondro-ectodermal dysplasia (Ellis–van Creveld syndrome).
- Reiger syndrome.

- Incontinentia pigmenti.
- Oro-facial-digital syndrome (Types I and II).

Ectodermal dysplasia

Ectodermal dysplasia describes a group of inherited disorders involving the ectodermally derived structures, i.e. the hair, teeth, nails, skin and sweat glands. The most common is the hypohydrotic X-linked form. The usual presentation is a male child with:
- Multiple congenital absence of teeth (Figure 7.1).
- Fine, sparse hair with shaft abnormalities (Figure 7.1B).
- Dry skin (Figure 7.1A).
- Frontal bossing.
- Maxillary hypoplasia.
- Lips showing little of the vermilion margin.

Heterozygous females are often diagnosed dentally. Teeth are small and conical, often with a large anterior diastema (Figure 7.2).

In some countries, dental care (including prevention, orthodontics and prosthetics) may be provided under government welfare schemes such as the Cleft Palate Scheme in Australia, which covers a range of craniofacial anomalies in addition to clefting.

Management

The aim of treatment is to provide adequate function, maintain the vertical dimension and restore aesthetic appeal. This can begin as soon as the child will allow an adequate impression to be taken. Often, the first set of dentures is worn in the pocket! As the child grows, however, there is a desire to have a more normal appearance. Ideally, treatment should begin at around 2–3 years of age. Provision of the upper denture before the lower may be one way of increasing acceptance. The aim is for these children to be wearing appliances that give them a dentition similar to their peers, and promote normal speech development by the time they are at kindergarten or primary school.

Treatment options

- Acid-etch composite buildups of conical teeth.
- Partial dentures: conventional or overdentures (Figure 7.2E, F).
- Surgical exposure of impacted teeth.
- Orthodontic adjustment of spaces.
- Laboratory-fabricated composite veneers, crowns and bridges.
- Osseo-integrated implants.

Clefting

Supernumerary teeth and oligodontia often occur adjacent to the cleft in children with such defects. Because of disruption of the dental lamina, there may be abnor-

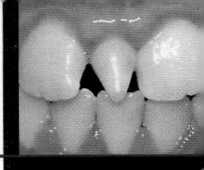

mal induction or proliferation, giving rise to either or both of these two abnormalities. Again, it is extremely rare for the canine tooth to be involved, as this tooth forms from ectoderm from the maxillary process rather than the frontonasal process (see Chapter 10).

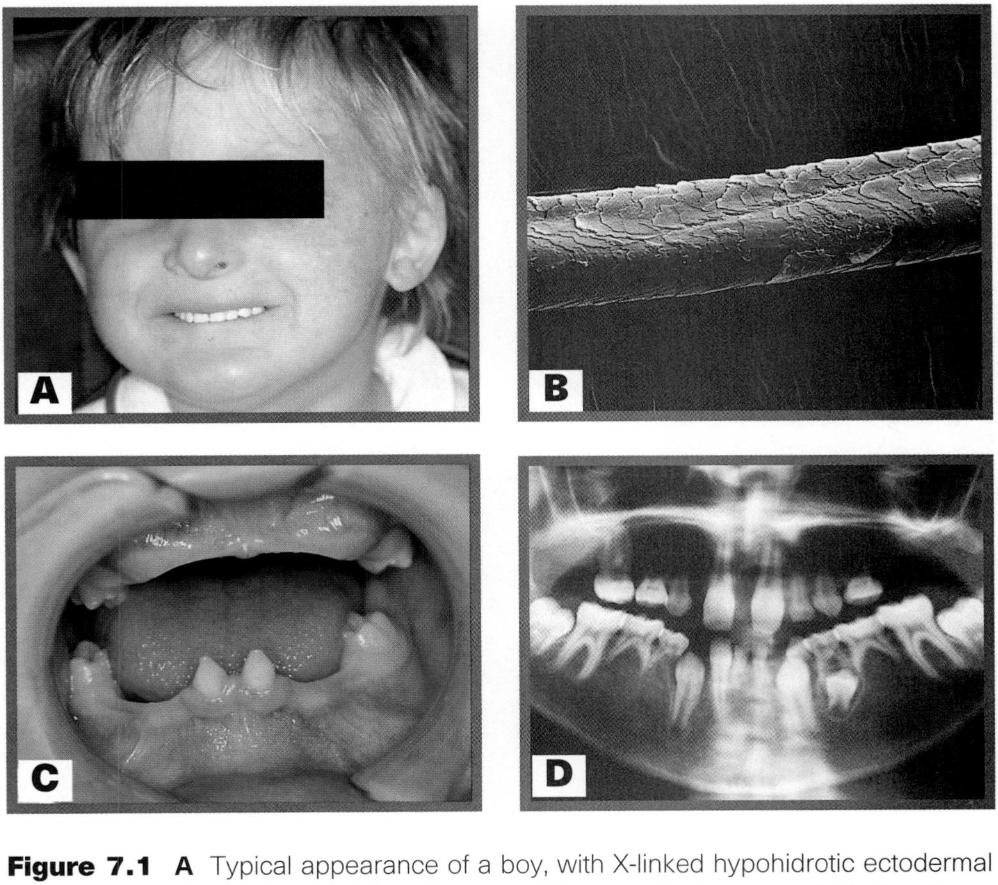

Figure 7.1 **A** Typical appearance of a boy, with X-linked hypohidrotic ectodermal dysplasia, wearing a denture. The skin around the eyes is dry and wrinkled and may be pigmented. **B** The hair is fine and sparse and often displays longitudinal grooves on the surface, as demonstrated under the scanning electron microscope. **C** Typical appearance of the dentition of a child with ectodermal dysplasia. Note the conical shaped teeth and also the large number of missing teeth. **D** Panoramic radiograph of a boy with autosomal dominant ectodermal dysplasia demonstrating congenital absence of primary and permanent teeth.

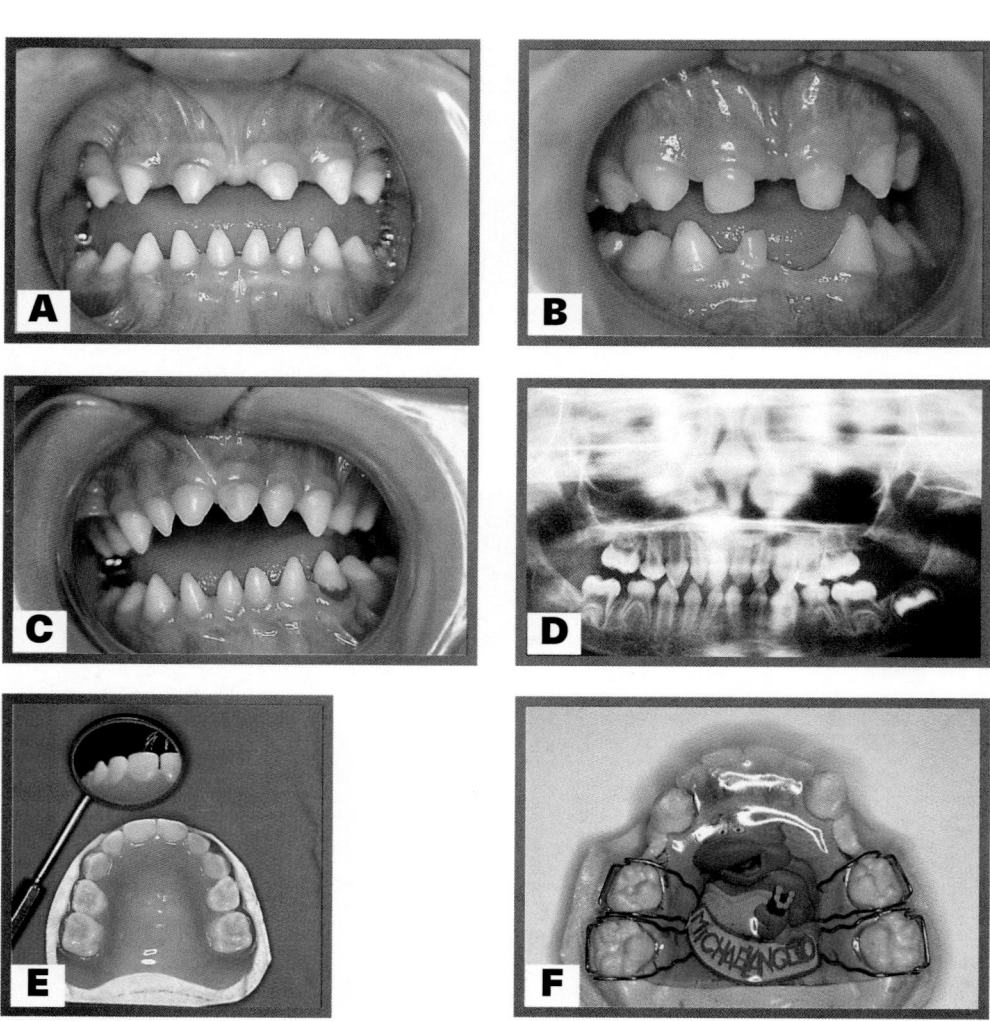

Figure 7.2 **A & B** Two patients diagnosed with ectodermal dysplasia both with many missing teeth and those that were present being small and conical in shape. Where teeth are congenitally missing, alveolar bone does not develop. Patient **B** is a heterozygous female with the X-linked form and is less severely affected than her brother who has anodontia. **C & D** Conical primary teeth are often associated with missing permanent teeth. This child had an autosomal recessive form of ectodermal dysplasia and was missing almost all of the permanent dentition. **E & F** Dentures for young children with ectodermal dysplasia. Young children tolerate dentures surprisingly well and Adams' cribs and ball retainers provide ideal retention around primary molars.

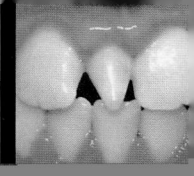

Single solitary incisor syndrome (monosuperocentroincisivodontic dwarfism) (Figure 7.3)

This is a syndrome that presents with a midline symmetrical upper-central incisor. The condition may also be associated with other midline disturbances such as cleft palate, choanal stenosis or atresia, imperforate anus or umbilical hernia and is part of the spectrum of the holoprosencephaly malformation complex. Of importance is the association with hypoplasia of the sella, pituitary dysfunction, growth hormone deficiency and subsequent short stature. The syndrome is diagnosed principally on the basis of the dental manifestations.

Osseo-integrated implants in children

There has been much controversy as to the timing of placement of osseo-integrated implants in young children. To date, there has been little published material about early placement and its long-term consequences. It is generally believed that implants act similarly to submerging ankylosed teeth and do not move with growing bone. Recent animal research has confirmed that most fixtures do become osseo-integrated in growing jaws; however, there was no evidence that the fixtures behaved like normal teeth during development. In the mandible the fixtures became displaced lingually, whereas in the maxilla they were displaced palatally and superiorly and did not follow the normal downwards and forwards growth of this bone. This latter point is important when considering the placement of implants in the anterior maxilla. Furthermore, fixtures locally retarded alveolar growth and changed the eruptive path of distally positioned tooth buds.

Implants should, in most cases, not be considered in children before the cessation of growth.

It should be noted, however, that in children with conditions such as ectodermal dysplasia, alveolar bone does not develop where teeth are congenitally absent. Consequently it may be possible to place implants much earlier in these children than in those with a normal alveolus.

Lyon hypothesis Before terminal cellular differentiation, the two X chromosomes in a female cell appear to be active; however, with differentiation, one is inactivated. The Lyon hypothesis relates to the inactivation of one of the X chromosomes in female cells. Recently, the proposed random nature of this inactivation has been challenged. This means that for female carriers of X-linked disorders approximately 50% of the cells will express the disorder whereas the others will have the normal phenotype. This is of particular importance in conditions such as ectodermal dysplasia, haemophilia and some forms of amelogenesis imperfecta. Heterozygous females with ectodermal dysplasia may have some missing teeth, although they are less affected than males. Similarly, in haemophilia A, heterozygous females often present with subclinical bleeding problems and a factor-VIII level less than 50%.

Disorders of proliferation

Supernumerary teeth

Budding of dental lamina, inherited as an autosomal dominant or X-linked trait.
- The shape may resemble a tooth of the normal series, in which case it can be incisiform, caniform or molariform; otherwise it may be conical or tuberculate.

Alternative terminology
- Mesiodens, paramolar, distomolar, hyperdontia, polydontism, supplementary teeth.

Frequency
- Primary teeth   0.3–0.8%   male:female   unknown
- Permanent teeth   1.0–3.5%   male:female   1:0.4
- 98% in maxilla, 75% of which are in the anterior palate.
- Present as conical or tuberculate forms.

Diagnosis
- Failed or ectopic eruption of permanent tooth (Figure 7.3B)
- Routine radiographic survey.
- As part of a syndrome such as cleidocranial dysplasia and Gardner's syndrome.

Management
- Conical teeth often erupt and are easily extracted (Figure 7.4A).
- Tubercular or inverted conical teeth require surgical removal (Figure 7.4D).
- Surgical removal as early as possible to allow uninhibited eruption of the permanent tooth.
- During surgical removal care should be taken to avoid disrupting the developing permanent teeth.
- Vertex occlusal films for horizontal and anteroposterior localization are the preferred radiographs (Figure 7.4C). If unavailable then use periapical films and tube-shift to locate.
- Before 10 years of age: if the unerupted central incisor is upright then surgically remove the supernumerary and allow normal eruption of the permanent tooth. Gingival exposure may be required later because of the surgical scar formation, which can inhibit final soft tissue emergence.
- After 10 years of age, or if the central incisor is malaligned: surgical exposure with or without bonding of brackets or chains and subsequent orthodontic traction may be required (Figure 7.6).

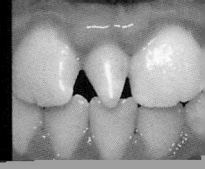

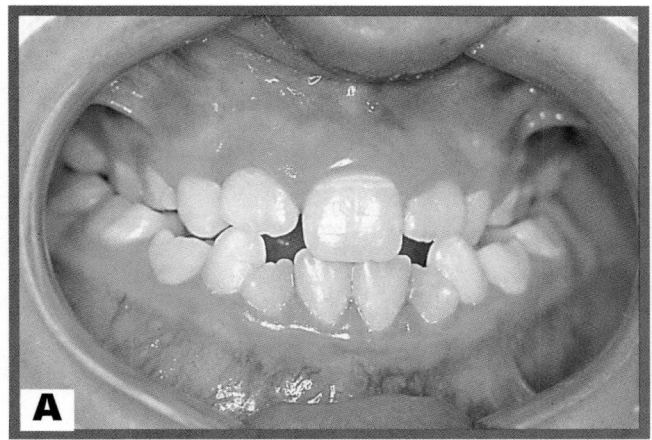
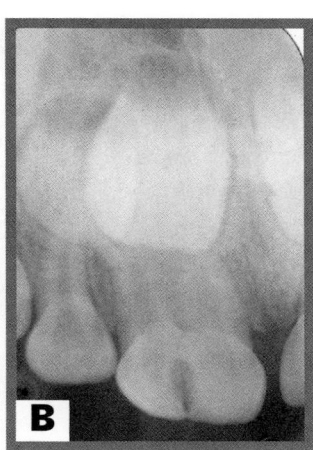

Figure 7.3 A Single solitary incisor syndrome, presenting with a symmetric incisor in the midline. This child had a mild growth hormone deficiency, with his height on the 10th percentile. **B** Periapical radiograph of the same patient in the primary dentition showing fused incisors. Note the caries in the groove between the two tooth units.

Cleidocranial dysplasia

This condition has an autosomal dominant mode of inheritance, with a high incidence of spontaneous mutation. The condition has been mapped to *6p21* (short arm of chromosome 6, locus 21).

Manifestations

- Short stature.
- Aplasia or hypoplasia of one or both clavicles.
- Delayed ossification of fontanelles and sutures.
- Frontal bossing.
- Hypertelorism and maxillary hypoplasia.
- Wormian bones in cranial sutures.
- Multiple supernumerary teeth (Figure 7.5).
- Delayed eruption of all teeth.
- Absent or altered cellular cementum.

It has now been shown that the supernumerary teeth are manifestations of a true third dentition, and consequently it is possible to predict when and where supernumeraries may form (Jensen and Kreiborg, 1990).

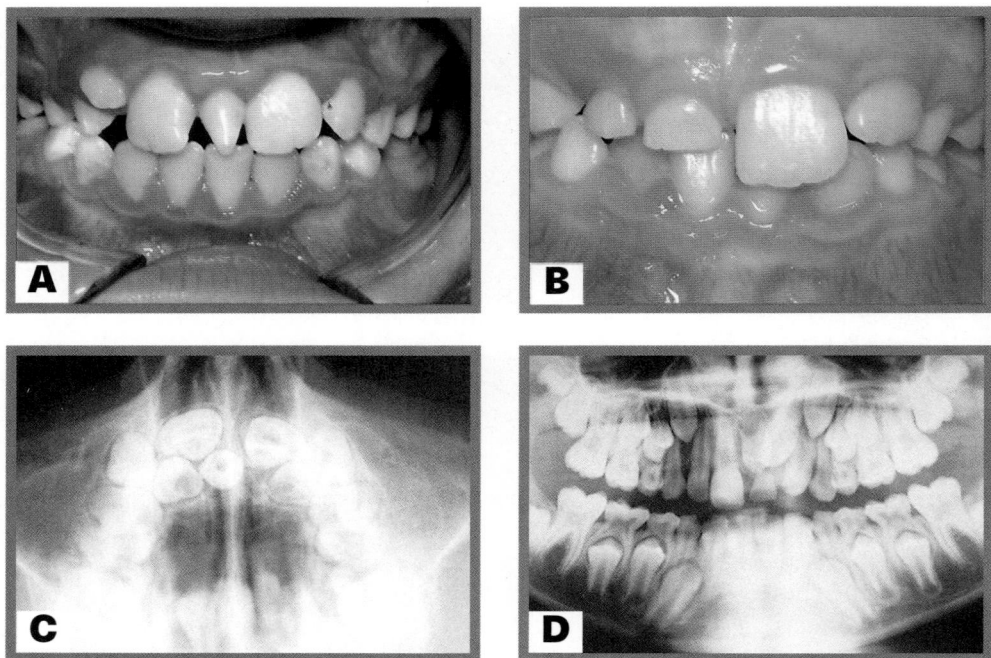

Figure 7.4 Common presentation of supernumerary teeth. **A** Conical teeth often erupt, except when inverted. **B** The late eruption of a permanent central incisor is most commonly caused by a supernumerary tooth. **C** A vertex-occlusal radiograph showing the true anteroposterior position of the supernumerary tooth. This radiograph was taken by an extra-oral technique which significantly reduces radiation exposure. **D** A panoramic radiograph is useful in determining the vertical orientation of the extra tooth and the degree of displacement of the permanent central incisor. In this case, after removal of the supernumerary, an upper denture was used as a space maintainer and the impacted tooth subsequently erupted into a normal position.

Management
- Early diagnosis and documentation.
- Planned removal of non-resorbing primary teeth.
- Surgical removal of supernumerary teeth.
- Surgical exposure of permanent teeth.
- Orthodontic alignment and consideration of orthognathic surgery when growth complete.

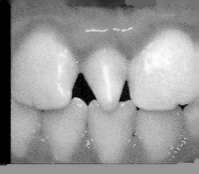

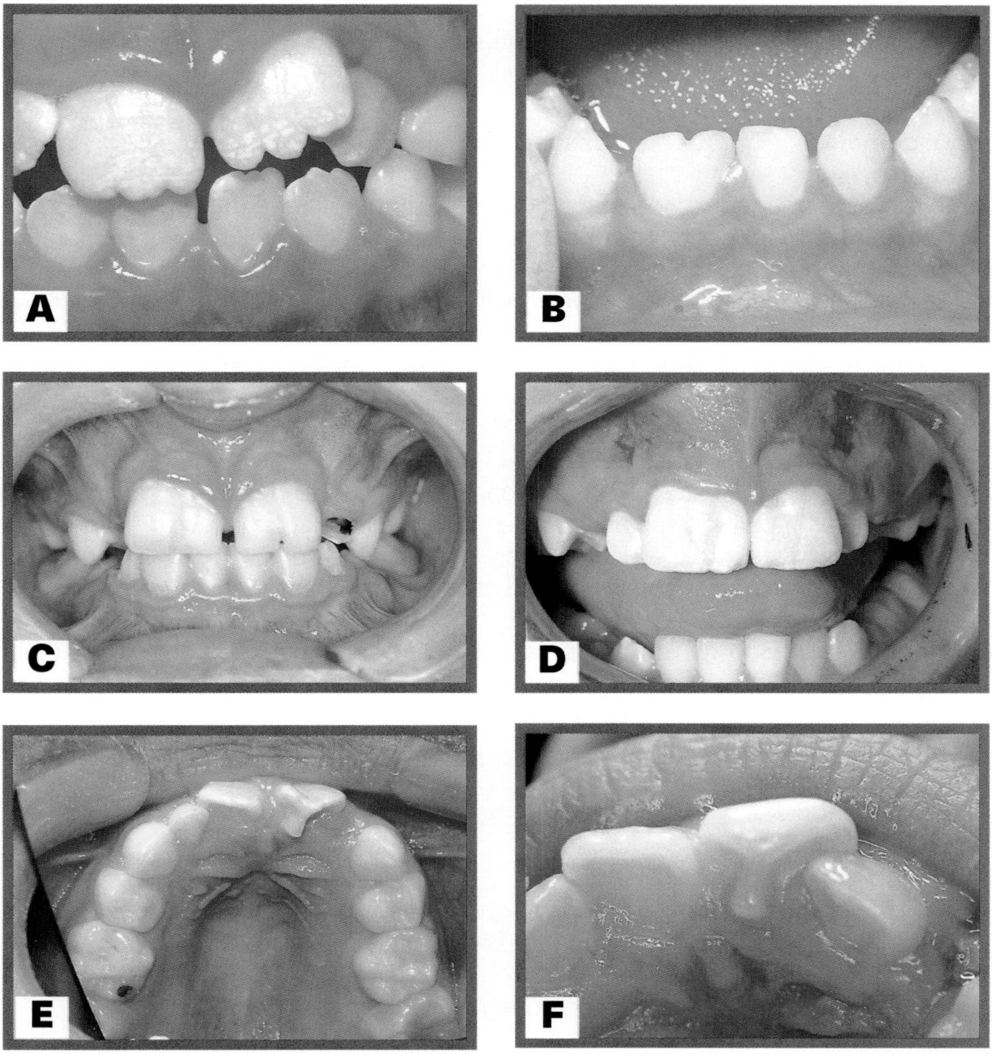

Figure 7.7 Morphological anomalies. **A** Mamelons, which are variations of normal anatomy. **B** Double tooth involving the right mandibular incisor, possibly caused by fusion of the normal lateral and central incisors. **C** Double tooth formed by fusion of the maxillary central incisors with two supernumerary teeth. Two root canals were present. **D** Bilateral double teeth in the maxillary central incisor region with single root canals. These teeth were extracted and the lateral incisors moved mesially with orthodontics. **E** Talon cusp. **F** T cingulum. The cingulum cusp has pulp horns and removal of the cusp will often result in an exposure of the pulp.

Germination

Budding of a second tooth from a single tooth germ. Usually one root canal is present. Hence the number of teeth in the arch is normal.

Management The groove on a double tooth is extremely prone to caries; therefore fissure sealing is essential.
- In the permanent dentition surgical separation of fused teeth may be possible with subsequent orthodontic alignment and restorative treatment as needed to reshape the crown.
- Reshaping or reduction of a double tooth with a single canal (geminated tooth) is usually impossible and extraction may be the only alternative. Orthodontic therapy and/or prosthetic replacement is then required. Implants may be an option for adolescents.

Dens invaginatus (Figure 7.8)

Maxillary lateral incisors may have a developmental invagination of the cingulum pit with often only a thin hard tissue barrier between the oral cavity and the pulp. Pulp necrosis often occurs soon after the eruption of the affected tooth, causing significant canine fossa cellulitis. This anomaly may occur in other teeth such as the first premolar.

Alternative terminology Dens in dente (used to describe the extreme variant, but is a misnomer), dilated composite odontome.

Frequency
- Primary dentition   0.1%
- Permanent dentition   4%   male>female

Management
- If newly erupted, the palatal surface should be fissure-sealed.
- If the root canal morphology is favourable then root-canal therapy should be undertaken.
- If internal anatomy is complex and unegotiable then extraction is necessary.

Dens evaginatus

An enamel-covered tubercule projecting from the occlusal surface of a premolar or, less commonly, from a canine or molar tooth. Usually bilateral and more common in the mandible. There is pulp tissue within the tubercle in 43% of cases.

Alternative terminology Leong's premolar, tuberculated premolar, axial core type odontome, occlusal enamel pearl, composite dilated odontome, cone-shaped supernumerary cusp, evaginated odontome, interstitial cusp.

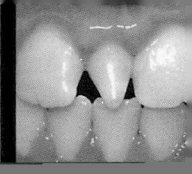

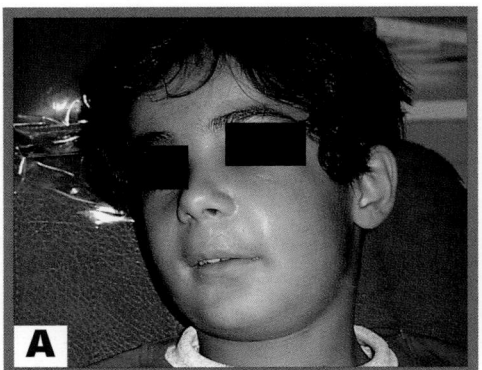

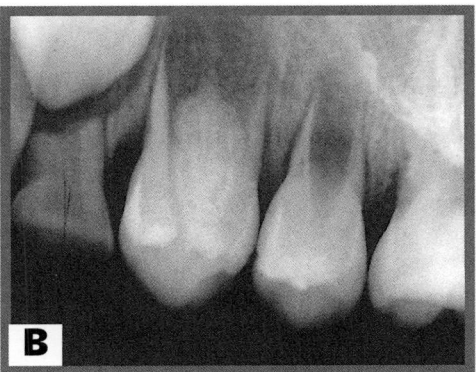

Figure 7.8 Maxillary canine fossa cellulitis from an infected dens invaginatus in a first premolar tooth. Because of root-canal morphology, and the severity of the infection, the tooth was removed. The patient required hospital admission with high-dose intravenous antibiotics, and surgical drainage of the abscess, under general anaesthesia.

Frequency
- Primary dentition almost unknown.
- Permanent dentition 4% (almost exclusively Mongoloid races).
- Possibly more common in females.

Management The tubercle can easily fracture because of occlusal interference, therefore grinding of the tubercle followed by sealing or applying fluoride varnish to reduce sensitivity can be of assistance. An alternative prophylactic measure is to support the sides of the tubercle with composite resin and then to recontour the occlusal surface to produce a central ridge. Ideally, this should be performed before the tooth comes into complete occlusion.

If fractured or abraded, pulp exposure commonly occurs. Because this exposure occurs soon after eruption, the apex of the tooth is often open and the long-term prognosis is poor. Extraction of the tooth should be performed after orthodontic consultation. A pulp dressing with calcium hydroxide may be required to stabilize the tooth if orthodontics is to commence later.

If diagnosed early, an elective Cvek pulpotomy can be performed to allow normal root formation.

Talon cusp (Figure 7.7E, F)
This is a horn-like projection of the cingulum of the maxillary incisor teeth. It may reach and contact the incisal edge of the tooth.

Alternative terminology T cingulum, Y-shaped cingulum, evaginated odontome, dens evaginatus.

Frequency
- Primary dentition   almost unknown
- Permanent dentition   1–2%

Management
- If there is no interference with the occlusion no treatment is required.
- If an interference is present, small reduction of enamel only, or elective Cvek pulpotomy to allow apexogenesis.

Taurodontism

Used to describe teeth with an enlarged pulp chamber. The distance from the cement-enamel junction to the bifurcation of the root is greater than the length of the roots. The tooth, therefore, has a long crown and short roots, similar to the teeth of cattle. The anomaly appears to be caused from a failure of Hertwig's epithelial root sheath to invaginate. Taurodontism may occur in a normal individual and may be inherited. Several syndromes and conditions have this anomaly.

Frequency Unknown.

Conditions with enlarged pulp chambers
- Vitamin-D-resistant rickets (hypophosphataemic rickets).
- Rickets (vitamin-D-dependent).
- Hypophosphatasia.
- Dentinogenesis imperfecta (some cases).
- Regional odontodysplasia.
- Klinefelter's syndrome.
- Shell teeth.

Congenital syphilis

Although very rare, congenital syphilis presents with several important diagnostic dental manifestations. Both primary and permanent incisors may have tapering crowns and medial notching of the incisal edge. This tapering or screwdriver-like appearance is important in the differential diagnosis as there are many causes of non-syphilitic notching of the incisal edge (e.g. trauma). Crowns of the molar teeth have a 'cobbled' or 'mulberry' appearance in congenital syphilis.

Developmental defects of enamel

Developmental defects of enamel can be inherited or acquired.

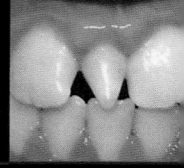

Chronological disturbances

Any severe systemic event during the development of the teeth (i.e. from 3 months *in utero* to 20 years) will result in some dental abnormality. Many of these anomalies are subclinical and can only be observed in hard-tissue sections with changes in incremental deposition lines. The neonatal line is manifest in all teeth, but unless there is severe hypoxia or fetal distress the disturbance will not be clinically evident. Different teeth will show defects at different levels of the crown depending on the stage of crown formation at the time the disturbance occurred. The resulting enamel may be reduced in quantity or in quality.

A defect is described as localized when only one tooth is affected and generalized when there is a symmetrical disturbance on teeth of the same type on both left and right sides.

Approximately 100 aetiological agents have been reported to cause developmental defects of enamel. Those causing localized defects are listed in Table 7.1 and those causing generalized defects in Table 7.2.

Developmental defects of enamel can be classified according to their clinical appearance:
- Discoloration.
- Opacities (hypomineralization).
- Hypoplasia.

In general, the aims of management are to treat pathology and pain, provide adequate aesthetic appeal, maintain occlusal function and maintain the vertical dimension.

Table 7.1 Aetiological agents that have been shown to produce developmental defects of enamel with a localized distribution

Aetiological agent	
Acute osteomyelitis	Gunshot wounds to jaws
Acute trauma to primary teeth	Irradiation
Ankylosis	Jaw fracture
Cleft palate	Laryngoscopy
Congenital epulis	Periapical infection of primary teeth
Electrical burn to mouth	Periodontal ligament injection
Extraction of primary teeth	

Tooth discoloration

Tooth discoloration may be extrinsic or intrinsic in nature. Extrinsic staining is superficial and occurs after tooth eruption. Intrinsic discoloration may result from a developmental defect of enamel or internal staining of the tooth (Figure 7.9). Although such internal staining is manifest as a change in enamel colour, the underlying defect may involve the dentine. See Table 7.3 for the differential diagnosis of tooth discoloration.

Opacities (hypomineralization)

A defect in the quality of the enamel. Hypocalcific defects or opacities are defects in the colour and translucency in enamel. Incomplete mineralization results in a change in the porosity of the enamel, causing opacity. This is located below the enamel surface, which remains intact.

Fluorosis (Figure 7.9E, F)

In its mildest forms, fluorosis is manifest as hypomineralization of the enamel, leading to opacities. These can range from tiny white flecks to confluent opacities throughout the enamel, making the crown totally lacking in translucency. Hypoplasia occurs at higher concentrations of fluoride. When the tooth first erupts the surface of the enamel may be intact; however, with attrition, areas of enamel are lost and stains are taken up into the porosities. At 1 ppm of fluoride in public water supplies, approximately 10% of the population will show very mild fluorosis. Severely affected cases require microabrasion or even composite resin or porcelain veneers. Many opacities are incorrectly labelled as fluorosis without adequate justification or investigation of fluoride history.

Management of stains and opacities

- Extrinsic stains can be removed simply with abrasives.
- Intrinsic stains, if superficial, may be removed with microabrasion techniques, i.e. 3% H_2O_2 and pumice.
- 18% HCl.

Rubber dam should always be used and must be ligated around individual teeth. $NaHCO_3$ paste applied to the gingival margin prior to dam placement, is used to protect soft tissue from any acid leakage. Apply the HCl to the affected area using a pledget of cotton wool for 10 seconds only, and then rinse thoroughly with water. This technique is potentially destructive to enamel and soft tissues and must be used with caution.

- Abrasion with pumice following etching with 37% phosphoric acid.
- Polishing labial surfaces with multi-fluted tungsten-carbide burr.

Deep intrinsic stains require removal of affected enamel and rebuilding with composite resin. Treatment using porcelain veneers and crowns should be delayed in adolescents until the gingival attachment is established at the cemento-enamel junction. Involvement in contact sports may be another reason for delaying

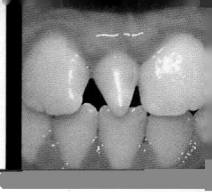

Table 7.2 Environmental aetiological agents that have been shown to produce developmental defects of enamel and discolouration with a generalized distribution

Prenatal	Perinatal	Postnatal	
Anaemia	Bile duct defects	Adrenal hyperfunction	Lead intoxication
Cardiac disease	Breech presentation	Cytotoxic medications	Measles
Congenital allergies	Caesarian section	Bulbar poliomyelitis	Mumps
Congenital syphilis	Erythroblastalis foetalis	Candida-endocrinopathy syndrome	Nephrotic syndrome
Cytomegalovirus	Haemolytic disorder	Chickenpox (varicella)	Neurological disorders
Diabetes	Hepatitis	Cholera	Otitis media
Fluoride	Intrapartum haemorrhage	Congenital cardiac disease	Pneumonia
Hypoxia	Low birthweight	Diphtheria	Pseudohypothyroidism
Renal disease	Neonatal asphyxia	Encephalitis	Renal dysfunction
Malnutrition	Neonatal hypocalcaemia	Fluoride	Scarlet fever
Pregnancy toxaemia	Placenta praevia	Gastrointestinal disturbances	Sickle-cell anaemia
Rubella	Prematurity	Hyperpituitarism	Tetracyclines
Stress	Prolonged labour	Hyperthyroidism	Tuberculosis
Thalidomide	Respiratory distress syndrome	Hypothyroidism	Typhus
Urinary tract infection	Tetanus	Hypoparathyroidism	Vitamin-A deficiency
Vitamin-A deficiency	Tetracyclines	Hypogonadism	Vitamin-C deficiency
Vitamin-D deficiency	Traumatic birth injuries	Intestinal lymphangiectasia	Vitamin-D deficiency
	Twinning	Smallpox	Vitamin-D intoxication
		Stress	

Table 7.3 Causes of tooth discoloration

Colour	Aetiology	Comments
Extrinsic discoloration		
Green	Chromogenic bacteria	Usually cervical and gingival areas
Yellow	Bile pigments from gingival crevicular fluid	Biliary atresia and jaundice
Black	Ferrous sulphate	Iron supplementation
Brown	Chromogenic bacteria	Arrested caries
Intrinsic discoloration with localized staining on one or several teeth		
Yellow/brown	Developmental defects	Usually after trauma or infection
White	Developmental defect	Subsurface decalcification in permanent teeth, after trauma or infection
Pink	Internal resorption	Seen before exfoliation of primary teeth or after trauma
Grey/black	Amalgam staining	Leakage of old amalgam restoration causing discoloration around the restoration
Chronological staining of dentition		
Bright yellow	Tetracycline	Unoxidized fluorophore, seen in newly erupted teeth
Yellow/grey–brown	Tetracycline	Erupted teeth, oxidized fluorophore (UV light) Colour also depends on the type of tetracycline
Yellow/brown	Systemic illness	Developmental defects of enamel affecting all teeth forming during illness
Generalized intrinsic staining of teeth, either single or complete dentition		
Grey–brown	Non-vitality	Usually after trauma
Yellow–brown to dark yellow	Amelogenesis imperfecta	Both dentitions are affected
Green–blue	Hyperbilirubinaemia	Seen in children with end-stage liver disease and premature infants
Blue–brown (opalescent)	Dentinogenesis imperfecta	All teeth uniformly affected, may be associated with osteogenesis imperfecta
Red–brown	Congenital porphyria	All teeth affected
White	Fluorosis/non-fluorotic	usually only permanent dentition

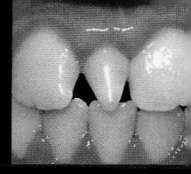

placement of complex restorations. The longevity of hybrid composite resins has improved substantially, along with colour stability, strength and translucency. These materials may be placed quickly and more cost-effectively than porcelain and other complex restorations such as crowns. It is important to always keep treatment options open.

Hypoplasia (Figure 7.9A, B)

A defect in quantity that causes a break in the surface continuity of the enamel. This is caused by failure of the apposition and protein matrix formation or an alteration in the mineralization of the matrix. In trauma cases, tissue may be lost after formation. Examples of hypoplastic defects are shown in Figure 7.9.

Management
- Localized hypoplastic defects may be restored with composite resin.
- It is important to maintain posterior support, and stainless-steel crowns may be required to restore grossly hypoplastic molars. These teeth are often exquisitely sensitive and treatment is made difficult by an inability to achieve good isolation for teeth that are only partially erupted. Glass–ionomers may be used temporarily to restore hypoplastic occlusal defects and prevent caries.
- Complex restorative treatment involving onlays and crowns should be delayed until late adolescence.

Amelogenesis imperfecta

The term amelogenesis imperfecta is usually applied to inherited defects of the enamel of both primary and permanent teeth. For practical purposes, it seems reasonable to extend this to include sporadic cases as well as those cases where the enamel defects are associated with extra-oral features, as found in some syndromes.

Amelogenesis imperfecta variants with Mendelian inheritance
- Autosomal dominant.
- Autosomal recessive.
- X-linked inheritance (gene locus: *Xp22*).
- Two genes have been identified, one on the X chromosome being the gene coding for amelogenin, which is the main structural protein of the enamel matrix. Another locus on chromosome 4 has been found to be involved in some cases of autosomal dominant amelogenesis imperfecta.

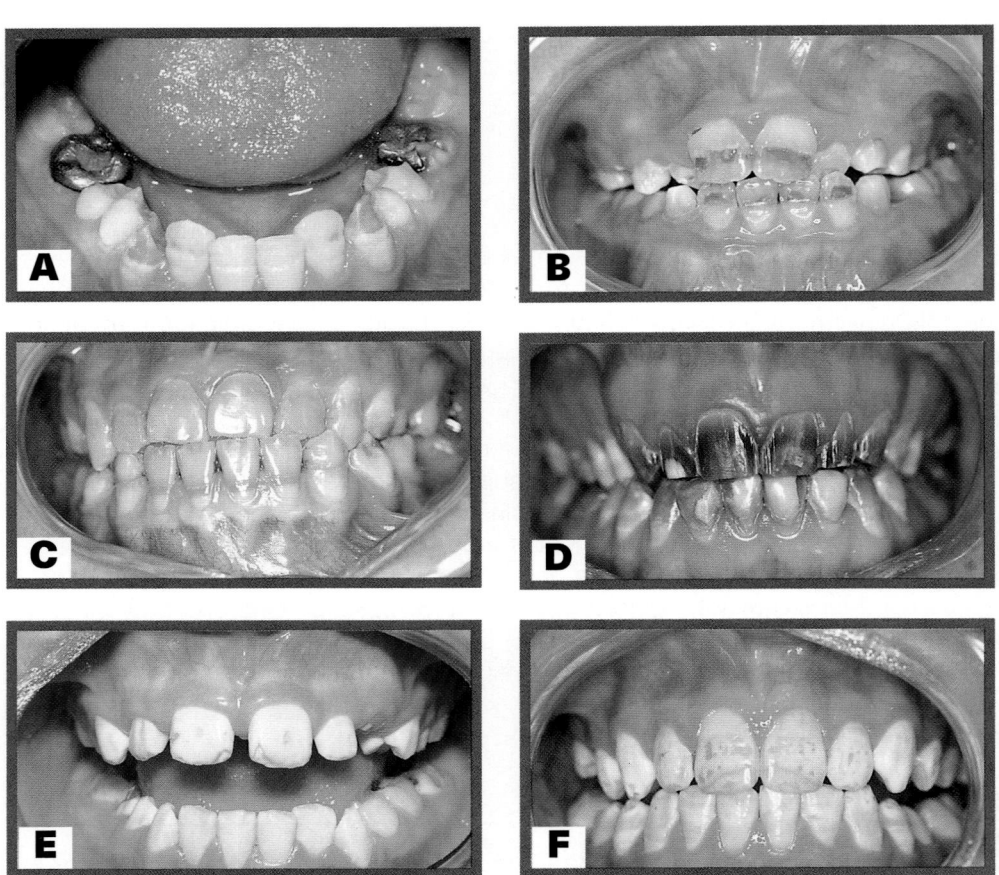

Figure 7.9 A Chronological enamel hypoplasia after severe measles at 18 months of age. **B** Vitamin-D deficiency from birth to 16 months of age. Note the different patterns of hypoplasia. **C** Tetracycline staining in an Asian child. Tetracyclines are available over the counter in some countries in South East Asia and this staining is primarily seen in this population group. **D** A severe case of tetracycline staining in a boy with cystic fibrosis. The anterior teeth have been prepared for porcelain veneers which were unsatisfactory. In these cases, intentional devitalization and non-vital bleaching with H_2O_2 may be a more conservative option, rather than crowning every tooth. **E & F** Fluorosis: **E** Uniform opacity throughout the crown. Some of the hypomineralized enamel has been lost on the incisal edge revealing normal enamel underneath. Stains have been taken up in porous enamel at the abraded margins. In patient **F**, white flecks are present which have only affected the upper incisor teeth to any significant degree. Where there has been attrition normal enamel is visible on the upper-left central incisor.

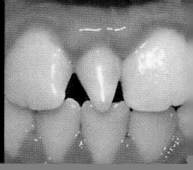

Frequency
- Estimated at 1:14000.
- Up to 1:800 reported in one Swedish paper.

Diagnosis
Based on the clinical and radiographic appearance and the mode of inheritance.

Phenotypes
Phenotypes range from hypoplastic (thin enamel) with spacing between adjacent teeth, to varying degrees of hypomineralization (poorly formed enamel) with altered colour and translucency, although in many cases both hypoplasia and hypomineralization are seen together. The colour of the enamel reflects the degree of hypomineralization—the darker the colour the more severe the degree of hypomineralization in general.

In X-linked amelogenesis imperfecta, females exhibit vertical bands of altered enamel manifesting Lyonization (see Lyon hypothesis). These bands may be thinner (because of hypoplasia) and/or altered in colour (because of hypomineralization). In such families there will be no male-to-male transmission, whereas the heterozygous females may pass on the trait to children of either sex (see Chapter 8: Genetic diseases).

In some forms of amelogenesis imperfecta the teeth fail to erupt, presumably due to a disturbance of the enamel organ, and they undergo replacement resorption of their crowns. In other forms, a skeletal anterior open bite is seen.

Hypoplastic forms
- Thin enamel (Figure 7.11).
- Account for the majority of cases.
- Lack of contact points between teeth in thin enamel type.
- Enamel may be rough, smooth, or randomly pitted (Figure 7.10).
- Female carriers of X-linked forms manifest Lyonization (see above) with vertical banding of normal and abnormal enamel.
- Teeth are delayed in eruption.
- Unerupted teeth may undergo replacement resorption.
- Anterior open bite associated with 60% of cases.

Hypomineralized forms
- Normal thickness of enamel initially.
- Dark yellow to brown in colour (Figure 7.10E).
- Enamel softer than normal, tends to chip and can be penetrated with an explorer. In severe forms the enamel may be scraped away with a scaler.
- Teeth erupt with normal thickness but enamel is soon lost, exposing rough, highly sensitive dentine.
- Large masses of supragingival calculus are present.

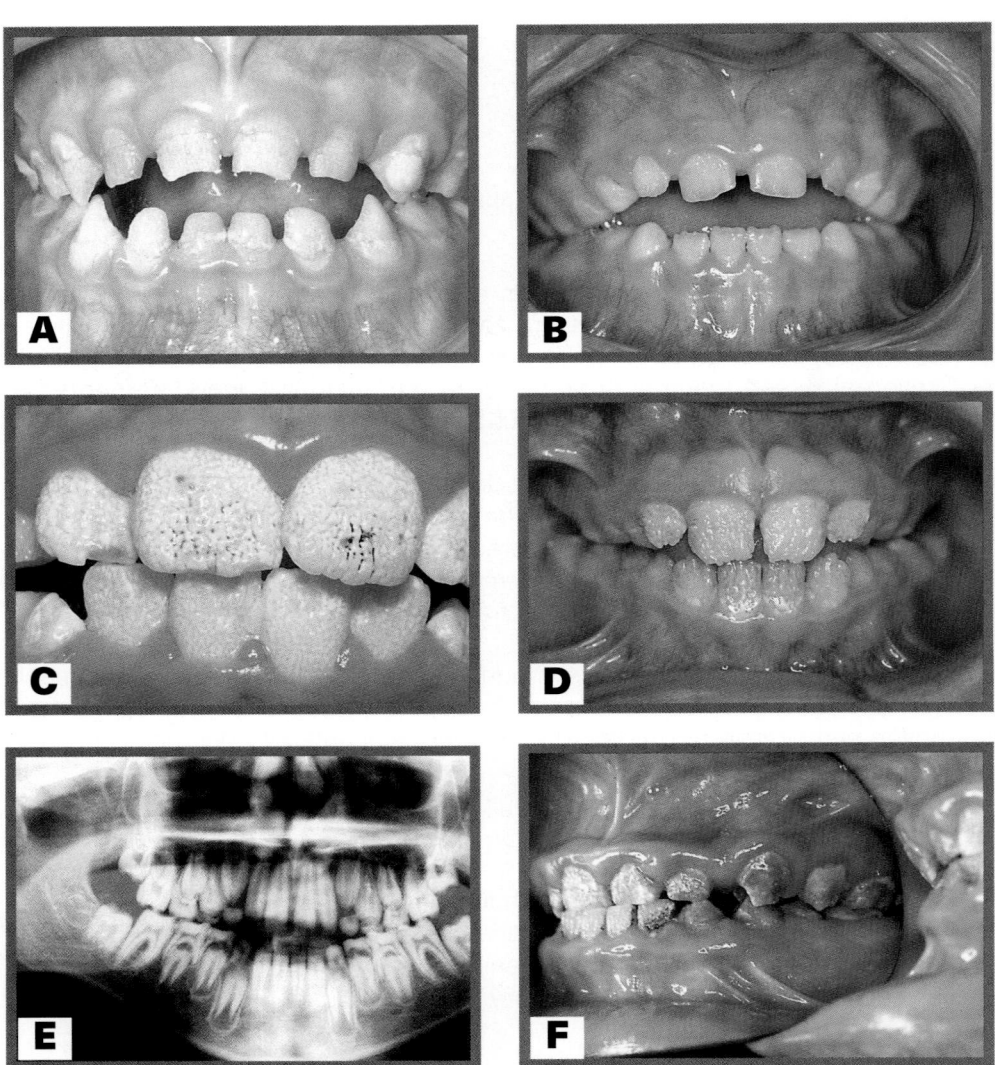

Figure 7.10 Different forms of amelogenesis imperfecta. **A** Autosomal recessive rough hypoplastic. **B** Autosomal dominant smooth hypoplastic with a marked anterior open bite. Note the open contact points in these two cases. **C** Autosomal-dominant pitting hypoplastic. **D** X-linked hypoplastic form in a female with vertical lines of abnormal and normal enamel. These represent enamel derived from different clones of ameloblasts that have undergone Lyonization. **E** OPG showing absent or very thin enamel in the hypoplastic forms. **F** Severe hypocalcified amelogenesis imperfecta. Note the discoloration and gross build-up of calculus on all surfaces.

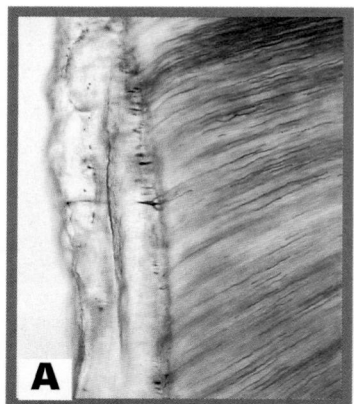 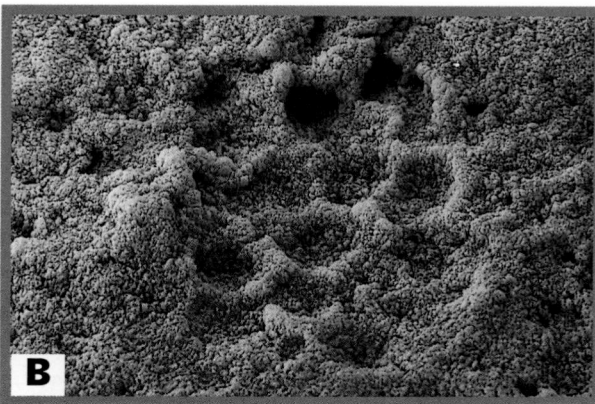

Figure 7.11 A Hard-tissue section of smooth hypoplastic amelogenesis imperfecta showing extremely thin enamel. **B** Scanning electron micrograph of similar patient with abnormal etching pattern of enamel. Crystalline structure of prisms is deficient.

- Radiographically, difficult to distinguish between enamel and dentine and may appear moth-eaten in severe cases.

Management
- Genetic counselling.
- Preservation of molar teeth with full coverage restorations to maintain vertical dimension. Overdentures may be an option in cases with small hypoplastic teeth (Figure 7.12E, F).
- Stainless-steel crowns or gold onlays on molars (Figure 7.13D).
- Care is required when trial fitting crowns, because defective enamel can be easily scraped or flaked off the tooth.
- Composite resin veneers over anterior teeth for aesthetics. It is possible to successfully bond composite to hypoplastic and hypomineralized enamel (Figure 7.12).
- Orthodontic and possible orthognathic surgery to correct anterior open bite in hypoplastic forms (Figure 7.13E).
- Delay definitive treatment with porcelain and precious metals until late adolescence.
- Adequate margins may be difficult to achieve because of the poor quality of the enamel (Figure 7.13C).

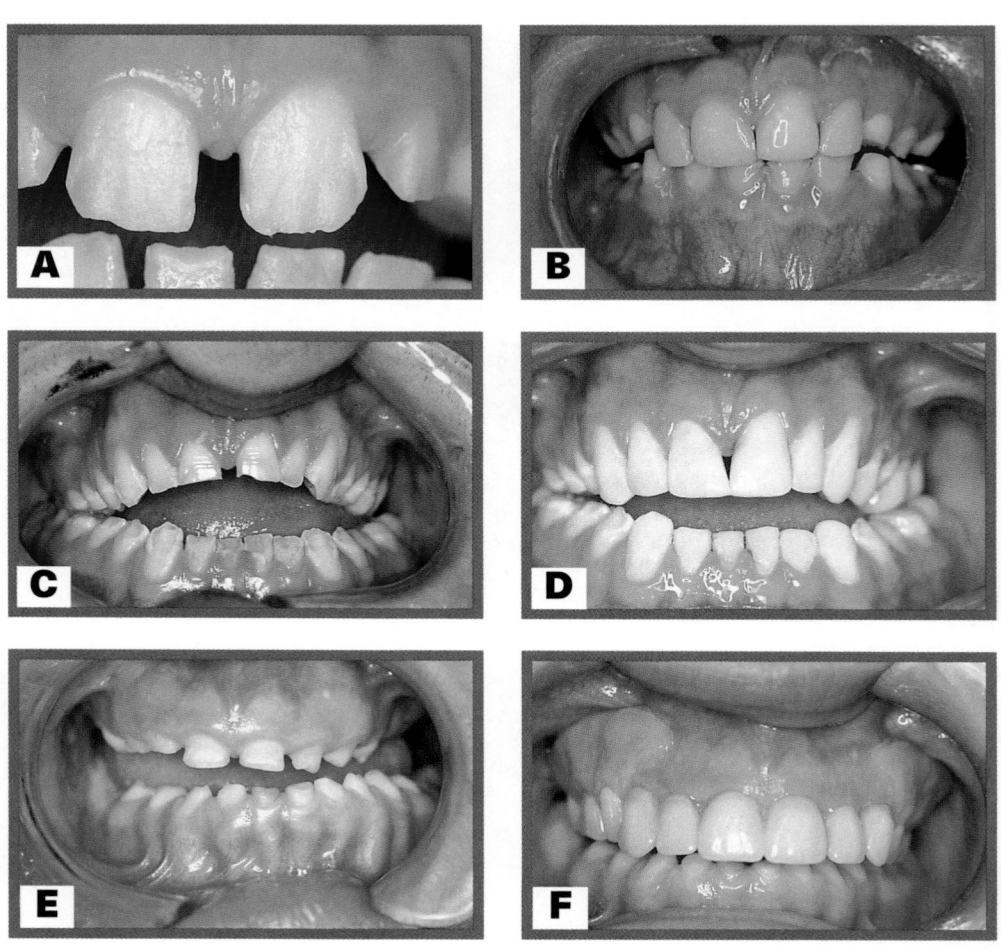

Figure 7.12 Different management options for amelogenesis imperfecta (AI): **A & B** Composite bonding to rough hypoplasia. Etching times should be slightly longer than usual; however, the roughness of the enamel surface aids in mechanical retention. **C & D** A case of smooth hypoplasia with a severe anterior and posterior open bite. The patient did not want orthodontics or orthognathic surgery and so the posterior occlusion was built up with composite resin, as were the anterior teeth. Because of the open bite, crown lengthening was easily achieved and the restorations have lasted for over 7 years without replacement. **E & F** A case of autosomal recessive AI associated with an autosomal recessive dystrophic epidermolysis bullosa. In this form of AI, posterior teeth fail to erupt and undergo spontaneous replacement resorption within the alveolus. The patient had no oral ulceration and, because of the small crown length and the prominent alveolus, an overdenture without a labial flange was constructed.

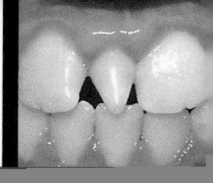

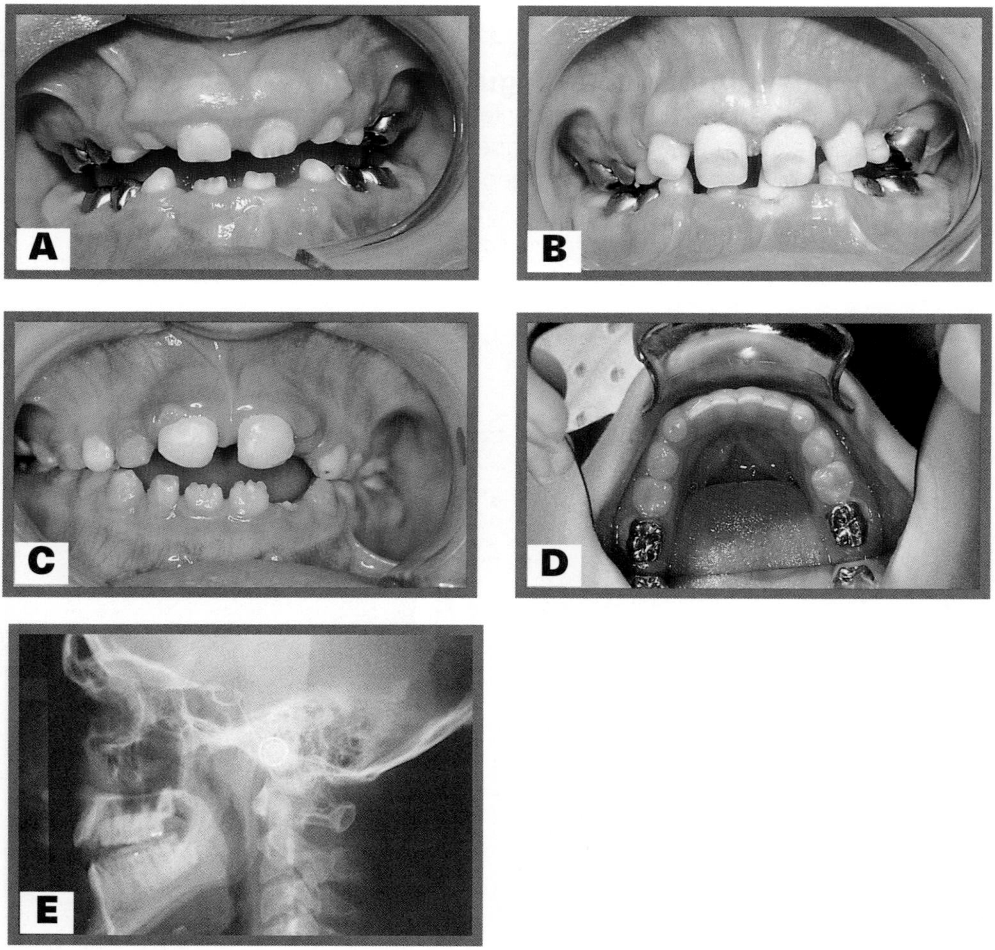

Figure 7.13 **A, B** A case of autosomal dominant smooth amelogenesis imperfecta (AI) with failure of eruption of the anterior teeth. Many of the posterior teeth are unerupted and undergoing resorption. Initial surgical exposure of the anterior segments did not aid their complete eruption. The gingivae contained small islands of calcification which may have impeded the eruption. Periodontal surgery with apically repositioned flaps was used to fully expose the crowns. **C** Not all cases using composite resin are successful. With progressive eruption of the teeth it is difficult for the patient to keep the gingival margins clean and often the restoration will fail. **D** Cast gold onlays are useful to protect the occlusal surfaces. No preparation of the crown was performed. Onlays were cemented with composite luting cement. **E** Severe open bite associated with autosomal-dominant hypoplastic AI.

Disorders of dentine

Dentinogenesis imperfecta (Figure 7.14)

Dentinogenesis imperfecta (DI) is an inherited disorder of dentine, which may or may not be associated with osteogenesis imperfecta. The term hereditary opalescent dentine is probably better than dentinogenesis imperfecta as it describes the general appearance. Osteogenesis imperfecta may also be present without DI; however,

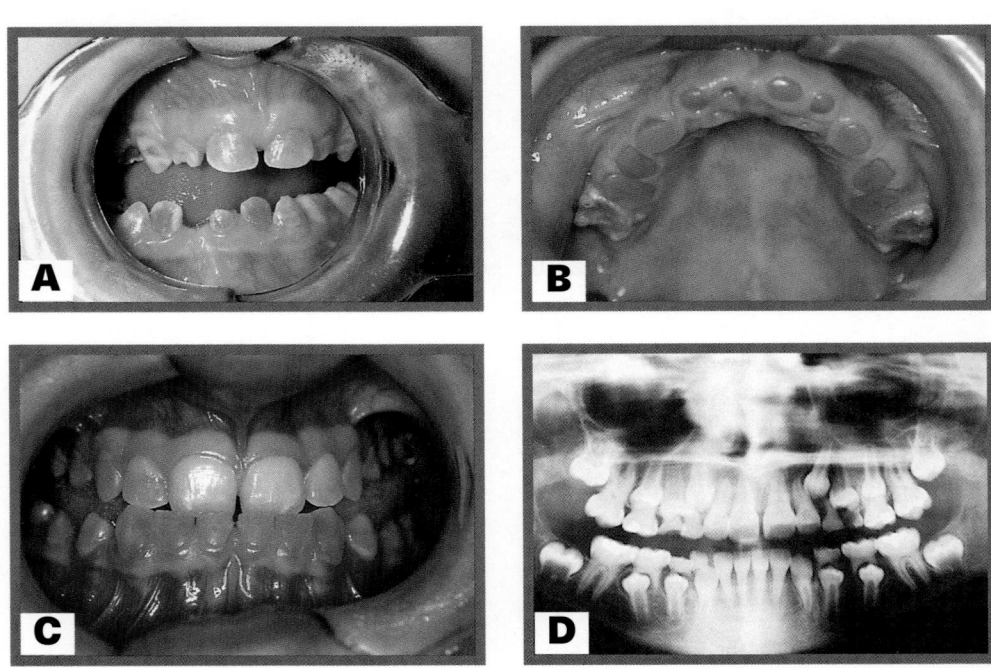

Figure 7.14 Manifestations of DI. **A** DI associated with osteogenesis imperfecta (OI). Dark discolouration of the crowns which appear clinically normal in size and shape. **B** Severe attrition in the primary dentition in a case of isolated DI. An overdenture was used to restore the vertical dimension and provide function as well as aesthetic appeal. **C** The permanent dentition is often not as severely affected when associated with OI, but not the severe skeletal Class-III malocclusion and the posterior open bite, which often requires a surgical solution. **D** Radiographic manifestations of DI, showing pulpal obliteration and short, bulbous crowns. The roots are thin and weak, so root-canal therapy is contraindicated. Periapical pathology is fortunately rare, however.

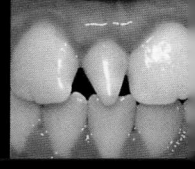

there is a possibility that, because of the same collagen defect, all children may manifest some form of dentinogenesis imperfecta, although it may be at a subclinical level. Both forms are transmitted as autosomal-dominant traits and are clinically indistinguishable dentally, although they have been mapped to different chromosomes. Osteogenesis imperfecta has been mapped to a mutation at *7q22*, whereas dentinogenesis imperfecta occurs at *4q13-21*. Children presenting with dentinogenesis imperfecta should be investigated for osteogenesis imperfecta by bone density measurement. The presence of blue sclera or a history of bone fractures should alert the clinician to osteogenesis imperfecta.

Dental manifestations
- Amber, grey to purple-bluish discolouration or opalescence. (Figure 7.14)
- Pulpal obliteration (Figure 7.14D).
- Short clinical bulbous crowns.
- Narrow roots.
- Enamel tends to chip or flake away 2–4 years after tooth eruption, exposing the soft dentine, which rapidly wears.

Recent research has indicated that the reason for the loss of enamel is that there are long lamellae in the enamel which become exposed with wear. This allows crack propagation and loss of the enamel in sheets.
- Mantle dentine appears normal.

Management
- Preservation of the vertical dimension of occlusion.
- Protection of posterior teeth from attrition.
- Provision of aesthetic appeal.
- Stainless-steel crowns for posterior teeth.
- Composite resin to build up anterior teeth.
- Overdentures in severe cases.

Osteogenesis imperfecta
An autosomal dominant inherited disorder of collagen with variable expression which affects bones.
- Multiple fractures of long bones with associated growth delay. Classified on the basis of the collagen defect, which appears to be a failure or alteration of cross-linking.

Type I
- Autosomal dominant inheritance, blue sclerae (*7q22*).
- Blue discoloration of sclerae.
- Variable bone fragility.
- Presenile hearing loss.

- Dentinogenesis imperfecta in 10% of children.

Type II
- Lethal perinatal trait.
- Autosomal recessive inheritance.
- Extreme bone fragility.
- Perinatal death.
- No dental anomaly.

Type III
- Progressive deformation.
- Autosomal recessive inheritance.
- Severe bone fragility.
- Normal sclerae.
- Severe growth retardation/skeletal deformity.
- With or without dentinogenesis imperfecta.

Type IV
- Autosomal dominant inheritance, normal sclerae.
- Bone fragility.
- Variable severe deformity of long bones and spine.
- Dentinogenesis imperfecta present in 80% of children.

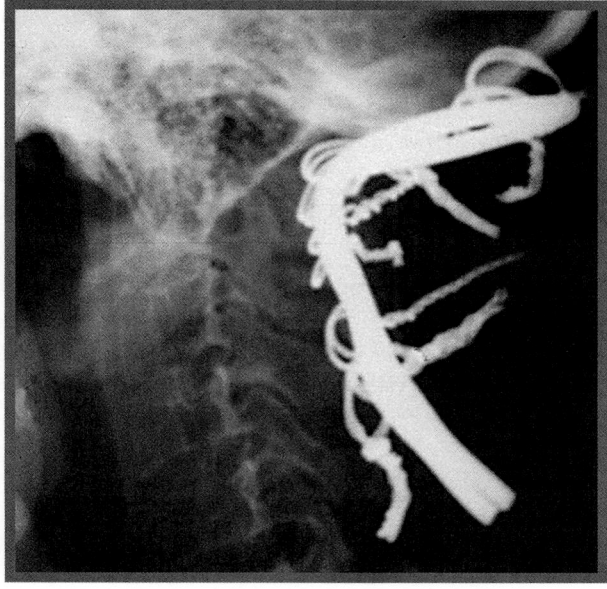

Figure 7.15 A 'Ransford Loop' used to stabilize the vertebral column in a child with Type-IV osteogenesis imperfecta and basilar impression. This life-saving procedure is performed by an anterior approach through the pharynx, splitting the palate and sectioning the odontoid process of C2. The vertebral column is then wired to the occipital bone. This child initially presented with trigeminal neuralgia caused by pressure from C2 on the pons.

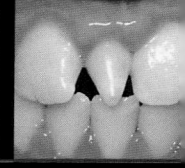

In severe cases there is spinal and vertebral collapse, and the child is often confined to a wheelchair. The collapse may also result in basilar compression as the odontoid process of C2 presses against the brainstem with neurological signs. This is a life-threatening condition (Figure 7.15).

There have been no reported cases of fracture of the mandible resulting from extraction of teeth in children with osteogenesis imperfecta.

Dentinal dysplasia
- Often described as rootless teeth.
- Autosomal-dominant transmission.
- Regional odontodysplasia.
- Very short or absent roots but clinically normal crowns.
- Pulpal obliteration similar to dentinogenesis imperfecta but with demilune on radiographs of molar teeth.
- Both dentitions affected.

Vitamin-D-resistant rickets (Figure 7.16)
- Also termed hereditary hypophosphataemic rickets.
- X-linked dominant disorder with rachitic changes in long bones associated with a failure of distal tubular reabsorption of phosphate in the kidneys. The rickets is unresponsive to vitamin D.
- Low serum phosphate.

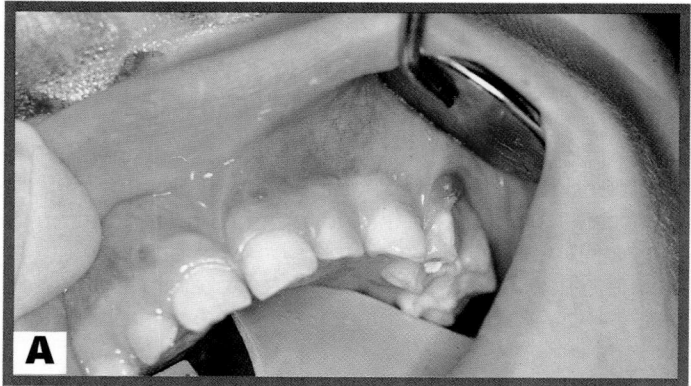
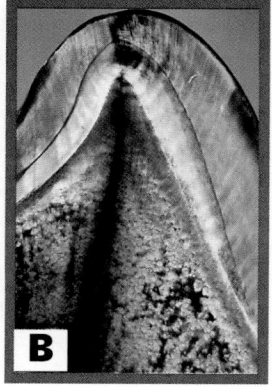

Figure 7.16 **A** Vitamin-D-resistant rickets presenting with multiple abscessed teeth in the absence of caries. **B** Under polarized light, the hard-tissue section demonstrates globular dentine and a pulp horn that extends to the dentino-enamel junction resulting in early exposure caused by attrition and subsequently pulpal necrosis.

- Short stature.
- Elevated alkaline phosphatase.

Dental manifestations
- Severe hypoplasia of incisal and occlusal enamel which is rapidly worn, exposing aberrant pulp horns, which are present up to the dentino-enamel junction.
- Multiple abscesses in the absence of caries.
- Large pulp chambers and delayed apical root closure.

Regional odontodysplasia (Figure 7.17)
- A sporadic defect in tooth formation of unknown aetiology.
- Presents initially with abscessed primary teeth before or soon after eruption.
- Localized to one or part of one quadrant but may cross the midline.
- Both enamel and dentine are affected, with gross hypoplasia of enamel and globular dentine.
- An anomaly of the microvasculature has been proposed as the cause, although this has not been proved. Capillary vascular malformations may be found on the skin overlying the area of the anomaly.

Alternative terminology Ghost teeth.

Management
- In spite of attempts to restore teeth with stainless-steel crowns or composite resin, most affected teeth require extraction. Permanent successors of affected primary teeth will also be affected.
- Partial dentures are required to restore the lost teeth.

Dentinal cysts (Figure 7.18)
An interesting but uncommon anomaly where a radiolucency is observed in the dentine of unerupted or partially erupted teeth. No enamel malformation is present and there is no caries. On opening into the lesion, it is often empty or filled with an amorphous tissue comprising small particles of tubular dentine and crystalline material. The cavity should subsequently be restored conservatively.

Dental effects of prematurity and low birthweight

Normal for gestational age	>2500 g
Low birthweight	>1500–2500 g
Very low birthweight	<1500 g
Extremely low birthweight	<1000 g

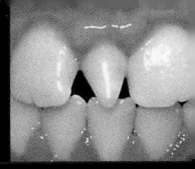

Problems in extreme prematurity

- Hyaline membrane disease and respiratory insufficiency.
- Hyperbilirubinaemia.
- Necrotizing enterocolitis.
- Intraventricular haemorrhage.
- Oxygen retinopathy.

The limiting factor in survival is based on lung development. Presently, in Australia, infants weighing less than 400 g at birth or that are born before a gestation of 24 weeks are not resuscitated. Hyaline membrane disease is now treated with

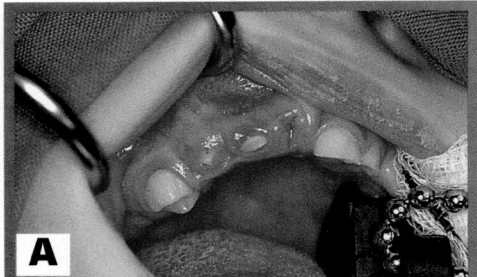

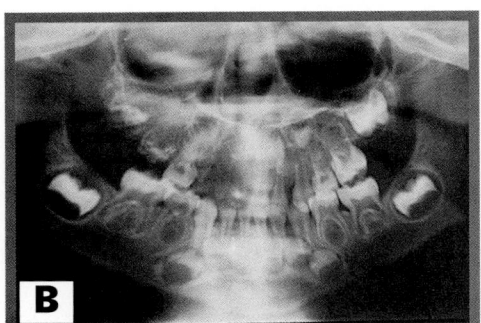

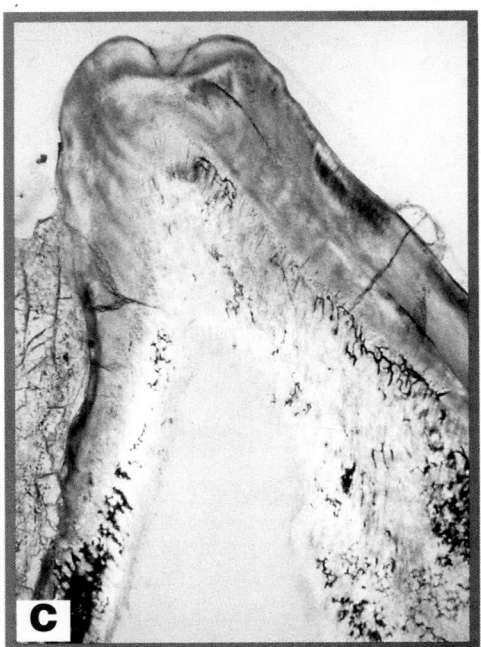

Figure 7.17 A Regional odontodysplasia presenting with abscessed incisors in the upper-right quadrant soon after eruption. **B** A hard-tissue section demonstrates the disruption of odontogenesis. **C** The panoramic radiograph shows involvement of all the teeth in this quadrant with the exception of the upper-right second primary molar tooth. The developing premolar above this tooth is normal. The child was treated by extraction of the affected teeth and placement of an upper partial denture. The upper-right premolar and upper-right second molar teeth have developed normally.

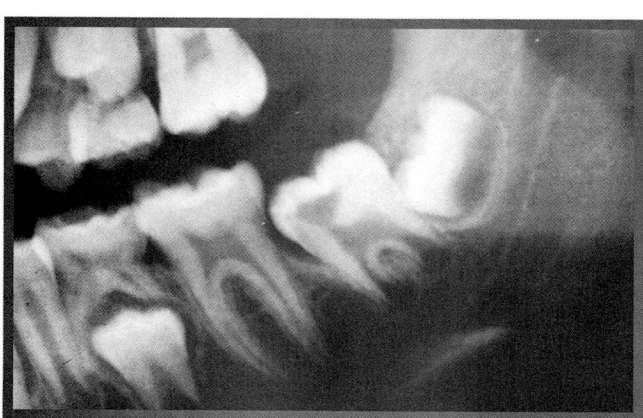

Figure 7.18 Dentine cyst in an unerupted lower second molar.

synthetic surfactant, although very young babies often develop pneumothoracies caused by the prematurity and fragility of the alveoli. Cerebral intraventricular bleeding and necrotizing enterocolitis with the resulting gut sepsis are common causes of mortality and morbidity. Surviving children are left with problems of growth retardation, delayed cognitive development and a range of other abnormalities.

Dental implications
- Hypoglycaemia.
- Hypocalcaemia with reactive pseudohyperparathyroidism.
- Hyperbilirubinaemia, causing green staining.
- Intubation trauma, causing enamel hypoplasia/hypocalification. Usually the maxillary left central incisor is affected. If the baby is intubated orally, palatal grooving may occur.
- Tooth eruption may be delayed, although it is often normal for the corrected age.
- Chronological opacities or hypoplasia.

Disorders of eruption

Eruption of teeth is not well correlated with somatic development. Children with growth disturbances may exhibit delayed eruption or the delay may be due to other causes, such as gingival overgrowth due to phenytoin. More importantly, premature exfoliation of teeth is associated with severe systemic disease (see Chapter 6) and requires investigation. Delayed eruption in the primary dentition requires no treatment other than determining that all teeth are present. It is uncommon for

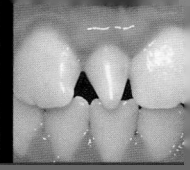

children to require surgical exposure of the teeth in infancy. Parents should be reassured that there is extreme variability in the eruption of teeth. In the permanent dentition, delayed eruption should be investigated for the presence of supernumeraries and other pathology. While the actual timing of tooth eruption is variable, tooth crown and root development and the eruption sequence are of much more relevance.

Natal and neonatal teeth (Figure 7.19)

Natal teeth are present at birth and in most cases are the normal primary incisor teeth erupting early. A neonatal tooth is one that erupts within 30 days of birth. The development of the tooth is consistent with age (i.e. only five-sixths of the crown is formed and no root will normally be present). This accounts for the mobility of the tooth. Babies with posterior natal teeth should be carefully investigated for other systemic conditions that may be associated with syndromes or other diseases.

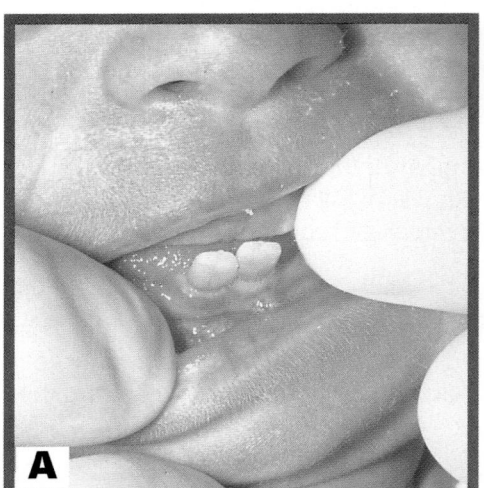

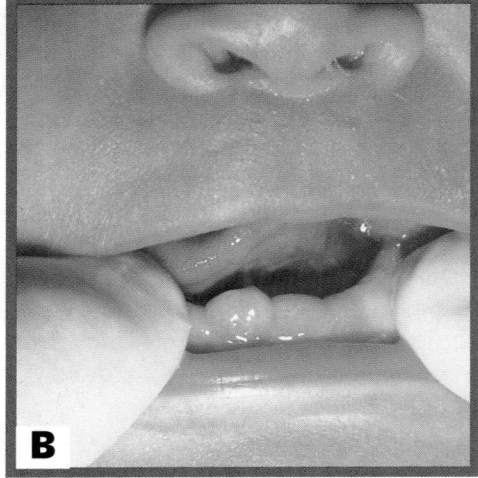

Figure 7.19 A Natal teeth in a 36-week premature infant. The teeth were extremely loose and, because of the respiratory difficulties experienced by the child, the teeth were removed. **B** A newborn infant with two lower incisors soon to erupt. The reduced enamel epithelium has fused with the gingivae and teeth will probably erupt within a few days.

Management
- If the teeth are not too mobile they should be retained as they will firm with time.
- If the tooth is excessively mobile then it may spontaneously exfoliate; however, because of the theoretical risk of aspiration or ingestion it should be electively removed.
- Care should be taken to extract the entire tooth, as often the crown is removed leaving behind the pulpal tissue. Dentine and a root will form subsequently; the root will require removal at a later date.
- The permanent teeth are unaffected by extraction of the primary tooth.

Ankylosis of primary molars (Figure 7.20)
It is quite common for primary molars to become ankylosed and never erupt or to appear to submerge into the alveolus following eruption. In fact, the tooth does not move while the bone grows around it. The timing of the removal of these teeth is based on the position of the first permanent molar and the extent of primary root resorption.

Management
- Orthodontic consultation (see Chapter 9).
- Surgical removal of the ankylosed tooth is to be avoided before eruption of the first permanent molar as this latter tooth will migrate mesially and space loss will occur with impaction of the second premolar. Once the permanent tooth has erupted, the primary tooth may be removed and a space maintainer inserted. If the premolar is congenitally absent early removal might be indicated.
- If there is radiographic evidence of resorption of the roots, then removal should be delayed as many of these teeth will exfoliate normally.
- Retain space and upright the permanent molar as required.

Root development (Figure 7.21)
Just as enamel can be affected by systemic illness, so too root development can be delayed, altered or arrested by systemic disease. This is most commonly seen when radiotherapy causes shortening and tapering of the roots of premolars (see Chapter 8.9).

Excessive orthodontic forces will also cause root resorption.

Dental age (maturity) determination
The paediatric dentist is often asked to help in age assessment, either at necropsy or for orphaned children. It is important to take into consideration ethnicity and somatic growth potential.

Tooth emergence is not as important as tooth crown calcification and root development. The most widely used and accepted method is that developed by

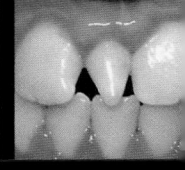

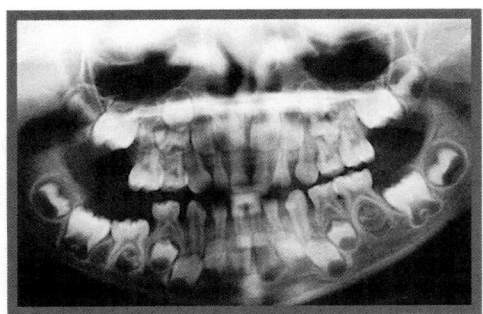

Figure 7.20 Ankylosis of the lower-right second primary molar. It is important to wait until the first permanent molar has erupted before surgical removal to avoid impaction of the lower-right second premolar. These teeth are often difficult to remove, especially if there is space loss, and they should be routinely sectioned and elevated to minimize excessive bone loss.

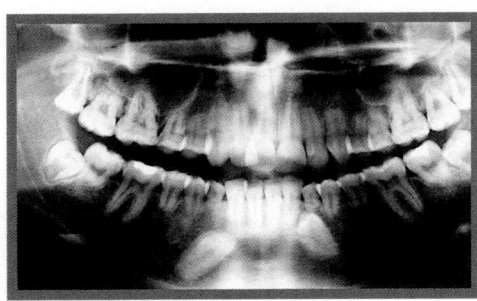

Figure 7.21 Arrested root development in a child who developed Stevens–Johnson syndrome at 10 years of age. Root development ceased at that time and all teeth except the third molars were affected. It is interesting that these molars, which were not undergoing calcification, were unaffected.

Demirjian and co-workers (1978). It is based on the panoramic radiographic appearance of tooth calcification at different stages.

While there remains little doubt that peak height velocity, skeletal development and sexual maturation are closely associated, dental development seems to be independent of general somatic development.

Loss of tooth structure

- Attrition.
- Erosion.
    Exogenous from diet, habits or environment.
    Gastro-oesophageal reflux.
- Abrasion.

Gastro-oesophageal reflux (Figure 7.23A)

When loss of enamel by erosion cannot be explained by dietary factors, reflux must be considered. Children with reflux will show enamel erosion, which is a smooth loss of tooth structure, often with amalgam restorations standing proud. Some children, however, have undiagnosed, asymptomatic reflux that presents first with enamel erosion.

Diagnosis
- Barium swallows may not demonstrate reflux.
- 24-hour pH manometery is required to assess the extent of reflux (Figure 7.23B).

Management
- Diagnosis and treatment of reflux condition before definitive restoration of the teeth.
- Histamine blockers (H_2 antagonists) such as ranitidine and cimetidine.
- Anti-emetics (prokinetic agents) such as metoclopramide.
- Composite resin or glass–ionomer coverings of posterior teeth.

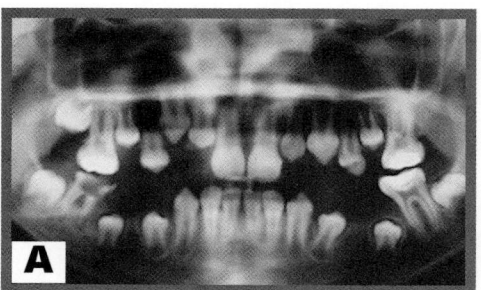 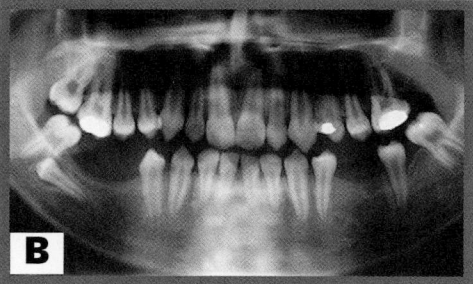

Figure 7.22 Teeth require guidance for normal eruption. In this case the lower-right first permanent molar was removed because of gross caries and pulpal necrosis. While the second molar has drifted slightly mesially, the second premolar has rotated and drifted distally and impacted against the second molar. Had the second primary molar not been removed it is unlikely that this premolar would have drifted.

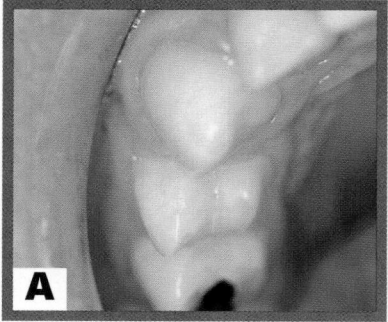 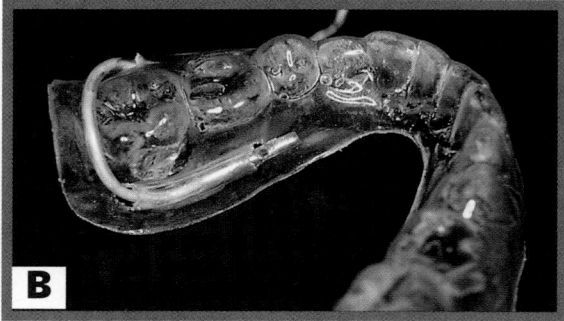

Figure 7.23 A Enamel erosion with asymptomatic gastro-oesophageal reflux. The first presentation of this child was to a dentist, because of the erosion. **B** A mouthguard containing a micro pH probe was worn in the mouth for a 24-hour period to measure the intra-oral pH. Another is placed in the lower oesophageal sphincter. **C** Some children have been measured with an intraoral pH of <1.

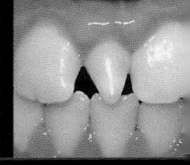

- Onlays on posterior teeth to protect occlusion.
- Nocturnal mouthguards with fluoride toothpaste as mechanical barriers against acid attack and fluoride to promote remineralization.

References

Oligodontia

BERGENDAL T, ECKERDAL O, HALLONSTEN A-L, KOCH G, KVINT S. Osseointegrated implants in the oral habilitation of a boy with ectodermal dysplasia: a case report. *Int Dent J* 1991, **41**:149–156.

FLEMING P, NELSON J, GORLIN RJ. Single maxillary central incisor in association with mid-line anomalies. *Br Dent J* 1990, **168**:476–479.

FREIRE-MAIA N, PINHEIRO M, eds. *Ectodermal dysplasias: a clinical and genetic study*. New York: Alan R Liss; 1984.

HALL RK. Congenitally missing teeth—diagnostic feature in many syndromes of the head and neck. *J Int Ass Dent Child* 1983, **14**:69–75.

LAI PY, SEOW WK. A controlled study of the association of various dental anomalies with hypodontia of permanent teeth. *J Pediatr Dent* 1989, **11**:291–295.

RAPPAPORT EB, ULSTROM R, GORLIN RJ, LUCKY AW, COLE E, MISER J. Solitary maxillary central incisor syndrome and short stature. *J Pediatr* 1977, **91**:924–928.

Supernumerary teeth

HOGSTROM A, ANDERSSON L. Complications related to surgical removal of anterior supernumerary teeth in children. *J Dent Child* 1987, **54**:341–343.

JENSEN BL, KREIBORG S. Development of the dentition in cleidocranial dysplasia. *J Oral Med Pathol* 1990, **19**:89–93.

JENSEN BL, KREIBORG S. Dental treatment strategies in cleidocranial dysplasia. *Br Dent J* 1992, **172**:243–247.

VON ARX T. Anterior maxillary supernumerary teeth. A clinical and radiographic study. *Aust Dent J* 1992, **37**:189–195.

Morphological anomalies

NAZIF MM, LAUGHLIN DF. Dens invaginatus in a geminated central incisor: case report. *J Pediatr Dent* 1990, **12**:250–251.

RAKES GM, AIELLO AS, KUSTER CG, LABART WA. Complications occurring resultant to dens invaginatus: a case report. *Pediatr Dent* 1988, **10**:53–56.

Enamel hypomineralization

CULLEN C. Erythroblastalis fetalis produced by Kell immunisation: dental findings. *J Pediatr Dent* 1990, **12**:393–396.

FLEMING P, WITKOP CJ, KUHLMANN WH. Staining and hypoplasia caused by tetracycline. *J Pediatr Dent* 1987, **9**:245–246.

J *Pediatr Dent* 1987, **9**:245-246.

Enamel hypoplasia

ELI H, SARNAT H, TALMI E. Effect of the birth process on the neonatal line in primary tooth enamel. J *Pediatr Dent* 11:220-223.

PENDRYS DG. 1991, Dental fluorosis in perspective. J Am Dent Assoc 1989, **122**:63-66.

CROLL TP. Enamel microabrasion for removal of superficial dysmineralization and decalcification defects. J Am Dent Assoc 1990, **129**:411-415.

Amelogenesis imperfecta

BÄCKMAN B, AMMEROTH G. Microradiographic study of amelogenesis imperfecta. Scand J Dent Res 1989, **97**:316-329.

SEOW WK. Clinical diagnosis and management strategies of amelogenesis imperfecta variants. *Pediatr Dent* 1993, **15**:384-393.

Dentine anomalies

COLE DEC, COHEN MM. Osteogenesis imperfecta: an update. J *Pediatr* 1991, **115**:73-74.

GAGE JP, SYMONS AL, ROUMANIUK K, DALEY T. Hereditary opalescent dentine: variation in expression. J Dent Child 1991, **58**:134-9.

ALDRED MJ, CRAWFORD PJM. Regional odontdysplasia: a bibliography. *Oral Pathol Med* 1989, **18**:251-263.

O'CARROLL MK, DUNCAN WK, PERKINS TM. Dentin dysplasia: review of the literature and a proposed subclassification based on radiographic findings. *Oral Surg Oral Med Oral Pathol* 1991, **72**:119-125.

SEOW WK, LATHAM SC. The spectrum of dental manifestations in vitamin D-resistant rickets: implication for management. *Pediatr Dent* 1991, **8**:245-250.

SEOW WK, BROWN JP, TUDEHOPE DA, O'CALLAGHAN M. Dental defects in the deciduous dentition of premature infants with low birth weight and neonatal rickets. *Pediatr Dent* 1984, **6**:88-92.

Eruption disorders

FRIEND GW, MINCER HM, CARRUTH KR, JONES JE. Natal primary molar: case report. J *Pediatr Dent* 1991, **13**:173-175.

MASATOMI Y, ABE K, OOSHIMA T. Unusual multiple natal teeth: case report. J *Pediatr Dent* 1991, **13**:170-172.

SAUK JJ. Genetic disorders involving tooth eruption anomalies. In: Davidovitch Z, ed. The *biological mechanisms of tooth eruption and root resorption*. Birmingham: EBSCO Media; 1988: 171-179.

Erosion

JARVINEN V, MUERMAN JH, HYVARINEN H, RYTOMAA I, MURTOMAA H. Dental erosion and upper gastrointestinal disorders. *Oral Surg Oral Med Oral Pathol* 1988, **65**:298-303.

Further reading

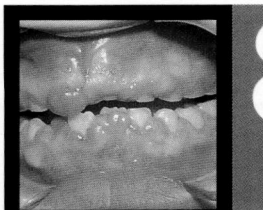

Medically compromised children

Contributors
Angus Cameron, Richard Widmer, James Lucas, Kerrod Hallett,
Peter Wong, Kareen Mekertichian, Sarah Raphael, David Isaacs,˙
Judy Kirk, Allison Kakakios, Peter King, Stephen O'Flaherty

Introduction

One of the main roles of the paediatric dentist is the coordination of management of children with medical problems. Terminology has changed recently, and in the USA, these patients are called 'children with special needs'. The term 'medically compromised' is useful, however, because it reminds the clinician that these children often have medical conditions that affect dental treatment or present with specific dental or oral manifestations. It is not the role of the specialist to treat all children with medical problems. Indeed, it is our belief that general practitioners should be active in the care of such children (Figure 8.1). The prevention of dental disease is of utmost importance for children with medical problems as simple dental problems may severely compromise a child's medical management.

Congenital cardiac disease

Children with congenital cardiac disease represent one of the largest groups of medically compromised patients the paediatric dentist manages. Although the majority of defects are sporadic, many lesions are a part of other syndromes or chromosomal abnormalities. The association of trisomy 21 (Down syndrome) and cardiac abnormality is well known, with over 70% of children being affected.

Congenital cardiac disease occurs in approximately 8–10 cases per 1000 live births and has an equal sex distribution. In the majority of cases, no aetiological agent or genetic factors are found. Risk factors associated with congenital cardiac disease include maternal rubella, diabetes, alcoholism, irradiation and drugs such as thalidomide, phenytoin and warfarin.

The degree of morbidity is dependent on the haemodynamics of the lesion. Flow disturbances are caused by structural abnormalities caused by shunting of blood flow, or obstructive defects. For convenience, defects are divided into cyanotic or acyanotic lesions depending on clinical presentation. The latter group may again be divided into obstructive or stenotic defects or those with

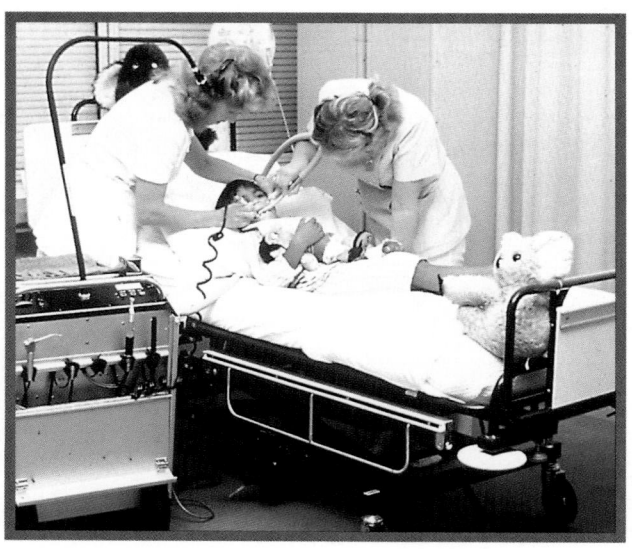

Figure 8.1 Dental treatment on a child in the wards. Not all children with medical problems require hospital admission, although treatment of such patients is often challenging. Mobile dental equipment is invaluable in providing quality dental care. The majority of hospital inpatients are treated in the dental surgery and usually only those in traction or in intensive-care units require bedside treatment.

left-to-right shunts. Those children with cyanotic heart disease are at significant risk during general anaesthesia and consultation with the cardiologist is essential.

Acyanotic defects with shunts

This group of conditions is characterized by a connection between systemic and pulmonary circulations. Such anomalies present as murmurs and, if large, cardiac enlargement, congestive heart failure and failure to thrive. Shunts are from the left to right.

Atrial septal defect A septal defect often located near the foramen ovale.

Ventricular septal defect Septal defect in the ventricular wall.

Patent ductus arteriosus Failure of closure of the ductus connecting the pulmonary artery with the aorta (normally closes soon after birth).

Anomalous pulmonary–venous return Failure of development of common pulmonary veins to left atrium.

Atrioventricular canal Defect in which the upper part of the ventricular septum and lower atrial septum are absent.

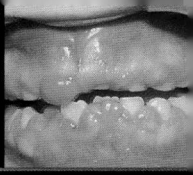

Acyanotic defects with obstruction

Coarctation of aorta Constriction of the aorta, distal or at the root of the subclavian artery.

Aortic stenosis Usually narrowing of the aortic valve itself but may be above (supra) or below (sub) the valve.

Pulmonary stenosis Narrowing of the pulmonary valve, and may involve the pulmonary arteries.

Cyanotic defects

The basic defect is one of right-to-left shunting of desaturated blood. Cyanotic defects are clinically evident if 50 g/L of desaturated haemoglobin is present in arterial blood. Infants with mild cyanosis may be pink at rest but show cyanosis during crying or on exertion.

Tetralogy of Fallot Ventricular septal defect, pulmonary stenosis or atresia, right-to-left shunt, overriding aorta, right ventricular hypertrophy.

Eisenmenger's syndrome Refers to cyanosis from any right-to-left shunt through a ventricular septal defect caused by increased pulmonary resistance.

Tricuspid atresia Absent tricuspid valve and absent right ventricle and pulmonary valve, the pulmonary circulation is maintained through a patent ductus arteriosus.

Pulmonary atresia Similar to tricuspid atresia except that the tricuspid valve is patent. Three-chambered heart.

Transposition of great vessels Aorta exits the heart from the right side, whereas the pulmonary artery exits from the left. The internal anatomy is normal.

Other cardiac diseases

Cardiomyopathies Dysfunction of the myocardium with associated cardiac failure.

Cardiac arrhythmias Accessory conduction pathways that bypass the atrioventricular node with premature excitation of the ventricle ahead of the atria, causing a disturbance of rate, rhythm or conduction (i.e. supraventricular tachycardia or SVT) Wolff–Parkinson–White syndrome (pre-excitation pattern).

Dental Implications

Clinical appearance

- Clubbing of fingers (see Figure 8.2).
- Cyanosis of mucosa.
- Shortness of breath.

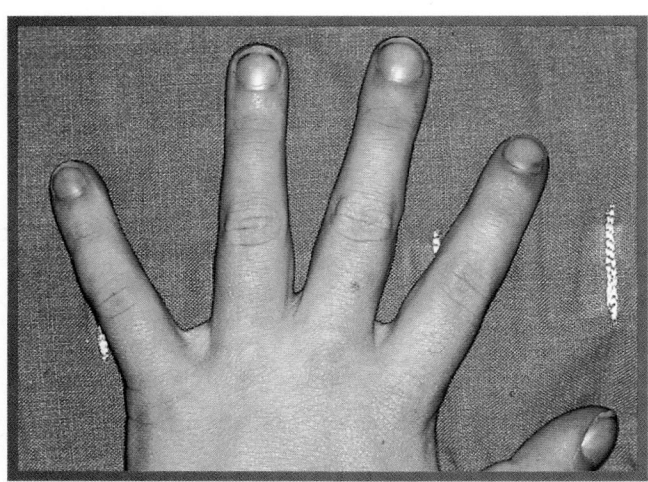

Figure 8.2 Clubbing of the fingers associated with complex cyanotic cardiac disease. Nailbeds also show cyanosis.

Dental management
- Risk of infective endocarditis—**all congenital cardiac anomalies require antibiotic cover as per protocols** (Appendix E).
- Pre-operative oral antiseptic mouthwash such as 0.2% chlorhexidine gluconate.
- Resistance of bacteria—some children have been prescribed long-term antibiotics and this merely builds up resistance organisms. In these cases it is important, when prescribing antibiotics for prophylaxis, that antibiotics from a different group be chosen.
- Bleeding tendency caused by consumption of clotting factors.
- Other medical conditions: congenital cardiac disease is associated with numerous other syndromes and medical conditions which may complicate dental treatment.
- Increased prevalence of enamel hypoplasia and dental caries in the primary dentition.
- Aggressive treatment of pulpally involved teeth. Pulpotomy is contraindicated in these patients because of the possibility of subsequent bacteraemias.
- Coordination of treatment. It is often better to treat a child with many carious teeth under general anaesthesia and complete all the work in one session. This removes the need to change antibiotics or to wait 1 month between visits. If a child is undergoing anaesthesia for other medical procedures try to coordinate the dental work to be performed at the same time.
- Vasoconstrictors—there is no contraindication to the use of vasoconstrictors in local anaesthetics.

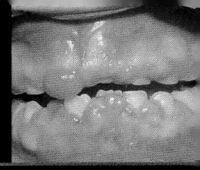

Bleeding disorders

Primary haemostasis is initiated after injury to a blood vessel with the formation of a primary platelet plug. This is mediated by interactions between the platelets, plasma-coagulation factors and the vessel wall. Secondary haemostasis, with fibrin as the end product, is also triggered by the initial injury and reaches its greatest intensity after the primary platelet plug is formed. It provides the framework for the formation of a stable clot.

Abnormal bleeding can occur when haemostasis is disturbed. The clinical manifestations of a disorder of haemostasis vary depending on the phase affected. Defects in primary haemostasis generally result in bleeding from the skin or mucosal surfaces, with the development of petechiae and purpura (ecchymosis). These disorders include von Willebrand's disease as well as defects in platelet function. In contrast, defects in secondary haemostasis, such as haemophilia, lead to bleeding that tends to be more deep-seated in muscles and joints. In both disorders, uncontrolled prolonged oral bleeding can occur from innocuous insults such as a tongue laceration or cheek biting.

Classification
- Platelet disorders.
- Thrombocytopenia.
- Thrombocytosis.
- Platelet-function disorders.
- von Willebrand's disease.
- Vitamin-C deficiency.
- Connective-tissue diseases.

Platelet disorders
Thrombocytopenia This may occur as an isolated entity of unknown cause (idiopathic thrombocytopenic purpura), as a result of marrow suppression by drugs or from other haematological diseases such as aplastic anaemia. Marrow replacement by neoplastic cells in haematological malignancies will also result in thrombocytopenia. Children undergoing chemotherapy and radiotherapy will have decreased platelet counts.

Thrombocytosis An increased number of platelets ($>500\times10^9$ per L) may be associated with bleeding caused by abnormal platelet function. Myeloproliferative disorders may present with thrombocytosis.

Platelet-function disorders These may be congenital or acquired. The most common cause of acquired decreased platelet function is the use of non-steroidal anti-inflammatory drugs. Administration of cycloxygenase inhibitors will result in blockage of the production of thromboxane A_2 for the life of the platelet (7–9 days).

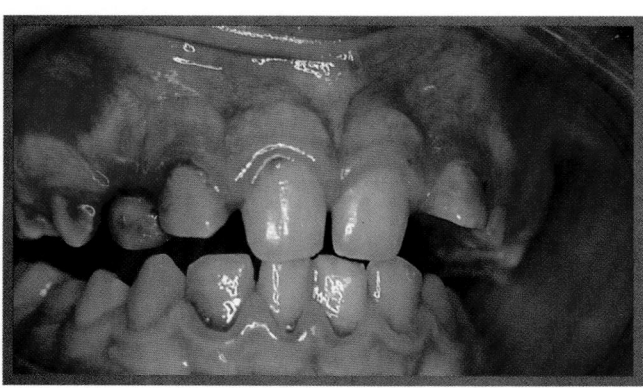

Figure 8.3 Gingival haemorrhage around an exfoliating upper-right primary canine in a child with Christmas disease (factor-IX deficiency). Normally, exfoliation of primary teeth is not of major concern and bleeding is locally controllable.

This results in a decrease in platelet aggregation. Some metabolic diseases, such as Gaucher's disease, also manifest with defects of platelet function.

Connective-tissue diseases
Diseases of connective tissue such as scurvy (vitamin-C deficiency) and Ehlers–Danlos syndrome result in bruising and purpura caused by vascular abnormalities and capillary fragility.

Von Willebrand's disease
As well as being a disorder of coagulation, platelet function is also decreased (see below).

Dental implications
A decrease in the number of platelets or platelet function will result in failure of initial clot formation. Children with thrombocytopenia will bleed immediately after trauma or surgery, unlike haemophiliacs who usually start to bleed 4 hours after the incident. The most common oral manifestations are petechiae and purpura. There may also be spontaneous gingival bleeding and prolonged episodes of bleeding after minor trauma or toothbrushing.

Dental management
- It is preferable to have platelet levels $>50 \times 10^9$ per L before extractions.
- Endodontic procedures may be preferable to extractions in order to avoid the need for platelet transfusion.
- Good surgical technique and local measures to control bleeding.
- Avoid block injections as these may be complicated by dissecting haematoma and airway obstruction.

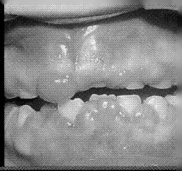

- Antifibrinolytics:
- Tranexamic acid (Cyklokapron) 25 mg/kg loading dose and 15–20 mg/kg three times a day for 5–7 days **OR**
- ε-aminocaproic acid (Amicar) 100 mg/kg loading dose and then 30 mg/kg four times a day for 7 days.
- During the time that antifibrinolytics are given, the patient should be instructed not to use straws, metal utensils, pacifiers or bottles.
- Avoid platelet transfusions, if possible, because of the development of antiplatelet antibodies and the risk of transmission of viral diseases such as hepatitis C and human immunodeficiency virus (HIV).

Coagulation disorders

Coagulation disorders result from a decrease in the amount of particular factors in the coagulation cascade. The most common disorders are haemophilia A and von Willebrand's disease, both manifesting a decrease in factor-VIII levels. This molecule is produced by endothelial cells and is composed of two portions. The largest part of the molecule is the von Willebrand's factor and is responsible for platelet aggregation. The coagulation part of the complex and factor IX are responsible for activation of factor X in the intrinsic pathway.

Haemophilia A
- X-linked recessive disorder with deficiency of factor VIII.
- 1:10 000 live male births, 30% spontaneous mutation.

Severe
- <1% factor VIII.
- Spontaneous bleeding into joints and muscles, including intracerebral haemorrhage.

Moderate
- 2–5% factor VIII.
- Less severe bleeding, which usually follows minor trauma.

Mild
- 5–25% factor VIII.
- May not manifest until middle or old age after significant trauma or surgery.

Normal
- 50–200% factor VIII from factor-VIII assay.

Von Willebrand's disease
- Autosomal dominant (gene locus *12p13*).
- Abnormality of factor VIII molecule complex.

- Platelet and factor VIII activity decreased, therefore both bleeding time and activated partial thromboplastin time (APTT) are elevated.
- The von Willebrand's factor is found in the plasma, platelets, megakaryocytes and endothelial cells and circulates as a major component of the factor VIII molecule complex. This disease is divided into subtypes, based on the platelet and plasma multimeric structure of the von Willebrand's factor. Treatment is dependent on the subtype.

Christmas disease (haemophilia B)
- Factor-IX deficiency.
- Elevated APTT.

Other disorders of coagulation
- Vitamin-K deficiency.
- Liver disease.
- Disseminated intravascular coagulation usually from overwhelming (Gram-negative) infection.

Tests
Bleeding
- Full-blood count (FBC) for platelet count: $150–400 \times 10^3/mL$
- Skin bleeding time: 9 minutes
- Platelet function tests in selected cases.

Coagulation
- Prothrombin-time test of extrinsic pathway   11–17 seconds
- APTT test of intrinsic pathway   24–38 seconds

Factor VIII assay
These assays are usually performed after the initial diagnosis of a coagulopathy.

Factor VIIIvon W Von Willebrand's cofactor, the main portion of the molecule, binds to platelets, carrier protein for factor-VIII concentrate (factor-VIIIc).

Factor VIIIc Procoagulation portion participates in the clotting cascade, deficient in haemophilia A.

Factor VIIIag Antigenic cofactor, antigenic component of FVIIIvonW.

Factor VIIIrcof Ristocetin cofactor, supports platelet aggregation.

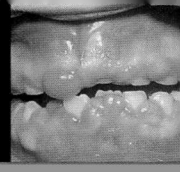

Dental implications
- Consultation with physician (haematologist).
- Local measures to control haemorrhage.
- Good local technique (i.e. minimal trauma during restorative and surgical work).
- No block anaesthesia without factor cover, due to risk of haematoma.
- Maxillary infiltration anaesthesia can generally be administered slowly without pretreatment with ε-aminocaproic acid and/or factor replacement. However, if the infiltration injection is into loose connective tissue or a highly vascular area, then factor replacement to achieve 40% activity levels is recommended.
- In the absence of factor replacement, intraperiodontal injections may be used but with great caution. The solution is placed under moderate pressure along the four axial surfaces of the tooth by inserting the needle into the gingival sulcus and the periodontal ligament space.
- Nitrous-oxide sedation can be effective for restorative procedures with the need for local anaesthesia. However, care must be taken when placing matrix bands.

Dental procedures
- Extractions must never be performed without first consulting the haematologist.
- Endodontics can be safely carried out without factor-cover.
- Periodontal therapy with scaling and subgingival curettage requires factor replacement.
- Multiple extractions require hospital admission in conjunction with the haematology team.
- Use rubber dam to protect soft tissues.

Haemophilia A
- Minor trauma may be life-threatening, especially with intracerebral bleeds; 15% of patients will form antibodies (inhibitors) to factor VIII, severely complicating management.
- Haemophiliacs are treated with replacement therapy.
- Severe haemorrhage is treated to 100% replacement, although minor bleeds can be controlled with replacement between 30 and 50%.
- One unit of factor VIIIc per kilogram will raise levels by 2%.
- Half-life of 10–12 hours.

Von Willebrand's disease
- Type I may be treated with 1-deamino (8-D-arginine) vasopressin (DDAVP).
- Types II and III require cryoprecipitate.

Christmas disease
- Prothrombinex, or fresh frozen plasma for mild cases.

Available factor replacements
- Factor VIIIc.
- Recombinant factor VIII.
- Cryoprecipitate.
- Prothrombinex (II, IX, X). Used for other clotting deficiencies.

Antifibrinolytics
- Tranexamic acid (Cyklokapron).
- ε-aminocaproic acid (Amicar).

DDAVP
- Used for mild haemophiliacs and those with von Willebrand's disease.
- Causes up to twofold release of factor VIII from endothelial cells—this is adequate if levels of factor VIII are >10%.

Problems in management

Characteristically, haemophilia bleeds are delayed 12-24 hours as primary haemostasis is not impaired, and local pressure has little effect. It is worth noting that mild haemophilia can go undiagnosed. The APTT is not sensitive enough to detect mild deficiencies of factor VIIIc and levels of factor VIIIc 25-30 IU/dL can be associated with a normal APTT. In addition, FVIIIc values in mild haemophilia are temporarily increased (as occurs in unaffected persons) by stress (exercise, bleeding). If there is a convincing history of a bleeding tendency always do a specific factor assay, even if screening tests are normal.

The normal regime for DDAVP is 0.3 µg/kg IV infusion over 1 hour before surgery followed by tranexamic acid, 15-20 mg/kg orally, every 8 hours for 7 days. After 9-12 hours, if the factor VIIIc levels are low (50-60%), the original dose of DDAVP may be repeated. This regime is useful in von Willebrand's disease and children on renal dialysis.
- DDAVP should **not** be used in cases of type-II von Willebrand's disease.

Questions commonly asked by parents

- Will my child's teeth erupt normally?

Usually yes, but there is often more bleeding from a traumatized operculum which may require active intervention.
- Do my child's teeth fall out normally (Figure 8.3)?

Yes, unless traumatized there is usually no abnormal bleeding associated with exfoliating primary teeth. If there is persistent mobility and oozing occurs then extraction may be necessary under appropriate factor cover.
- Can a child with a bleeding disorder have orthodontic treatment?

Yes, provided extractions are performed after appropriate consultation with the haematologist and there is vigilant maintenance of the appliances.

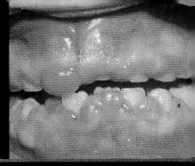

Management of children on anticoagulants

The management of these children is often extremely difficult. Anticoagulants are usually prescribed for children with valvular heart disease and prosthetic valves. If extractions or surgery are required, it is necessary to decrease the clotting times to allow adequate coagulation but not to such an extent to cause emboli or clotting around the valves. These children's management is of course complicated by their congenital cardiac defect and antibiotics are required for prophylaxis against endocarditis.

Therapeutic drugs used
- Warfarin (coumarin)
    Vitamin-K antagonist (factors II, VII, IX and X are depleted).
    3–4 days required for full anticoagulation onset.
    Assessed by prothrombin level (factor-VII levels)
    International normalization ratio (INR) 2.0–2.5.
- Heparin
    Shorter acting, immediate onset, given intravenously.
    Inhibits factors IX, X and XII.

Dental management
- Prevention.
- Consultation with physician (haematologist).
- Local measures by application of topical thrombin, packing with microfibrillar collagen haemostat, or oxidized cellulose and suturing of wounds. Splints or Stomahesive bandages may also be of benefit. There have been recent reports of the efficacy of 'fibrin glue' in the dental management of coagulopathies.
- Admission of patient to hospital.
- Cessation of Warfarin and commencement of heparin infusion to decrease the INR to just above normal.
- Recommencement of Warfarin 48 hours after surgery and re-establish correct prothrombin and APTT.
- In emergency situations, with prolonged bleeding from oral wounds post-surgery, following recommencement of Warfarin, fresh frozen plasma may be required. Topical thrombin may also be of benefit.

Management of oral haemorrhage

Bleeding from the mouth can occur at any time. There may have been a slow ooze for several days or, at the other extreme, there may be a significant sudden oral bleed. Such bleeding can occur without warning and may not be associated with any prior investigative or operative work. As well, haemorrhage from the mouth can occur after such procedures as biopsy, restorative work, or tooth extraction.

The initial management of such cases involves identifying the exact site of haemorrhage, controlling the haemorrhage and then preventing recurrence. In cases of haemorrhage from the mouth, that has not been associated with any dental activity, clinicians should take an accurate history of the bleeding, its duration, volume and any causative factors. Such bleeding may occur around an erupting tooth or from an exfoliating tooth site or may be associated with trauma or congenital malformations such as arteriovenous malformations (see Chapter 6: 'Pigmented, vascular and erythematous lesions').

In cases of oral haemorrhage, following dental procedures, the the steps listed below should be taken. It is important to prevent or minimize bleeding in the first instance. This can be achieved by:

- A sensible limitation of surgical trauma.
- Compression of the alveolus following extraction.
- Being aware of previous bleeding episodes and packing sockets with resorbable gels, as indicated.
- Adequate suturing of extraction sites (only if wound healing enhanced).
- Apply pressure to the extraction site postoperatively via gauze packs or removable-type appliances.
- Definitive postoperative instructions regarding adequate rest, limitation of nicotine and alcohol intake, avoidance of excessively hot foods, and prescription of appropriate medication.

In cases of massive haemorrhage following tooth extraction which can occur because of arteriovenous malformations, remember that the best method of controlling the haemorrhage is to replace the extracted tooth in the first instance.

Red-cell disorders

Anaemia (Figure 8.4)
Anaemia is usually an incidental finding in paediatric dental practice. A full blood count is usually ordered when children present with acute infections, undiagnosed systemic or oral pathology, after major trauma associated with blood loss, or on work-up before surgery for medically compromised patients. When unexpected anaemia is discovered, follow-up by the paediatrician is required.

Haemolytic anaemia
Haemolytic disease of the newborn or erythroblastosis fetalis is caused by Rhesus (Rh) incompatibility. Discoloration of those primary teeth which are calcifying at the time of birth will occur. The cusp tips of the first permanent molars may also be affected. A yellow to green staining is most commonly seen as a result of high levels of unconjugated (unbound) bilirubin (see Fig. 8.4 for differential diagnosis).

Glucose-6-phosphate dehydrogenase deficiency This inborn error of metabolism results in haemolytic anaemia when the child is exposed to certain drugs or

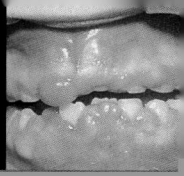

infection. The important drugs include:
- Sulphonamides.
- Chloramphenicol.
- Aspirin.
- Prilocaine—in high doses, Citanest may induce methaemoglobinaemia and should be avoided.

Thalassaemia The thalassaemias are a group of disorders where one of the globin chains of the haemoglobin complex are absent or reduced. Adult blood contains haemoglobin A, which is composed of two globin chains (HbA, $\alpha_2\beta_2$), and a small amount of haemoglobin A_2 (HbA$_2$, $\alpha_2\gamma_2$). Children also produce some fetal haemoglobin (HbF, $\alpha_2\delta_2$). Homozygous thalassaemia (deletion of the α chain) is incompatible with life, while the heterozygous phenotype has few clinically significant symptoms.

Of more significance is homozygous β-thalassaemia or thalassaemia major (Cooley's anaemia). Because of the absence of the β chain, there is a compensatory increased production of HbA$_2$ and HbF. As erythropoiesis is inadequate the bone marrow is reactive and there is recruitment overgrowth of bone, such as the maxilla and diploe of the skull. There may be severe anaemia with marked associated hepatosplenomegaly.

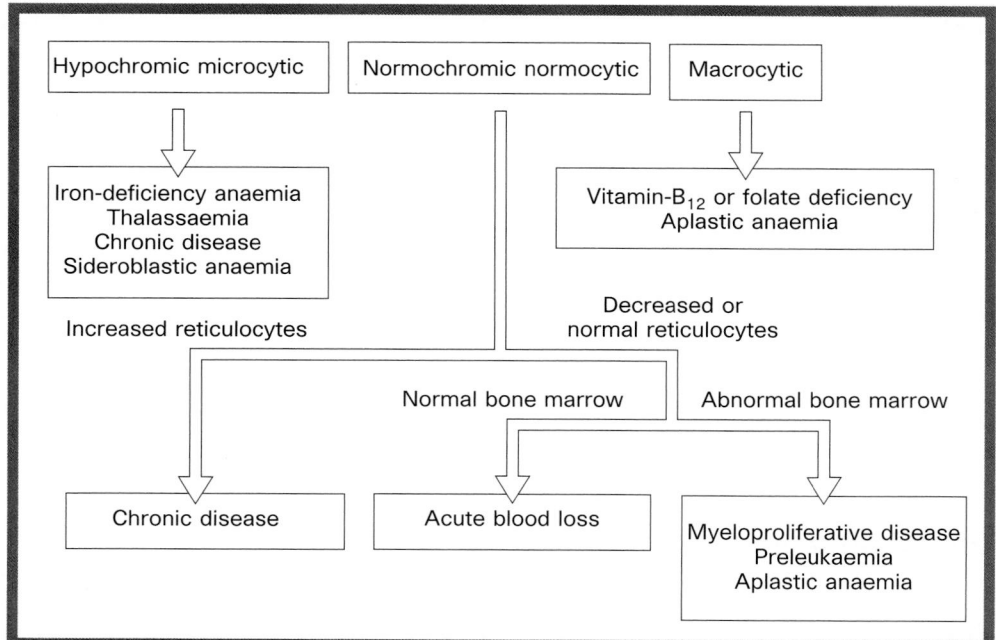

Figure 8.4 Differential diagnosis of anaemia.

Dental implications

Because of maxillary and zygomatic overgrowth there is often a severe class-II division-1 malocclusion with separation of teeth and widening of the periodontal-ligament space. Lateral skull radiographs demonstrate a 'hair-on-end' appearance. Children are managed with regular blood transfusions and desferrioxamine—an iron-chelating agent.

Dental management

- Consultation with haematologist.
- Schedule dental treatment shortly after blood transfusions.
- Avoid treatment if haemoglobin <100 g/L.
- Antibiotic prophylaxis, especially if child has had splenectomy.
- Orthodontic treatment may be undertaken and teeth will move quickly through the bone. Retention may, however, be difficult.

Immunodeficiency

Immunodeficiency may be caused by quantitative or qualitative defects in neutrophils, primary immunodeficiencies, involving T cells, B cells, complement, or combined defects and acquired disorders. Prevention is the key to successful management. Antibiotics should be used for the prevention of infection.

Qualitative neutrophil disorders (Figure 8.5)
Chemotactic disorders
- Chediak–Higashi syndrome.
- Lazy-leucocyte syndrome.
- Leucocyte-adhesion defect.

Phagocytic disorders
- Agammaglobulinaemia.

Defects in microbial killing
- Chronic granulomatous disease.
- Recurrent skin infections with *Staphylococcus aureus*.

Quantitative neutrophil disorders
- Neutropenia <1.8×10^9 cells per L.
- Chemo- and radiotherapy. Cytotoxic drugs used for childhood neoplasia.
- Cyclic neutropenia 21–28-day cycling of neutrophils.
- Leukaemia infiltration of bone marrow by other cells.
- Agranulocytosis.
- Aplastic anaemia.

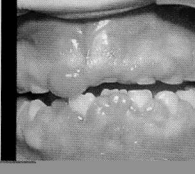

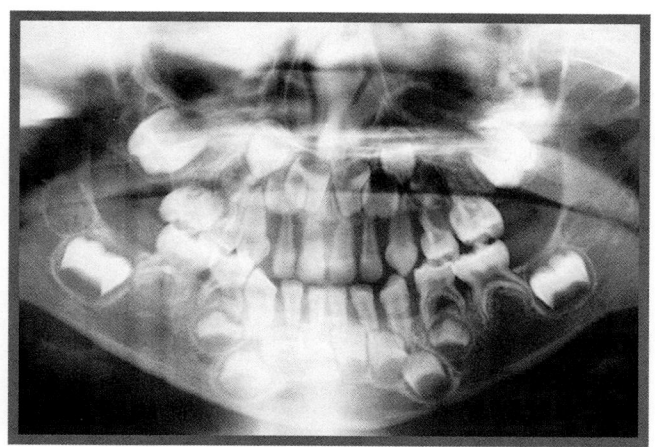

Figure 8.5 Leucocyte-adhesion defect in a 4-year-old manifesting severe periodontal disease and marginal bone loss. The upper and lower anterior teeth exfoliated within months of this radiograph being taken.

- Drug-induced neutropenia.

Life-threatening sepsis is associated with a level of neutrophils $<0.5 \times 10^9$ cells per L.

Primary immunodeficiencies
B cell defects
- Selective IgA deficiency.
- Agammaglobulinaemia.

T cell defects
- Di George syndrome with thymic aplasia.
- Chronic mucocutaneous candidiasis.

Combined immunodeficiency
- Severe combined immunodeficiency.
- Wiskott–Aldrich syndrome.
- Ataxia telangiectasia.

Acquired immunodeficiency
- HIV.
- Drug-induced—cytotoxics/corticosteroids/cyclosporin A.
- Chemotherapy and radiotherapy.

Dental implications
Neutrophil deficiencies and T-cell defects
- Candidosis (see Figure 8.6B).
- Severe gingivitis/prepubertal periodontitis (Figure 8.5).
- Gingivostomatitis.

- Recurrent aphthous ulceration.
- Recurrent herpes simplex virus infection.
- Premature exfoliation of primary teeth.

B-cell deficiencies
- Few oral complications.
- Recurrent bacterial infections, especially pneumonia and skin lesions.

Dental management
- Prevention and regular review.
- Prophylactic antibiotics.
- Extraction of pulpally involved teeth.
- Acyclovir for recurrent herpes simplex virus.
- Antifungals—Nystatin
         Amphotericin B
         may require systemic administration.
- Chlorhexidine 0.2% mouthwashes.

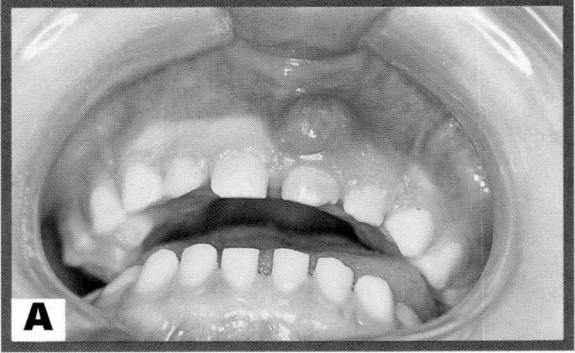 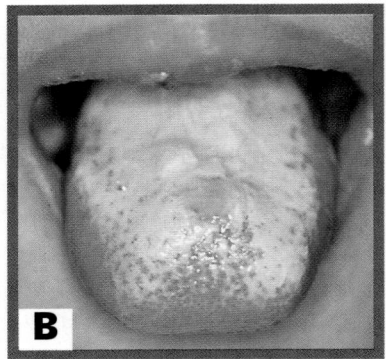

Figure 8.6 Two manifestations of immunodeficiency. **A** Abscess formation, above the upper-right primary lateral incisor tooth after administration of high-dose steroids for asthma, in an area that was previously quiescent. **B** Candidal infection of the tongue in an immunocompromised child.

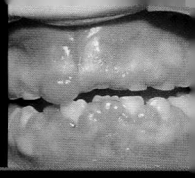

HIV infection and AIDS

Spread
Over the past 12 years, acquired immunodeficiency syndrome (AIDS) has emerged as a disease with social, political, medical and economic implications. By the end of the decade, there could be at least ten million HIV-infected children. By September 1992, 11 182 adult women and 3577 children from 31 European countries had been diagnosed with AIDS. More than 50% of the women acquired the infection through intravenous drug use, although 30% had become infected through heterosexual contact. Increased availability of travel, changing sexual mores, increased use of blood products, and increased drug abuse have all contributed to the worldwide increase in HIV infection.

Transmission
The main transmission media are body fluids, such as blood and semen. Saliva contains low and inconsistent levels of the HIV virus and is unlikely to provide a significant mode of transmission. Consequently, the two major routes of transmission in children are vertical (from an infected mother) and from blood products, with haemophiliacs being most at risk. Vertical transmission rates are up to 39% and occur before, during or after birth. Infection from breast feeding may be up to 29%.

Serodiagnosis
The screening enzyme-linked immunoadsorbent assay (ELISA) test for HIV antibodies is liable to give false negatives and any apparently positive results must be confirmed by the Western blot assay. Antigen assays are far more reliable, but a failure to detect virus or antigen in a young antibody-positive child does not exclude infection. A positive virus or antigen test is likely to indicate infection.

Occupational transmission
Because of the long incubation period and the limitations of histories and serodiagnosis it must be assumed that all blood derivatives may be infectious.

Immune function
The HIV virus attaches to the CD4 variant of the T4-helper lymphocyte and remains within infected cells throughout their life, being transmitted to other cells mainly by cell-to-cell contact. Other cells that may be affected include macrophages, and possibly endothelial, neuroglial, epithelial and dendritic cells.

The principal effect of HIV infection on the immune system is depletion of CD4 lymphocytes (helper cells) which results in a drop in the absolute CD4 count and a reversal of the CD4:CD8 ratio. These are immune indicators of disease progression.

Oral diseases associated with HIV infection (Figure 8.7)

Oral lesions are often early warning signs of HIV infection. Common disorders may manifest in different ways in the presence of HIV. In children, the most common lesions are candidiasis, gingivitis and parotid swelling.

Herpes simplex Recurrences are frequent and are typically intra-oral and circumoral. Other parts of the body may also be affected. Treatment is by acyclovir.

Aphthous-type ulcers These are persistent and very common. Treatment is palliative.

Salivary gland enlargement Occurs in both paediatric and adult patients and is similar to the presentation of mumps. It may be unilateral or bilateral and results in xerostomia and pain. Reduced salivary flow may lead to candidosis and dental caries. Treatment involves the use of saliva replacements, mouth sprays and salivary stimulants such as chewing gum.

Hairy leucoplakia Uncommon in children, with only four reported cases. Occurs predominantly on the lateral border of the tongue and occasionally the buccal mucosa and the soft palate. Langerhans' cells are reduced in hairy leucoplakia. There is no suggestion that this is a premalignant lesion and no treatment is required.

Oral candidosis The most common oral lesion in HIV infection is acute pseudomembranous candidiasis. It is an early lesion and suggests the presence of other opportunistic infections. The severity of the candidal infection may be related to the T4:T8 ratio and occurs when CD4 counts are less than 300 per mL. Oesophageal candidiasis occurs when CD4 counts drop below 100 per mL. Fungal infections can be related to reduced salivary flow and S-IgA. It responds well to treatment with systemic antifungals and an improvement in oral hygiene.

HIV gingivitis Manifests as red erythematous gingival tissues and can extend to the free gingival margin. There is often spontaneous gingival haemorrhage and petechiae within the gingival margin, either localized or generalized. Consideration must be given to a fungal component. Treatment involves improved oral hygiene and the use of chlorhexidine gluconate, 0.2%, mouthwashes and gels.

HIV periodontitis HIV periodontitis manifests with deep pain and spontaneous bleeding, interproximal necrosis and cratering, and intense erythema far greater than in acute necrotizing ulcerative gingivitis. HIV periodontitis appears more frequently in HIV-infected patients who have reduced T4:T8 ratios and symptomatic infection, such as thrush or a severe opportunistic infection.

Organisms such as black-pigmented bacteroides and Gram-positive rods which

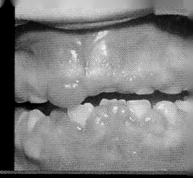

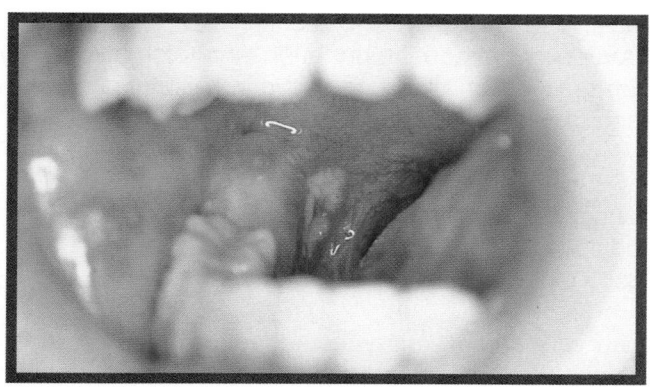

Figure 8.7 Severe oral ulceration in a child in the terminal stages of AIDS. The ulceration was most likely due to disseminated HSV infection to which the child succumbed 7 days after this photograph was taken.

are similar to those found in adult periodontitis have been identified in HIV periodontitis. Treatment is similar to that for acute necrotizing ulcerative gingivitis with the use of metronidazole.

Kaposi's sarcoma Uncommon in children and adolescents. It affects the palate especially, but also the gingivae and the tongue. Treatment is by chemotherapy, radiotherapy, or laser excision.

Natural history of vertically acquired paediatric HIV infection

Human immunodeficiency virus infection has been identified in increasing numbers of children with otherwise unexplained immune deficiency and opportunistic infections of the type found in adults with AIDS. For the limited purposes of epidemiological surveillance, the Centres for Disease Control (CDC) characterizes a case of paediatric HIV infection as a reliably diagnosed disease in children that is at least moderately indicative of underlying cellular immunodeficiency, and with which no known cause of underlying cellular immunodeficiency or any other reduced resistance is reported to be associated.

By the end of 1994, 123 children under 13 years, had been diagnosed as HIV-positive in Australia. Of this group, 28% were diagnosed with AIDS and 80% of these children had died. The majority of children (44%) acquired the infection as haemophiliacs or children with coagulopathies, whereas vertical transmission from an HIV mother accounted for 29% of infections. In 1994, however, perinatal exposure was solely responsible for new cases of childhood HIV infection in Australia (McDonald *et al.*, 1995)

The risk factors for paediatric HIV infection vary depending on the age group. Most children with AIDS are under 5 years of age. The primary risk factors are perinatal. Infants born to women who are intravenous drug users or who have bisexual partners comprise the largest group. About a third of the infants weigh less than 2500 g at birth and are small for gestational age.

- 25–30% of children develop AIDS in the first year of life.
- Lymphocytic interstitial pneumonitis is frequent, but often asymptomatic.
- Primary infection, rather than reactivation of opportunistic infections, occurs (cytomegalovirus, retinitis and toxoplasmosis are rare).
- Bacterial infections are rare, in particular *Streptococcus pneumoniae* and *Haemophilus influenzae*.
- The presenting pattern of encephalopathy varies with age.
- Growth failure occurs in addition to failure to thrive.
- Kaposi's sarcoma is rare but lymphomas, especially with central nervous system involvement, occur.

The progression of disease can vary and, in many instances, oral and physical symptoms do not present for years after infection with the virus. Consequently, many patients may lead very normal and effective lives.

Paediatric oncology

Childhood cancer accounts for about 1% of all cancer cases in the population. In Australia, an annual-incidence rate of malignant tumours in children under 15 years is approximately 11 per 100 000. Approximately 600–700 children aged between birth and 15 years develop cancer each year.

Whereas most adult cancers are carcinomas with strong aetiological associations, childhood cancers are a wide range of different histological types of tumour with less aetiological connection. The incidence, either in childhood cancer as a whole or in individual types of cancer, varies little from one country to the next and no racial group is exempt. Among more than 50 types of childhood cancers the most common forms include leukaemias, lymphomas, central nervous system tumours, primary sarcomas of bone and soft tissues (Figure 8.8), Wilms' tumours, neuroblastomas and retinoblastomas. Acute leukaemias and tumours of the central nervous system accounted for approximately one-half of the cases.

- Multimodal therapy (chemotherapy, radiotherapy and surgery) has resulted in an overall cure rate for childhood cancer of approximately 70%.

Leukaemia
A heterogenous group of haematological malignancies caused by clonal proliferation of primitive white blood cells.

Acute lymphoblastic leukaemia
- Accounts for 80–85% of acute childhood leukaemias.
- Defined by the presence of 30% lymphoblasts in the bone marrow.
- Therapy is tailored to the risk of relapse and includes combination induction chemotherapy, central nervous system and maintenance chemotherapy.
- Approximately 2 years for total therapy.

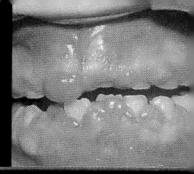

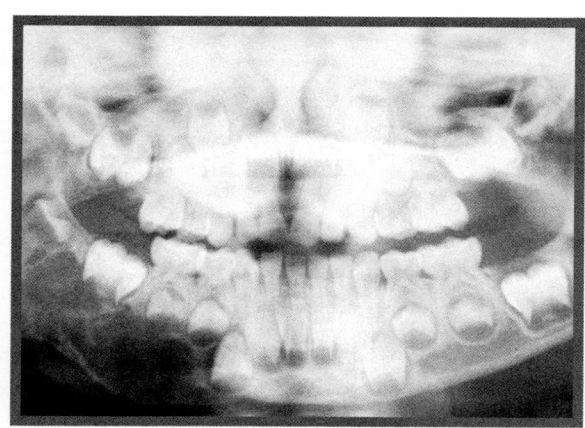

Figure 8.8 Neoplasms may arise as primary lesions within the jaws, invade from local tumours or may seed as metastases from distant primaries. The panoramic radiograph shows an extensive primary neoplasm of the right mandible involving the infratemporal fossa. Histologically, this lesion was a desmoplastic fibroma and required a hemimandibulectomy.

- Recently intrathecal therapy (commonly methotrexate) has been used to replace cranial irradiation.
- Generally 70% of patients are cured with standard therapy.
- Prognosis depends on age, initial white cell count, cytogenetic abnormalities and other features.
- Bone-marrow transplantation reserved for high-risk or relapsed patients.

Acute myeloid leukaemia
- 15–20% of acute childhood leukaemias.
- Bone marrow infiltrated with primitive myeloid cells, classified by morphological appearance.
- Clinical features similar to other leukaemias.
- Acute myeloid leukaemia with monocytic morphology (M4/M5) is associated with gingival infiltration and promyelocytic morphology (M3) is associated with disseminated intravascular coagulation.
- Induction therapy may be followed by bone-marrow transplantation (autogenous or allogenic).
- Cure rate is less than acute lymphoblastic leukemia—approximately 50% with modern therapy.

Chronic myeloid leukaemia
- Rare in childhood, accounts for <5% of cases.
- Two types—one is identical to adult chronic myeloid leukemia and is characterized by the presence of the Philadelphia chromosome (Ph) in malignant cells. The second or juvenile form occurs earlier in infancy with a rapid course, infection, haemorrhage and poor survival.

- Bone-marrow biopsy reveals granulocytic proliferation without an excess of blasts.
- Chronic phase treated with hydroxyurea or interferon and lasts for an average of 3 years, but inevitably proceeds to an acute blast phase resembling acute leukaemia.
- Preferred therapy: allogenic bone-marrow transplant within 1 year of diagnosis.

Clinical features
- Fatigue and weight loss.
- Anaemia.
- Purpura.
- Infection and febrile episodes.
- Hepatosplenomegaly and lymphadenopathy.
- Bone pain.

Investigations
- Full-blood count:
    anaemia
    neutropenia
    thrombocytopenia.
- Leucocytosis plus circulating blasts.
- Bone-marrow biopsy required to confirm diagnosis.
- Lumbar puncture to exclude central nervous system involvement.

Problems in medical management
Bone-marrow suppression
- Suppression of the bone marrow will appear at diagnosis from malignant infiltration and later caused by therapy.
- Subsequent anaemia, infection and bleeding.
- Infection in the immunocompromised child is life-threatening and may be caused by bacteria, viral agents, fungi or parasites. Broad-spectrum antibiotic treatment is usually required.

Disease relapse
- May occur in the marrow, central nervous system or other organs (i.e. testes).
- Treatment is individualized.

Late effects of therapy See below.

Solid tumours in childhood
Brain tumours
- Most frequent solid tumours of childhood.

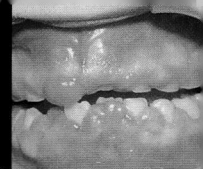

- 70% are gliomas, mostly low-grade astrocytomas or medulloblastoma
- More than 50% of paediatric intracranial tumours occur in the posterior cranial fossa (infratentorial).
- Surgical excision, combined with radiotherapy, (with or without chemotherapy) is the standard approach to treatment.
- Chemotherapy is used to delay or avoid cranial radiotherapy in infants.
- Overall survival approximately 40% at 10 years.

Non-Hodgkin's lymphoma
- Arises from transformed B or T lymphocytes in lymph nodes and lymphoreticular tissue.
- Primary tumour may be abdominal (B cell) or in the neck /thorax (T cell).
- Tumour spread is local or to bone marrow/central nervous system.
- Primary mode of therapy is chemotherapy.
- Up to 90% cure rate for localized non-Hodgkin's lymphoma.

Wilms' tumour
- Arises from kidney around 3–4 years of age.
- Usually presents as asymptomatic abdominal mass.
- Associated with aniridia and other congenital anomalies.
- Excellent response to combined therapy; surgery/chemotherapy, with or without radiotherapy, depending on disease stage.
- Commonly lung, hepatic and skeletal metastases.

Neuroblastoma
- Arises from neural crest cells anywhere along sympathetic chain.
- Most common site is abdominal, either in adrenal gland or paraspinal ganglia. Other sites include thorax, neck or pelvis.
- Majority of patients present with tumour spread to lymph nodes, bone marrow, liver or subcutaneous tissues.
- Diagnosis confirmed by raised levels of urinary catecholamines and tissue biopsy.
- May have elevated α-fetoprotein levels.
- Prognosis poor for advanced disease.

Rhabdomyosarcoma
- Arises from embryonal mesenchymal tissue with potential of differentiating to skeletal (striated) muscle.
- Patients present with a painless, usually rapidly enlarging subcutaneous lump, almost anywhere in the body. Common sites include head and neck, genitourinary tract and extremities. Large lesions in the head and neck invade bone, and jaw lesions are common.

- Treatment includes surgery with adjuvant chemotherapy and/or radiotherapy.
- Prognosis influenced by site and stage at diagnosis.

Hodgkin's disease
- Lymphoid malignancy characterized by presence of Reed–Sternberg cells.
- Usually teenagers and young adults.
- Presents most commonly with painless enlargements of lower cervical and/or mediastinal lymph nodes accompanied by fever and weight loss.
- Excellent response to chemotherapy. Radiotherapy is required for more advanced disease.
- Cure rate approaches 90%.

Retinoblastoma
- Tumour of the retinoblasts in children <5 years.
- May have a strong hereditary component.
- Usually white or yellow pupillary reflex (normally red reflex).
- Treatment often requires enucleation of the globe and radiotherapy.

Osteosarcoma
- Rare malignant tumour of bone, mostly in the metaphyseal region of long bones with distal femur the most common site.
- Teenagers most common age affected.
- Metastasizes mostly to lung and bone.
- Requires wide resection of tumour plus multi-agent chemotherapy.

Ewing's sarcoma
- Malignant tumour of bone in teenagers. It commonly involves the midshaft of long bones, although any bone may be involved.
- Most common in proximal femur or pelvis.
- Characterized by densely packed, small, round cells.
- Requires surgery, chemotherapy, and local irradiation.
- Worse prognosis with pelvic primary or metastatic disease.

Langerhans' cell histiocytosis
- Rare neoplasm that presents with premature exfoliation of primary teeth.
- Prognosis depends on the extent of disease at diagnosis and the age and progression of lesions (see Chapter 6).

Dental management
- As for immunocompromised children.
- Supportive therapy.
- Extraction of carious teeth.

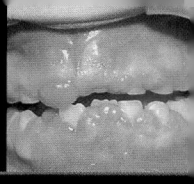

- Meticulous oral hygiene.
- Chlorhexidine 0.2% mouthwashes.
- Topical Xylocaine (Xylocaine viscous 2%).
- Topical and systemic antifungals.
- Prophylactic antibiotics.
- Systemic antiviral medications.

Late effects of childhood neoplasia

Dramatic advances in the treatment of childhood cancer in the past three decades have led to the long-term cures of at least half of patients diagnosed today. Because about one child in 600 develops cancer before the age of 15 years, almost one child in every thousand will be a survivor of cancer. As the number of survivors of a variety of paediatric cancers increases, the delayed adverse sequelae of treatment in these patients are emerging. They are unique because of the impairment of active growth and development during cancer therapy.

Adverse sequelae caused by the cancer treatment include:

Surgery
- Results in disfigurement (Figure 8.9B).
- Loss of function.
- Stenosis and nerve damage.

Radiotherapy
- Skin hyperpigmentation.
- Cutaneous telangiectasia.
- Subcutaneous tissue atrophy.
- Permanent thinning or loss of hair (Figure 8.9A).
- Second malignancy.
- Growth impairment.
- Disturbances of intellectual, endocrine, liver, lung, kidney and germ-cell functions.

Chemotherapy
- Cytotoxic drugs can cause damage to several organs: liver, kidney, germ cells of the testis, lung, heart, and brain.
- Increases incidence of second neoplasm.

The effects of chemotherapy and radiotherapy appear to be synergistic. Because craniofacial and dental development are not complete until the adolescent period it is not surprising that dental late effects are commonly found in survivors of childhood cancer. Chronic problems involving target tissues lead to impairment of growth and development of hard and soft tissues, which may result in orofacial asymmetry, xerostomia, dental caries, trismus and a variety of dental abnormalities. Generally, the nature and degree of these complications vary widely and

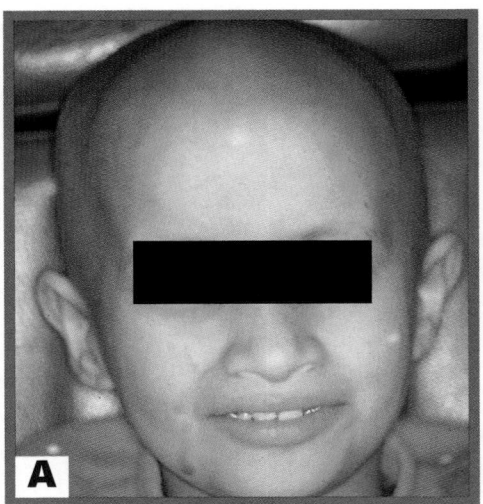
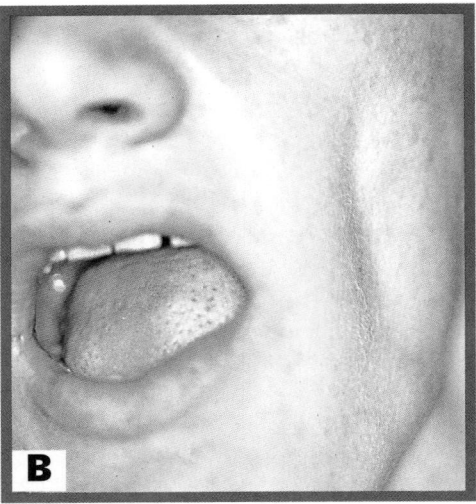

Figure 8.9 **A** A child in remission for acute lymphoblastic leukaemia with typical alopecia resulting from chemotherapy. **B** Late effects of surgery and radiotherapy for a rhabdomyosarcoma of the left masseter involving the parotid and the ramus of mandible. Note the limited oral opening and the facial deformity. Access for restorative work on the carious molars was extremely difficult. Caries resulted from reduced salivary flow after removal of the parotid gland.

depend on a number of factors:
- Type and location of malignancy.
- Age of the patient.
- Site and amount of surgery.
- Location and dosage of radiotherapy.
- Fractionated versus whole-dose radiation.
- Type, total dosage and timing of chemotherapeutic agents.
- Oral health status and
- Level of dental care before, during and after therapy.

Dental late effects (Figure 8.11)
Radiation
- Salivary gland damage and xerostomia is temporary in children, because of the lower dosage of radiation and greater regenerative capacity.
- Lower incidence of radiation caries.
- Enamel hypoplasia.

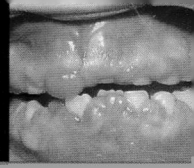

- Altered crown morphology.
- Microdontia.
- Shortness and tapering of roots, abnormal root curvature.
- Rootless teeth and tooth agenesis.
- Mean dental age of the children within the normal range.
- Micrognathia and retrognathia due to effects of cranial irradiation.

Children younger than 5 years of age are affected more severely than older patients. The altered craniofacial growth, a diminished mandibular growth, is associated with the field of irradiation which includes a portion of ascending ramus and the entire condyle of the mandible.

Chemotherapy complications The lack of specificity of cytotoxic agents in terms of differentiating neoplastic cells from metabolically active normal cells, such as ameloblasts and odontoblasts, might result in abnormalities of dental development. Microdontia, enlarged pulp chambers, shortening, thinning and blunting of root, and delayed eruption have been frequently found in patients receiving chemotherapy. Enamel opacities, hypocalcification and a high caries rate have also been noted in several studies, however, it remains unclear whether these findings are due to direct alteration of enamel formation or maturation, or to alterations in oral environment (saliva and flora), diet, and home-care among the patients who were on chemotherapy.

Because most childhood cancers are treated by combined chemotherapy and head and neck irradiation it is difficult to know the exact effect of each treatment. In general, dental late effects are more severe in patients who receive a higher dosage of either chemotherapy or radiotherapy. Dental aberrations are more severe and extensive in patients younger than 6 years of ages. Total body irradiation in bone-marrow transplantation appears to worsen the dental disturbances.

Renal disease

End-stage renal failure leads to a drop in glomerular filtration rate which results in progressive hypertension, fluid retention, and build-up of metabolites that are not excreted normally.

Conditions affecting the kidneys
- Ureteric reflux causing reflux nephropathy or hypoplasia.
- Obstructive uropathy.
- Glomerulonephritis/glomerulosclerosis.
- Medullary cystic disease.
- Systemic lupus erythematosus.
- Cystinosis.

Dental implications

- Children usually exhibit growth retardation.
- Pale and anaemic.
- Bleeding tendency due to capillary fragility and thrombocytopenia.
- Children on dialysis are anticoagulated.
- Caries rate is lower in children with end-stage renal disease, possibly caused by ammonia being released in saliva.
- Uraemic stomatitis may develop when serum urea is over 300 mg/mL. Occurs as ulcerated or non-ulcerative forms. Both have a tendency to bleed and are open to secondary infection.

Dental changes

These are dependent on the time of onset of disease. Those teeth calcifying during renal failure will exhibit chronological hypoplasia or hypomineralization. Teeth are often green or brown because of the incorporation of blood products such as biliverdin. Caries is often low in these children, but calculus formation is increased.

Renal osteodystrophy (Figure 8.10A)

Hypocalcaemia is present because of phosphate retention and decreased calcium absorption. This active absorption from the gut is dependent on vitamin D_3. However, vitamin D metabolism is impaired due to failure of the hydroxylation of 25-hydroxycholecalciferol (vitamin D_3) to 1,25-dihydroxy vitamin D_3 in the diseased kidney. In an attempt to raise serum calcium there is a secondary hyperpara-

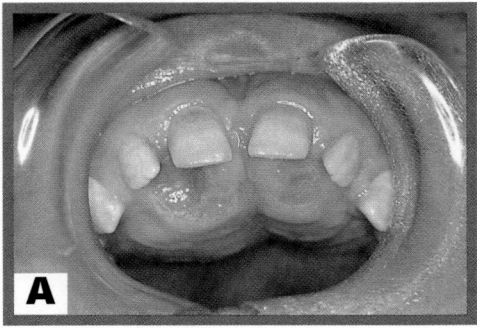
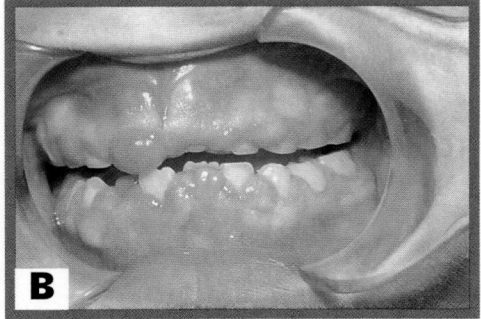

Figure 8.10 A Severe renal osteodystrophy in a child in end-stage renal failure. There has been gross expansion of the maxilla in an attempt to produce red blood cells because of failure of erythropoiesis. This is similar to events in β thalassaemia. **B** Gingival overgrowth from cyclosporin A after kidney transplantation. The teeth are also hypoplastic and small because of renal disease in infancy.

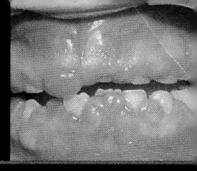

thyroidism. Calcium is removed from bone giving rise to the characteristic radiographic appearance (see 'Hyperparathyroidism' below).

Dental management
- Consultation with renal physician.
- Prevention. This is of great importance before transplantation.
- Extraction of pulpally involved teeth. Treatment should be aggressive.
- Admission is required for general anaesthesia.

Dialysis
Children on haemodialysis receive anticoagulants but may be successfully managed with DDAVP. Any treatment, and especially extractions, should be performed the day after dialysis. Sockets should be packed and sutured. Platelet transfusions are to be avoided if possible. Children managed with continuous ambulatory peritoneal dialysis (CAPD) can be managed more conservatively.
- Antibiotic prophylaxis is required.

Drug interactions
Patients with end-stage renal failure are managed with antihypertensives and steroids and are therefore anaemic and significantly immunocompromised. Medications that are metabolized in the kidney should be used only after consultation with the child's physician. Dentists should also be aware that renal excretion of drugs is also impaired.

Drugs to avoid in patients with renal insufficiency
- Paracetamol.
- Penicillin.
- Tetracycline.
- If patients are adequately haemodialysed it may be necessary to increase dosage of drugs.
- Additional doses should be given after haemodialysis is complete.

Liver disease

Biliary atresia
Congenital obliteration or hypoplasia of the bile ducts resulting in biliary cirrhosis and portal hypertension. In severe cases, transplantation is necessary.

α_1-Antitrypsin deficiency
- Deficiency in hepatic secretion of α_1-globulin.
- Leads to progressive hepatomegaly and cirrhosis.
- Treated by transplantation.

Liver function tests
- Full-blood count and coagulation profile should be routinely tested
- Alanine aminotransferase (ALT)   7–47 U/L.
- Alkaline phosphatase   60–391 U/L.
- γ-Glutamyl transpeptidase (γGT)   5–43 U/L.
- Total bilirubin.
- Albumin (a decrease may reflect impaired protein synthesis).

Dental implications
Coagulation problems are of major concern due to the reduction in production of vitamin-K dependent clotting factors (II, VII, IX, X).

Patients are usually managed with high-dose steroids and are immunocompromised. Children are usually mildly anaemic due to destruction of red blood cells. High levels of circulating red-blood-cell degradation products may become incorporated in developing enamel. High unconjugated bilirubin will cause green developmental staining of enamel.

Dental management
- Consultation with paediatric gastroenterologist and haematologist.
- Aggressive management of caries with extraction of suspect teeth, especially prior to transplantation.
- Coagulopathies are usually managed with fresh frozen plasma to replace deficient clotting factors.
- Antibiotic prophylaxis required.

Hepatitis A (infectious hepatitis)
Transmission period is very short (3 weeks). The important point to note is that there is no carrier state. If a patient is hepatitis-A positive treatment should be delayed for at least 4 weeks.

Hepatitis B (serum hepatitis)
Hepatitis B results If the HBsAg test is positive the blood is automatically tested for the 'e' antigen. If 'e' is negative, the patient is a chronic healthy carrier. If the 'e' antigen is positive the patient is a chronic active carrier.

Chronic healthy carrier (HBsAg +ve, e –ve) The degree of infectivity of these patients, although significant, is thought to be less than that of chronic active carriers. The liver function test for this patient should be normal.

Chronic active carrier (HBsAg +ve, e+ve) The chronic active carrier has active viral replication and is very infective. These patients have active liver disease, their liver function tests will be abnormal. (this is usually reflected by a decreased albumin which is important because this protein is involved with the production of clotting factors).

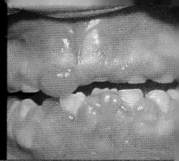

It is important to liaise directly with the patient's physician in the first instance when planning dental treatment and to do so again at regular intervals while the patient is under the care of the paediatric dental unit.

Liver function tests Useful with chronic active carrier (HBsAg +ve, e+ve).

In cases of chronic healthy carriers (HBsAg +ve, e –ve), if recently diagnosed, or just recently become negative for HBsAg then liver function tests should be considered.

Also if a patient has just recovered from Hepatitis A then liver function tests may be considered.

Hepatitis C (non-A, non-B hepatitis)

The hepatitis C virus (HCV) is the cause of what was previously termed non-A, non-B hepatitis. Patients with antibodies to HCV are chronic carriers and are potentially infectious. They are usually asymptomatic although their liver enzymes may be intermittently abnormal. Transmission of HCV is primarily by blood or blood products; however, the virus can be detected, by polymerase chain reaction (PCR), in the saliva of chronic carriers.

Organ transplantation (Figure 8.10B)

Transplantation of kidney, liver, cornea, heart and heart/lung are now routine procedures in major paediatric facilities. Unfortunately, there is an acute shortage of organs for transplantation and many children succumb to their illness before a donor organ is found. The main management problem with children undergoing organ transplantation is that of immunodeficiency. There are late effects of the transplantation including ongoing immune suppression, graft-versus-host disease (GVHD) and the effects of total body irradiation (TBI) in bone-marrow transplantation. It should be said, however, that most children are more easily treated after transplantation because of the cure of their original disease. This is especially true of children with end-stage hepatic or renal failure.

Dental implications

Immunosuppressive therapy includes corticosteroids and cyclosporin A. Cyclosporin is nephrotoxic and hepatotoxic and also causes hypertension. Gingival overgrowth results from treatment with cyclosporin and nifedipine.

Dental management

- Elimination of all possible sites of infection.
- Teeth with large carious lesions, even if not pulpally involved, should be extracted. Primary teeth soon to exfoliate should also be removed.
- Meticulous oral hygiene programme.
- Gingivectomy if required.

- Antibiotics for invasive treatment.

Bone-marrow transplantation

Varying with the institution, bone-marrow transplantation is used to treat children suffering from a number of conditions. These are:

- First or second relapse of acute lymphoblastic leukemia.
- Acute myeloid leukemia in first remission.
- Aplastic anaemia.
- Grade-IV neuroblastoma.
- Burkitt's lymphoma.

Dental management

- Dental treatment should be performed at lest 2 weeks prior to induction of chemotherapy or total body irradiation (TBI) to allow adequate healing.
- Chlorhexidine 0.2% mouthwashes and gels applied to the mucosa with toothettes qid to reduce mucositis.
- Prophylactic systemic aciclovir and antifungals during immunosuppression.
- Local haemorrhage controlled with topical thrombin, ε-aminocaproic acid.
- Topical fluoride gel application with neutral NaF gel in custom trays.
- Artificial saliva during periods of xerostomia.
- Antibiotic coverage for all procedures.

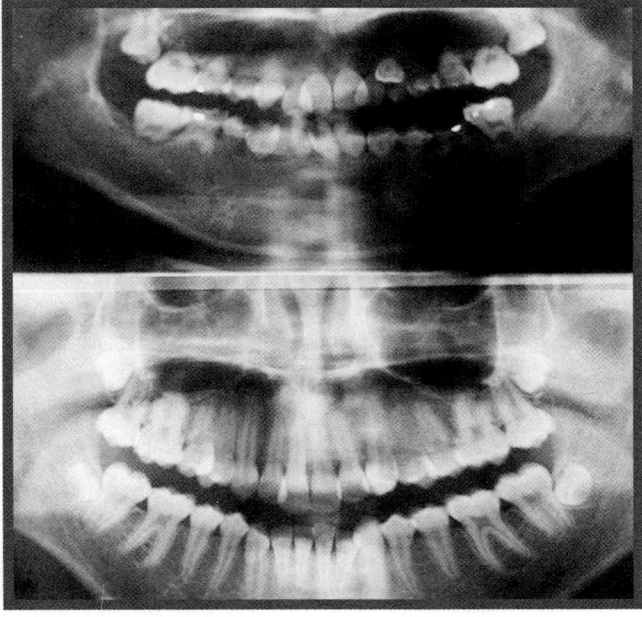

Figure 8.11 Effects of radiation to the head and neck. A set of identical twins, the first of which had acute lymphoblastic leukaemia diagnosed at 18 months. She relapsed during the first remission and received a bone-marrow transplant and TBI. The comparison with her sister at 15 years of age is dramatic. There is agenesis of some permanent teeth, arrested root development of the incisors and first permanent molars and mircrodontia.

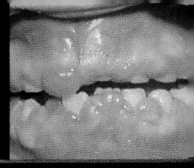

Graft-versus-host disease

Graft-versus-host disease (GVHD) occurs when transplanted T cells recognize the tissues of the host as being foreign. It is a major problem in bone-marrow transplantation with significant manifestations in up to 50% of patients. The acute form usually appears within a few weeks of transplantation with signs of fever, rash, diarrhoea and abnormal liver function leading to jaundice. Chronic GVHD often follows some months later and is characterized by lichenoid or scleroderma-like changes to the skin and mucosa, keratoconjunctivitis, pulmonary insufficiency, abnormal liver function, and intestinal problems.

Oral manifestations

These vary with the severity of the condition, but often include:
- Mild oral mucosal erythema.
- Painful desquamative gingivitis.
- Angular chelitis.
- Loss of lingual papillae.
- Lichenoid maculae and striae.
- Xerostomia.

Diagnosis Biopsy mucosa of lower lip, which should include two minor salivary glands. Histological changes will be evident both in stratified squamous epithelium, with a chronic lymphocytic inflammatory infiltrate and in the minor salivary glands showing chronic sialadenitis.

Endocrinopathies

Diabetes mellitus

Type-I or insulin-dependent diabetes mellitus is the most common form in children. Approximately 2 in 1000 children between the ages of 5 and 18 years have the disease. The development of type-I diabetes results from viral or toxic insults to the pancreatic islets of those children genetically predisposed to developing the disorder. An autoimmune mechanism has also been suggested in the destruction of the insulin-producing β cells. The goal of treatment is to maintain blood glucose at a normal level and thereby reduce the potential complication of hyperglycaemia and ketoacidosis. This generally involves administration of an intermediate-acting insulin. Pancreatic transplantation is now offering new hope and is currently under critical investigation.

Evaluation
- Family history—relatives of patients with diabetes are two times more likely to develop the disease than the population at large.

- Symptoms—polydipsia, polyuria, weight loss with polyphagia, enuresis, recurrent infections and candidiasis.
- Glycosuria may be present.
- Ketoacidosis and coma are possible.

Diagnosis
- Fasting blood-glucose level above 120 mg/dL.
- Abnormal oral glucose tolerance test.
- Elevated glycosylated haemoglobin test values.

Dental implications
- Periodontal disease is the most consistent oral finding in patients with poorly controlled diabetes. These patients exhibit increased alveolar bone resorption and inflammatory gingival changes. This may mimic the clinical manifestation of juvenile periodontitis.
- Xerostomia and recurrent intra-oral abscesses may be present.
- Enamel hypocalcification and hypoplasia along with reduced salivary flow can predispose these patients to an increased frequency of caries.
- Altered flora with an increase in *Candida albicans*, haemolytic streptococci and staphylococci.

Dental management
- Children with well-controlled diabetes can receive dental treatment in the normal way, except when a general anaesthesia is required. For routine dental appointments, the patient should eat a normal meal before the dental procedure, but a glucose source should always be available to treat the onset of hypoglycaemia.
- Fasting before a general anaesthesia requires careful adjustment of hypoglycaemia therapy because hypoglycaemia related to anaesthesia can be fatal.
- Healing can be delayed, particularly in surgical cases, and oral sepsis can be an additional risk in the delicate control of a diabetic child.
- All children treated under general anaesthesia should be admitted to hospital and their care supervised by the paediatric endocrine team. It is standard practice to start a dextrose and insulin infusion to avoid complications with fasting.
- Prophylactic antibiotics.

Pituitary disorders
Hypopituitarism Hypopituitary dwarfism, resulting from anterior pituitary insufficiency is either idiopathic or secondary to pituitary or hypothalamic disease (craniopharyngioma, infections, granulomatous disease, trauma). Although other pituitary hormones may be deficient, usually there is an isolated deficiency in growth hormone. Treatment consists of supplemental growth hormone which stimulates

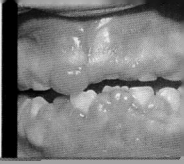

the differentiation of epiphyseal growth plate precursor cells and induces clonal expansion of cartilage cells.

Early detection and therapeutic management are essential to diminish the growth disturbance. Although treatment will prevent loss of stature proportional to age, it cannot make up for any deficiency present at diagnosis.

Dental implications
- Decreased linear facial measurements (particularly in the posterior facial height) and decreased linear cranial base measurements.
- Often an open bite accompanied by the typical immature hypopituitary face.
- Skeletal development is consistently more retarded than craniofacial development, but tooth eruption and root formation can be delayed or incomplete.
- Hypopituitarism has effects on adrenal-gland activity that may lead to hypothyroidism and produce a risk of hypopituitary coma. This may be precipitated by any stressful event including trauma, surgery, general anaesthesia or infection.

Hyperpituitarism
- Gigantism/acromegaly resulting from primary hypersecretion of pituitary hormones and pituitary hyperplasia is usually associated with pituitary neoplasms, which are extremely rare in children. Hypersecretion of hormones, however, may be a secondary finding in conditions like hypogonadism, hypoadrenalism and hypothyroidism due to a decreased hormonal negative feedback.
- Severity of the craniofacial manifestations of hyperpituitarism is dependent on the time of onset and the duration of hypersecretion. In children with open epiphyses, hypersecretion of growth hormone results in gigantism. This leads to generalized overgrowth of skeletal and soft tissues with marked increase in height and size.
- Gigantism, although rare, is usually associated with an eosinophilic adenoma but can be also associated with a hypothalamic tumour. In adolescents and adults with closed epiphyses, hypersecretion leads to acromegaly which consists chiefly of enlargement of the distal parts of the body with little, if any, increase in height.

Dental implications
- Precocious and accelerated development of the craniofacial skeleton.
- Prognathism.
- Accelerated dental development and eruption, enlarged crenated tongue and facial features.
- Marked thickening of the cranium and cortical bone of the mandible.
- Overdevelopment of osseous structures with poor maturation and quality (osteoporosis) with hypercementosis.

Dental management Dental management of patients with pituitary disorders focuses mainly on the craniofacial malformations. Treatment needs to be planned carefully and coordinated with other medical disciplines. No contraindications exist for comprehensive dental health care.

Thyroid disorders

Hypothyroidism Hypothyroidism may be either congenital (cretinism) or acquired (juvenile myxoedema). Thyroid hormone deficiency is most often secondary to a primary disease of the thyroid and less commonly associated with hypothalamic and/or pituitary insufficiency. Cretinism is rare in those states where antenatal testing is performed. It can be attributed to aplasia, hypoplasia or maldescent of the gland, familial inborn metabolic errors, maternal intrauterine teratogens, iodide deficiency and idiopathic causes. Juvenile myxoedema can stem from a multitude of causes—thyroidectomy, thyroid irradiation, autoimmune diseases, infection or medication.

Hypothyroidic changes include growth retardation, diminished physical activity, decreased circulation, poor muscle tone, speech disorders, delayed mental development and craniofacial manifestation.

These changes are obviously dependent on the age of onset of the disease, the degree of thyroid hormone production lag, and the timing of diagnosis and treatment. Treatment focuses on supplementing this hormone by synthetic hormone (thyroxine) or animal thyroprotein and in most developed countries, thyroid function is now tested soon after birth by measurement of thyroid hormone levels (T_3 and T_4).

Dental implications
- Decreased vertical facial growth, decreased cranial-base length and flexure, maxillary protrusion and open bite with immature facial patterns.
- Delayed eruption and increased spacing of teeth.
- Developmental retardation and hypoplasia.

Hyperthyroidism Although of undetermined aetiology, hyperthyroidism has an association with immunological deficiencies, infectious diseases, heredity and neoplasms. The most common associations are Graves' disease, toxic multinodular goitre, toxic adenoma and subacute thyroiditis. This condition is five times more common in females and is most likely to appear between 12 and 14 years of age. It is usually associated with a goitre and has a cyclic clinical course.

Hyperthyroidic changes can mimic a state of overactivity of the sympathetic nervous system (nervousness, emotional instability, heat intolerance, loss of weight despite increased appetite, insomnia, marked perspiration, changes in skin, hair and nails, and gastrointestinal disturbances). Ocular abnormalities, such as lid lag, exophthalmos and widening of the palpebral fissures, are often found as are cardiovascular abnormalities.

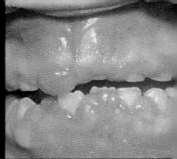

Dental manifestations

- Accelerated growth and development of the craniofacial complex and skeleton.
- Precocious eruption of teeth.
- Periodontal/periapical destruction and osteoporosis.
- Increased vertical facial height with open bite and mild prognathism.

Dental management The principle risk in children with thyroid disorders is associated with general anaesthesia. The hypothyroid patient is at risk of developing congestive cardiac failure which may be precipitated by general anaesthesia. Anaemia, if present, further increases the hazards as does cardiomegaly which may result in sudden hypertension during anaesthetic induction. The cardiac effects of hyperthyroidism also increase the risks of general anaesthesia, particularly in patients with chronic rhythm disturbances. The untreated patient is also at risk from infection or surgical procedures since a thyroid crisis may be precipitated.

Oral infections seem to have an injurious effect on the thyroid gland, either directly or through toxic substances, and may aggravate hyperthyroidism or exacerbate symptoms associated with hyperfunction. Oral infections should be treated aggressively in conjunction with the help of the child's physician and endocrinologist. Antithyroid drugs may produce parotitis and agranulocytosis, which predispose the patient to bleeding episodes, ulceronecrotic lesions and oral infections.

The general management of such patients is analogous to that of patients with hypertensive disease. Dental appointments should be of short duration and as simple as possible.

Parathyroid disorders

Hypoparathyroidism Usually results from structural or functional deficiencies occurring during childhood, parathyroidectomy occurring during thyroidectomy, irradiation of the gland, neoplasm or autoimmune disease. Treatment focuses on maintaining serum calcium through medication, diet supplementation and vitamin-D therapy. Hypoparathyroidic changes include prolonged hypocalcaemia with a resultant hyperphosphataemia, neuromuscular excitability and tetany. Cardiovascular dysfunction, idiopathic epilepsy, ectodermal defects and craniofacial manifestation can also be found with permanent physical and mental retardation occurring if diagnosis and treatment are delayed.

Dental implications

- Circumoral paraesthesia and spasm of the facial muscles.
- Hypoplasia of enamel, hypodontia and root anomalies.
- Delayed or arrested tooth eruption.
- Acute and chronic oral candidiasis.

Pseudohypoparathyroidism Albright's hereditary osteodystrophy is a familial X-linked dominant disease in which there are adequate parathyroid hormone levels but inadequate response to the hormone in bone and kidney. In general, males are more severely affected than females although females are more commonly encountered.

Dental implications
- Round full faces with short neck.
- Delayed or incomplete eruption of teeth.
- Enamel hypoplasia and short roots.

Hyperparathyroidism Excessive production of parathyroid hormone may result from a primary defect in the gland (adenoma hyperplasia, hypertrophy) or secondarily as a compensatory phenomenon, usually correcting hypocalcaemia states caused by rickets or by chronic renal disease. Primary disease results in hypercalcaemia and hypercalciuria, leading to muscle weakness, gastrointestinal disturbances, polyuria, kidney stones, soft-tissue calcification, osseous malformation (osteoporosis and osteomalacia) and pain.

Whitlock summarized these changes as 'stones, bones, abdominal groans and psychic moans'. In infants and young children there may be failure to thrive, poor feeding and muscular hypotonia, leading to mental retardation, convulsions and blindness.

Bony lesions are called brown tumours because they contain areas of haemorrhage, containing an abundance of multinucleated giant cells, fibroblasts and haemosiderin. Generalized osteoporosis with cortical resorption is the most common bone lesion and radiographic signs include rarefactions, loss of trabeculation, ground-glass appearance, total or partial loss of lamina dura, lytic lesions and metastatic calcifications.

Dental implications
- Increasing mobility and drifting of teeth with no apparent pathologic periodontal pocketing.
- Malocclusion.
- Metastatic soft-tissue calcification.
- Periapical radiolucencies and root resorption.
- Loss of lamina dura and generalized loss of radiodensity.

Dental management Generally, routine dental treatment involves no modifications unless there are associated medical complications present. Manifestations of Addison's disease may accompany hypoparathyroidism and thus the patient may be at risk from stressful procedures such as surgery and general anaesthesia. Hyperparathyroidism may be associated with cardiac arrhythmias which increase the risk of serious problems during general anaesthesia. Risk of pathological fractures in advanced disease may be a theoretical complication of oral surgical procedures. Splinting of mobile teeth is a useful adjunct to prevent pain and further drifting.

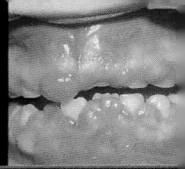
Neurological disease

Epilepsy
Febrile convulsions A term used to describe a child under 5 years of age who suffers a seizure in response to febrile illness. Usually can be diagnosed when the temperature is over 38°C and no other cause of the convulsions has been found.

Classification
- Generalized either tonic–clonic (*grand mal*) or absence (*petit mal*).
- Partial, simple or complex.

Dental implications The major problems with epileptic children is gingival enlargement and the precipitation of a seizure in the surgery.

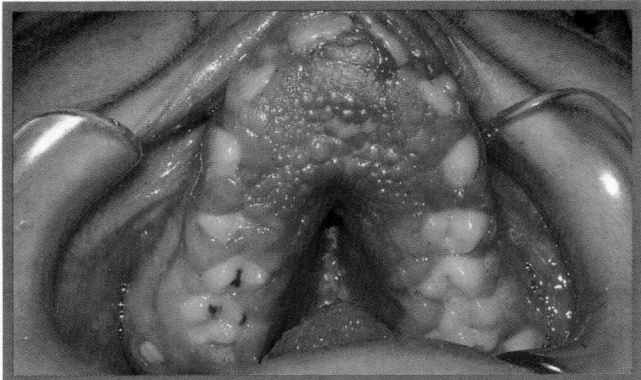

Figure 8.12 Severe phenytoin gingival enlargement in a child with cerebral palsy. The hypertonicity of the oral musculature has caused the protrusion of the anterior teeth and the orthopaedic compression of the maxilla.

Dental management Management of gingival overgrowth is dependent on oral hygiene. In severe cases, full-mouth gingivectomy may be required but overgrowth will recur if oral hygiene is not maintained. This may be especially difficult in children with intellectual handicaps and is often dependent on the motivation and skill of the parents and caregivers. It is important to always keep the interests of the child in mind—in which case aggressive surgical treatment may not benefit the child in the long term (Figure 8.12).

Cerebral palsy
The cognitive ability of a child with cerebral palsy (CP) cannot be determined quickly. Take time with these children to assess their abilities. Many patients with CP have no mental impairment. They may use verbal communication that requires some patience or a communication aid. Do not change the voice tone or level of

language when addressing these children. Reflex limb extension patterns may be triggered during dental visits if care is not taken. These contractions may occur during transfer of the patient from wheelchair to the dental chair. Discuss the transfer with the parent or caregivers before offering assistance. The reflex may also be stimulated if the patient's head is loose or unsupported. Ensure that the child is stabilized in the chair with blankets or pillows. If a reflex pattern occurs where the limbs are in extension:

- Raise the chair.
- Stabilize the head in the midline.
- Bring the arms forward.
- Reassure the child.

Gag, cough, bite and swallowing reflexes may be impaired or abnormal in children with cerebral palsy. If the gag reflex is more exaggerated treat the patient in a more upright position with the neck in slight flexion and the knees bent upwards, if possible. Use short bursts of the triplex with good high-speed suction.

Mouth props may be used; however, for those patients with impaired swallowing there is an increased risk of aspiration. Rubber dam is especially useful.

If the patient's bite reflex to oral stimulation is still present introduce instruments from the side rather than the front. To allow examination, apply gentle pressure with the forefinger on the anterior border of the ascending ramus and in the retromolar triangle. This avoids the risk of having a bitten finger.

For those children with hydrocephalus, shunts that empty into the vasculature require antibiotic prophylaxis against endocarditis (i.e. superior vena cava). It is generally considered that ventriculoperitoneal shunts do not require prophylactic cover.

Respiratory disease

Asthma

Australia has one of the highest rates of childhood asthma in the world with one in five children and one in seven adolescents affected. It is a condition characterized by hyper-responsiveness of the airways and bronchial inflammation, leading to attacks of wheezing and coughing in response to certain triggers. Currently, there is an emphasis on prophylactic medications to prevent episodes rather than simply treating acute attacks.

Dental implications

- The major risk is acute attack in the dental surgery (see Appendix D).
- Steroid medications may cause extrinsic staining of the teeth due to changes in oral flora and may also predispose to candidiasis.
- Children on high-dose corticosteroids may be immunocompromised.
- Previously, many oral medications contained large amounts of sugar and hence caries rates were much higher in these children.

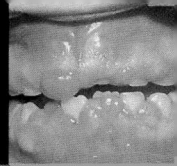

Dental management
- Regular prophylaxis if extrinsic staining present.
- Children who have been admitted for their asthma in the last 12 months and/or those managed with steroids are not suitable for day-stay anaesthesia and should be admitted pre-operatively to be jointly managed by the paediatric respiratory team.
- There are no contraindications to the use of N_2O.

Cystic fibrosis
- Autosomal recessive disorder of mucus-secreting exocrine glands.
- Airway and pancreatic diseases with resulting respiratory illness, malabsorption and growth retardation.
- Major cause of death is respiratory failure from recurrent chest infections.

Dental implications
- Some children were previously treated with broad-spectrum tetracyclines and so may exhibit staining in the secondary dentition.
- Increased and altered parotid flow rates appear not to predispose to caries, possibly because of long-term use of antibiotics.

Dental management
- Prevention.
- Any use of relative analgesia or general anaesthesia must be discussed with the respiratory paediatrician. Physiotherapy is required preoperatively and post-operatively.
- Long appointments should be avoided.
- Although life expectancy has increased with current therapies, there should be a rational and pragmatic approach to treatment planning.

Other patients with special needs

Children with special needs require dental appointments that are tailored to make best use of their abilities. The clinician who understands how to accommodate a child's disability will provide the secure environment required to successfully treat these children.

Visual impairment
- Allow the child to make full use of their tactile sense and their sense of smell when familiarizing them to the dental environment and dental procedures.
- Offer verbal and physical reassurance to the child once a rapport has been established. They cannot see your smile.
- Paint a picture in the mind of your patients by describing the treatment and the environment throughout the procedure. A startle reflex may occur if patients

are not warned before different instruments are introduced into the mouth without warning.
- Many visually impaired people are photophobic. It is important to ask parents and children about light sensitivity. Safety glasses should preferably be tinted.

Deafness
- Investigate how the child communicates.
- A common fault is to talk loudly rather than slowly. If the patient lip reads, face the child and speak clearly and slowly.
- It is useful to learn basic sign language. It should be noted that even within the English-speaking world, there are different signing languages for each country.
- Make it easy for patients to maintain visual contact because these children may be startled if they are touched without visual contact.
- Deaf children may be very sensitive to vibration and so introduce high-speed and low-speed drills carefully.
- If a hearing aid is worn the volume may need adjustment. Try to avoid blocking the ears and the hearing aid with the forearms when operating, as this will create feedback.

Developmental disability
- As in many cases of treating medically compromised children, the first appointment is often one in which to familiarize both the dentist with the child's condition and the child with the dental environment. Find out the patient's likes, dislikes and behaviour patterns. Offer verbal support and allow time to develop a rapport with the child.
- Support of the parent or caregivers is extremely important in reinforcing and administering preventive advice, oral hygiene practices and diet modification. Consultation with the school or institution may be required to modify diet.
- Take a thorough medical history. Developmental delay is a broad term covering children with a range of medical conditions and syndromes. It is essential that obscure syndromes be researched before performing treatment.
- Photocopy relevant information for the child's file.

Genetic diseases

Although generally uncommon, many children with genetic abnormalities will present to the paediatric dentist with specific dental anomalies associated with their condition or medical problems which complicate their dental management. Never assume that all children have been diagnosed before they present, as many children are diagnosed with significant genetic disease late in childhood, either because the disease has late manifestations or because conditions have been

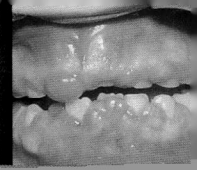

Table 8.1 Classification of genetic abnormalities

	Defect	Examples
Chromosomal structure	Aneuplodies (abnormal number of chromosomes)	Down's syndrome, trisomy 21 Klinefelter's syndrome XXY Turner's syndrome XO
	Chromosomal deletions and translocations	*18q*-deletion of part of long arm of chromosome 18
Single-gene defects	Autosomal dominant	Cleidocranial dysplasia Osteogenesis imperfecta
	Autosomal recessive	Cystic fibrosis
	X-linked recessive	Haemophilia Ectodermal dysplasia
Polygenic disorders	Multiple minor gene abnormalities interacting with environmental influences	Cleft palate Diabetes mellitus Allergic conditions Schizophrenia

Adapted from: Jones KL. *Smith's recognizable patterns of human malformation.* 4th. ed. Philadelphia: WB Saunders; 1988.

missed (Table 8.1). When taking the history it is always useful to draw a simple family pedigree (Figure 8.13).

Terms used in morphogenesis

Usually structural defects occur early in development with single problems that create secondary anomalies and manifest with multiple defects at birth or later. These sequences may be divided into three basic groups:

Malformation
- Poor formation of tissue.
- May be single or multiple but are primary structural abnormalities.
- Poor prognosis for normal growth in the areas affected.
- Recurrence rate of 1–5% e.g.:
  cleft palate
  enamel anomaly in amelogenesis imperfecta.

Deformation
- Unusual forces acting on normal tissues, usually from abnormal interuterine pressures.
- Good prognosis for normal growth and a low risk of recurrence e.g.:
  club foot
  micrognathia associated with Robin sequence.

Disruption
- Destruction or breakdown of normal tissue, which may result from vascular, infective, or physical causes.
- Low risk of recurrence, poor prognosis for normal growth in affected areas e.g.:
    deafness from congenital rubella
    bizarre facial clefting from amniotic bands
    hemifacial microsomia (from stapedial artery haemorrhage).

Syndrome
- A recognizable pattern of malformation.
- Multiple defects that cannot be explained on the basis of a single initiating defect.

Sequence
- A pattern of multiple anomalies arising from a single structural defect or event. Also termed anomalad.

Risk of recurrence in genetic disorders (Figure 8.13)
Autosomal dominant
- 50% of offspring will be affected from a single affected parent.
- Many dominant conditions have variable penetrance and so the manifestations may be increased or reduced.
Autosomal recessive
- If both parents are carriers, the risk of the child being a carrier is 50% and a 25% chance that the child will be homozygous for the condition (i.e. the trait will be expressed).
- If one parent is a carrier there is a 25% chance of the child being a carrier.

X-linked recessive
- Fifty percent transmission from female carriers.
- No male-to-male transmission from affected fathers, but all girls will be carriers.

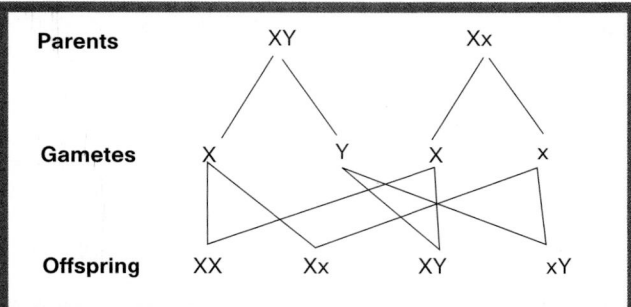

Figure 8.13
Calculation of risk in an X-linked recessive disorder. 50% of the boys are affected and 50% of the girls will be carriers.

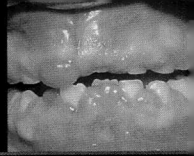

X-linked dominant
- Twice as many girls affected.
- 50% of offspring affected from mother.
- All girls affected from father, but no male to male transmission.

References

Cardiac disease
BARCO CT. Prevention of infective endocarditis: a review of medical and dental literature
J Periodontol 1991, **62**:510–523.
DURACK DT, KAPLAN EL, BISNO AL. Apparent failures of endocarditis prophylaxis. Analysis of 52 cases submitted to a national registry. J*AMA* 1983, **250**:2318–2322.
SAIMAN L, PRINCE A, GERSONY WM. Pediatric infective endocarditis in the modern era. *J Pediatr* 1993, **122**:847–853.
WAHL MJ. Myths of dental-induced endocarditis. *Arch Intern Med* 1994, **154**:137–144.

Bleeding disorders
HOTER LW. HEMOPHILIA A. *N Engl J Med* 1994, **330**:38–47.
JOHNSON WT, LEARY JM. Management of dental patients with bleeding disorders: review and update. *Oral Surg Oral Med Oral Pathol* 1988, **66**:297–303.
WARRIER AI, LUSHER JM. DDAVP: a useful alternative to blood components in moderate hemophilia A and von Willebrand disease. *J Pediatr* 1983, **102**:228.

Immunodeficiency
DONLON WC. Immunology in pediatric dentistry. *Pediatr Dent* 1983,**5**:195–199.
MOYER IN, KOBAYASHI RH, CANNON ML, SIMON JF, COOLEY RO, RICH K. Dental treatment of children with severe combined immunodeficiency. *Pediatr Dent* 1983, **5**:79.
PORTER SR, SCULLY C. Orofacial manifestations in the primary immunodeficiency disorders. *Oral Surg Oral Med Oral Pathol* 1994, **78**:4–13.
WALDMAN HB, WALDMAN ME. Increasing numbers of pediatric AIDS patients. *J Dent Child* 1991, 58:400–404.

Oncology
BERG JH, BLEYER WA. Pediatric dentistry in care of the cancer patient. *J Pediatr Dent* 1995, 17:257–258.
BERKOWIT RI, STRANOFJORD S, JONES P, *et al.* Stomatologic complications of bone marrow transplantation in a pediatric population. *Pediatr Dent* 1987, **9**:105–110.
DAHLLÖF G, BARR M, BOLME P, *et al.* Disturbances in dental development fter total body irradiation in bone marrow transplant recipients. *Oral Surg Oral Med Oral Pathol* 1988, **65**:41–44.
DAHLLÖF G, MODÉER T, BOLME P, RINGDEN O, HEIMDAHL A. Oral health in children treated with bone marrow transplantation: a one year follow-up. *J Dent Child* 1988, **55**:196–200.
FERRETTI GA. Chlorohexidine prophylaxis for chemotherapy and radiotherapy induced stamatitis:

a randomized double-blind trial. *Oral Surg Oral Med Oral Pathol* 1990, **I69**:331–338.

GOHO C. Chemo radiation therapy: effect on dental development. *Pediatr Dent* 1993, **15**:6–12.

National Cancer Monographs. *Oral complications of cancer therapy.* NCI Monographs Vol 9; 1990. National Institutes of Health, Washington USA.

HIV

D'ANGELO LJ, GETSON P, LUBAN NL, GAYLE HD. Human immunodeficiency virus infection in urban adolescents: Can we predict who is at risk? *Pediatrics* 1991, **88**:982–986.

LITTLE JW, MELNICK SL, RHAME FS, BALFOUR HH JR, DECHER L, RHODUS NL, MERRY JW *et al*. Prevalence of oral lesions in symptomatic and asymptomatic HIV patients. *Gen Dent* 1994, **42**:446–450.

MACDONALD AM, CROFTS N, BLUMER CE, GERTIG DM, PATTEN JJ, ROBERTS M, DAVEY T, MULLINS SE, CHUAH JC, BAILEY KA, *et al*. The pattern of diagnosed HIV infection in Australia, 1984–1992. *AIDS* 1994,**8**:513–519.

Liver/Kidney disease

BUCKLEY DJ, KOUTTS J, STEWART JH. Control of severely uremic patients undergoing oral surgery. *Oral Surg Oral Med Oral Pathol* 1986, **61**:546–549.

LITTLE JW, RHODUS NL. Dental treatment of the liver transplant patient. *Oral Surg* 1992, **73**:419–426.

SEOW WK, SHEPHERD RW, THONG Y. Oral changes associated with end-stage liver disease and liver transplantation: implications for dental management. *J Dent Child* 1991, **58**:474.

WISNOM CJ, LEE RJ. Increased seroprevalence of hepatitis B in dental personnel necessitates awareness of revised pediatric hepatitis B vaccine recommendations. *J Public Health Dent* 1993, **53**:231–234.

Endocrine disorders

DAHMS WT. An update in diabetes mellitus. *Pediatr Dent* 1991, **13**:79.

Neurological disorders

NELSON LP, URELES SD, HOLMES G. An update in paediatric seizure disorders. *Pediatr Dent* 1991, **13**:128.

Genetics

GORLIN RRJ, COHEN MM, LEVIN LS. *Syndromes of the head and neck*, 3rd ed. Oxford: Oxford University Press; 1990.

JONES, KL. *Smith's recognizable patterns of human malformation*, 4th ed. Philadelphia: WB Saunders; 1988.

PEARN J, GAGE J. Genetics and oral health. *Aust Dent J* 1987, **32**:1–10.

Further reading

HALL R. *Pediatric orofacial medicine and pathology*. London: Chapman and Hall Medical; 1994.

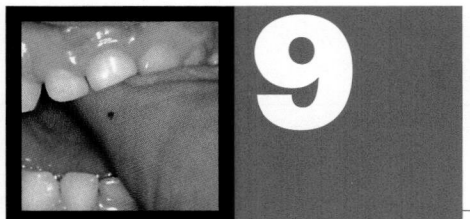

9 Orthodontic diagnosis and treatment in the mixed dentition

Contributors

John Fricker, Tissa Jayasekera

Introduction

The primary aims of orthodontic treatment in the mixed dentition are to correct dental arch irregularities, occlusal and jaw relation abnormalities and to eliminate functional interferences. These may be classified as preventive or interceptive. The term 'preventive' applies to the elimination of factors that may lead to malocclusion in an otherwise normally developing dentition. 'Interceptive' implies that corrective measures may be necessary to prevent a potential irregularity from progressing into a more severe malocclusion.

It is essential to have a sound understanding of the time sequence in the development of the child's dentition, and the ability to recognize the rate and direction of the general physical maturation of the child. Many cases of apparent malocclusion in the mixed dentition are actually part of the normal process of dental development. Incisor irregularities, spacing and apparent ectopic eruption of teeth may present early in the mixed dentition yet self-correct with growth and development. Neither the appliances used nor the treatment itself should interfere with the often rapid changes in eruption of permanent teeth and the dynamic nature of occlusal adjustment.

Indications for treatment

- Crowding.
- Space opening or regaining.
- Digit sucking.
- Missing teeth.
    Congenital absence.
    Traumatic loss.
- Elimination of supernumerary teeth.
- Eruption of teeth.
    Ectopic teeth.
    Impaction.
    Transposition, ankylosis.

- Class-II malocclusion.
  - Increased overbite.
  - Increased overjet.
- Class-III malocclusion.
  - Anterior cross-bite.
  - Posterior cross-bite.
  - Open bites.

Crowding

Mixed dentition analysis

The purpose of a mixed dentition analysis is to determine the space available in the dental arch for the permanent successors to erupt. To complete this analysis it is necessary to first record the arch perimeter length and the mesiodistal widths of the mandibular permanent incisors.

Measurement of arch length The most accurate way to determine arch length is to measure directly from a set of study casts. Soft wire can be adapted from the mesial of the first permanent molar to follow the arch perimeter of the distal of the contralateral second primary molar. The wire should be shaped to the ideal arch form and not follow any teeth out of alignment. Once the arch length has been determined, it is then necessary to estimate the space required for the permanent successors. There are two methods for this:

- Using radiographs with allowances for magnification.
- Using tooth prediction formulas.

Moyers' analysis A Moyers' prediction chart will indicate the level of confidence in predicting whether the space available is sufficient to accommodate the unerupted teeth. In this analysis the width of each mandibular permanent incisor is measured and then added. Using this value in the Moyers' table (at a 75% confidence level) it is possible to determine if the space available in the arch will be sufficient for posterior tooth eruption.

Arch prediction There is a high correlation between the sizes of the permanent mandibular incisors and the combined sizes of premolars and permanent canines. Thus, it is possible to forecast the amount of space required for the unerupted teeth and to plan interceptive and or preventive space management requirements (Figure 9.1).

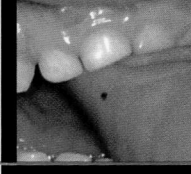
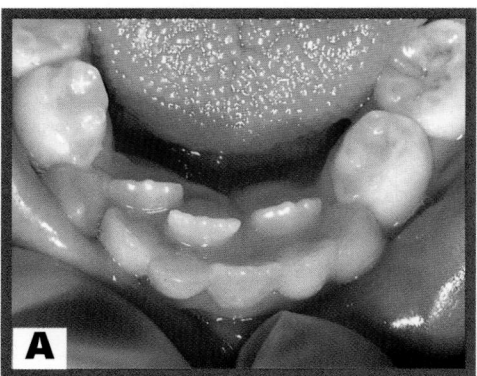
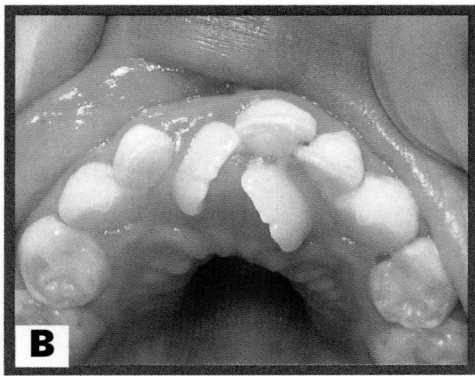

Figure 9.1 Common presentations of anterior crowding. It is important to inform parents and children of where teeth will erupt. **A** Lower permanent incisors form lingually to the primary teeth and in patients with tooth to base-bone discrepancy, they will erupt behind the primaries. It is often wise to facilitate removal of such teeth as in **B** to avoid the development of a cross-bite.

Space maintenance

Factors to consider for placement of space maintainer

- The loss of one or more primary incisor teeth (maxillary or mandibular) results in little space loss if canines and molars are present.
- Premature loss of a mandibular primary canine will result in the collapse of the incisal segment lingually and a midline shift to that side, resulting in loss of arch length. This can be very rapid, particularly where there is a strong muscle sling from the lower lip.
- Whenever a primary second molar is lost prematurely, whether before or after the eruption of the permanent first molar, there will be a loss of arch length caused by the mesial drift of the permanent molar.
- Where arch length is adequate before loss of a primary first or second molar, a space maintainer should be fitted in order to preserve available space.

Space-maintaining devices

The best space maintenance therapy is the preservation of the primary molars until natural exfoliation. Although dental health education and improved caries prevention have lowered the number of children who develop malocclusion because of premature loss of primary teeth, it is still one of the most common controllable causes of malocclusion.

Types of space maintainers

Removable
- Removable space maintainers have the shortcomings of all removable appliances.
- They may be worn at the whim of the patient.
- May be broken.
- Easily lost when removed by the patient.
- A removable space maintainer that is only worn at night is often sufficient to hold space and prevent the mesial drift of permanent molars. Night-only wearing of the appliance also reduces the risk of loss or breakage by the patient. The appliance should be washed and inserted immediately before going to bed, then removed, washed and placed in a safe place when not worn.

Fixed appliances Fixed appliances have the advantage that they are worn continuously and their action cannot be affected by patient intervention.

It should be noted that the placement of a fixed appliance in a child at high risk of caries may compromise those teeth which are banded, or even adjacent teeth.

Common appliances
- Acrylic Hawley retainer.
- Band and loop (Figure 9.2).
- Distal shoe appliance.

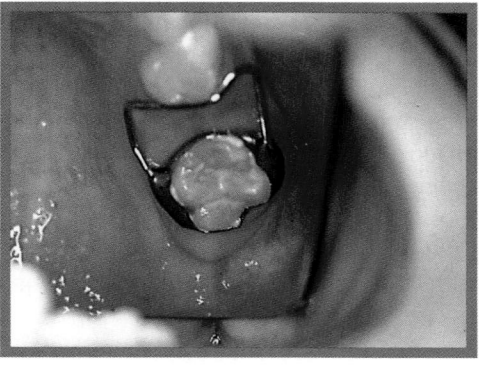

Figure 9.2 A band-and-loop space maintainer. The placement of a space maintainer must not compromise the permanent tooth. Bands should be cemented with a luting glass–ionomer as a protection against caries and the appliance reviewed regularly. As the premolar erupts, the appliance is removed when there is interference with normal emergence.

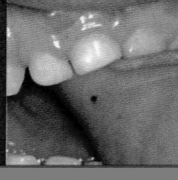

Regaining space

Space regaining is most successful where there is a dental and skeletal class-I pattern with normal vertical proportions. Where there is a class-II or class-III pattern with deep overbite or open bite, it is likely that space loss is not a simple dento-alveolar problem.

Radiographs and study models

These are essential aids in assessing space needs. It is important to note whether teeth have moved bodily into the space or have tipped as tipping mechanics is much easier to control than bodily tooth movement. Radiographic examination should also locate the permanent second molars and establish space available for distalization of the first permanent molars.

Premature loss

When a primary second molar is lost prematurely due to caries or to the ectopic eruption of the first permanent molar, the first permanent molar will drift mesially. This is most pronounced in the maxilla with a more rapid shift of the molar.

The earlier the loss of the second primary molar and the less the root development of the permanent molar, the greater will be the amount of bodily mesial shift of the permanent molar.

- Removable appliances are efficient in regaining spaces where uprighting of tilted permanent molars is required.
- Where bodily movement is needed, fixed appliances are used.

Thumb and finger sucking

One of the most common oral activities of the infant and young child is thumb and finger sucking. Sucking habits are perfectly normal in infancy. The infant will suck on any object brought into contact with the lips. This reflex behaviour lasts for the first several months of postnatal life. It is an adaptive reflex common to mammals.

Because it is a normal activity, thumb and finger sucking may be ignored in infancy. Thumb or finger sucking that is discontinued by age 2–3 years produces no permanent malformation of the jaws or displacement of the teeth. Continued beyond the time that the permanent incisor teeth erupt, it is almost always a factor in producing malocclusion in the anterior portion of the mouth.

- Children who begin thumbsucking again later in childhood often have underlying social or psychological problems.

Malocclusion from thumb sucking

- Anterior open bite.
- Protrusion of the upper incisor teeth.
- The lower incisor teeth may or may not be displaced by the abnormal sucking habit.
- Tendency for the tongue to perpetuate open bite with anterior tongue thrust. Protruding maxillary incisors and an anterior open bite favour the forward positioning of the tongue.
- Posterior cross-bite due to overactivity of buccinator compressing the maxilla.

Control of thumb or finger sucking (Figure 9.3)

Chemical means

The chemical therapy employs either hot-tasting, bitter-flavoured preparations or distasteful agents that are applied to the fingers or thumbs. Such things as cayenne pepper, quinine and asafetida have been used to make the thumb or fingers so distasteful that the child will keep them out of his mouth. These preparations are effective with a limited number of children, and only when the habit is not firmly entrenched.

Mechanical means

- A simple device for controlling thumb or finger sucking is the application of adhesive tape to the thumb or finger. In many instances this changes the character of the finger sufficiently to call the child's attention to the fact that it is being placed in the mouth.
- A Hawley appliance with a palatal bar may be fitted as a habit reminder. This is important because in many instances thumb and finger sucking habits are at the subconscious level of the individual's attention. Even though there may be some desire on the part of the child to discontinue the act, they may find it difficult to do so unless made aware when they are sucking the thumb or finger.
- Often the child will respond to simple encouragement and explanation of the effect of digit sucking on the teeth. The child's own desire to break the habit means they react positively to such encouragement.
- The critical time for the elimination of digit sucking is as the permanent incisors erupt. This generally coincides with entry into school, where peer pressure can be a powerful inducement to discontinue the habit.
- Psychological assessment is often beneficial in older children.

Congenitally absent teeth

Congenitally absent teeth are teeth that have not developed from the initiation stage of tooth development (see Chapter 7).

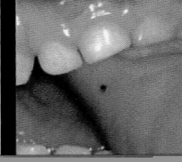

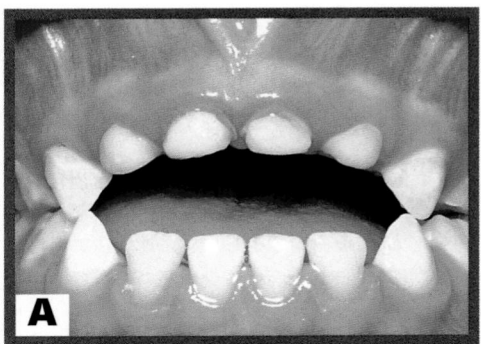
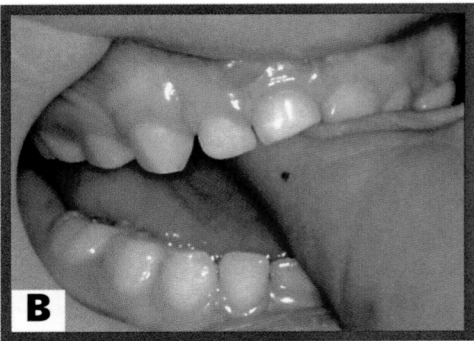

Figure 9.3 **A** An anterior open bite caused by a dummy sucking habit. Even a malocclusion of this size will improve once the habit has stopped and requires no active treatment. Notice the anterior teeth have been restored, due to nursing the caries associated with the dummy and a bottle at night. **B** Position of a thumb exerting orthopaedic as well as orthodontic forces.

Investigation

An understanding of the normal sequence and average age of eruption of permanent teeth will alert the practitioner to the possibility of congenital absence. Any delay in the normal eruption time of permanent teeth or exfoliation of primary teeth should be investigated radiographically. The panoramic film will provide the best view for investigation of premolars and molars but is often unclear in the incisor region because of the narrow focal trough. It may be necessary to supplement this with either periapical films or, in the maxilla, a vertex occlusal film.

A radiographic survey at age 5 years of age will demonstrate the presence or absence of all permanent teeth except for third molars. Third molars are generally not radiographically visible before the age of 9 years. Generally, a radiograph will show the tooth follicle before calcification begins, although there is a range in development time for second premolars between the presentation of the follicle and calcification commencing.

Management

Where a permanent tooth is diagnosed as congenitally absent, there are two choices in management:
- Retain the space after loss of the primary tooth and insert a prosthetic replacement.
- Orthodontically close the space.

Where premolars are absent the preferred method is the orthodontic closure of spaces; however, where a maxillary lateral incisor or a central incisor is absent a decision on whether to open a space or close a space depends on the skeletal balance between maxilla and mandible.

Class-III patterns Where the maxilla is proportionally smaller than the mandible there can be a dental cross-bite either anteriorly or posteriorly. Orthodontic correction will involve maxillary expansion, although it is extremely difficult to close spaces in the maxillary anterior segment without constricting the maxillary dental arch more than it would already be constricted.
- Prosthetic replacement of the absent incisor is usually the treatment of choice.

Class-II pattern This malocclusion is characterized by a smaller mandible with an increased overjet. The preferred option for a missing lateral incisor is to reduce the overjet by closing anterior spaces, placing the permanent canines in the position of the lateral incisors. Restorative techniques using resin veneers and acid-etch technology can be applied to reshape the canines as lateral incisors, restoring the anatomy of the substituted teeth and providing a balanced smile.
- Traumatic loss of a maxillary incisor can be treated orthodontically within the same guidelines as those for congenital absence of teeth.

Orthodontic aspects of supernumerary teeth

Development and aetiology
Location Supernumerary teeth may be found in any part of the dental arch; however, the most frequent sites are in the regions of the maxillary midline and the third molars. Tubercular and inverted supernumerary teeth are most often unerupted, and they commonly delay or inhibit the eruption of the central incisors. Because the supernumerary teeth develop late, they are not often found in the primary dentition and when they do develop with the primary teeth they usually erupt. Supernumerary teeth in the region of the lateral incisors, either in the primary or permanent dentition, usually erupt into the arch.

Orthodontic effects
Delay or failure of eruption The failure of a permanent tooth to erupt leads to malocclusion as adjacent teeth shift into the area that should be occupied by the permanent tooth. Moreover, the supernumerary tooth can be a cause of ectopic eruption of other teeth, producing a malocclusion.

Displacement of permanent teeth
- Rotation.
- Diastemas.
- Mesiodistal or labiolingual deflections.
- Axial malposition.
- Development of dentigerous cysts.
- Resorption of roots of adjoining teeth.

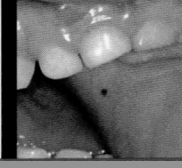

Treatment planning

- Even though supernumerary teeth may not produce a malocclusion, they should be removed as soon as possible after detection to avoid future problems.
- A supernumerary primary incisor may be retained if there is sufficient room for it. The tooth should be extracted when the permanent lateral incisor is ready to erupt.
- If there is an extra permanent lateral present with the primary supernumerary, it may be removed at the same time. Usually, the more distal of the two teeth is the supernumerary tooth.

Identification of a supernumerary tooth that is similar in form and size to the adjacent tooth can be made by comparing the teeth with those on the opposite side of the dental arch. The tooth that more closely resembles the size and shape the normal lateral incisor should be retained.

Timed extraction

The total amount of arch length deficiency is the key to planning of timed extractions. For this to be beneficial a cephalometric analysis should show the child to be growing within a normal pattern and that all the permanent teeth are present radiographically and in the normal order of eruption.

Canine extraction

- An arch length discrepancy of <4mm in the mandible can result in the loss of a primary canine as the lateral incisor erupts, and in midline shift to this side.
- The other primary canine should be removed and a fixed lingual arch appliance placed to support the incisors as the midlines correct themselves.
- As the permanent canines erupt it may be necessary to reduce the mesial of the primary first molars and then, as the first premolars erupt, reduce the mesial of the second primary molar.

Arch deficiency Where there is an arch deficiency of <4mm, serial extraction may be considered. The purpose of this treatment is to encourage the early eruption of the first premolars ahead of the permanent canines. The premolars are then removed, allowing room for the canines to erupt spontaneously.

Treatment stages in serial extraction

- First, the primary canines are removed to allow spontaneous alignment of the incisors.
- The primary first molars are removed to allow the eruption of the first premolars.

- Once the first premolars are erupted, they are removed and a space maintainer is issued to allow the permanent canines to erupt.
- Further orthodontic treatment is usually required to achieve correct root angulation and incisor torque.
- Well-aligned lower incisors.
- Thus serial extraction is a planned procedure which demands a minimum of 5 years' supervision by the dentist of the developing occlusion. Without such a commitment, the objectives will not be achieved and the patient may well be left worse off than before.

Indications
The following points are essential when considering a serial extraction programme:
- Class-I molar relationship.
- Class-I skeletal base.
- Minimal overbite, overjet or open bite.
- Radiographic and/or clinical evidence of all permanent teeth.

Contraindications to serial extraction
Serial extraction should not be performed in the following circumstances:
- Class-I malocclusions where the lack of space is slight and the teeth show only slight crowding.
- When there are permanent teeth congenitally absent from the dental arch.
- When there is a deep overbite or an open bite, these should be treated before undertaking serial extraction.
- Where there is a skeletal discrepancy in the dental arches.

Ectopic eruption of first permanent molars (Figure 9.4)

This can be an indication of an inadequate arch length, and a radiographic survey is required to confirm the presence of premolar teeth. The permanent teeth may resorb the distal margins of the second primary molars; this is more common in the maxilla.

Management
- Where there is impaction of the permanent molar against the distal of the second primary molar, disking of the primary molar will allow the spontaneous eruption of the permanent molar.
- Placement of orthodontic separators or brass ligature wire is usually difficult and uncomfortable, and has mixed success.
- Where the resorption of the primary molar is advanced, the loss of this tooth is indicated and space-regaining mechanics should be considered once the permanent molar has erupted.

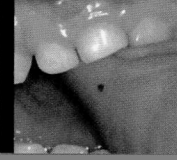

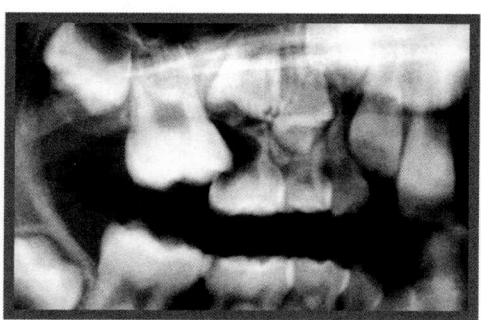

Figure 9.4 Ectopic eruption of the first permanent molars, causing resorption of the primary teeth. In this position, it is unlikely that the first permanent molars would erupt and space loss had already occurred. The primary molars were extracted and a space-regaining appliance constructed.

- Parents should be warned that further orthodontic treatment is usually required because of arch-length deficiencies.

Extraction of first permanent molars (Figure 9.5)

Gross caries involving the first permanent molars poses a difficult dilemma in treatment planning. The early presentation of the patient is essential in obtaining favourable results. The basic questions as to whether these teeth should be removed or restored are:
- What is the long-term prognosis for the tooth?
- Is it preferable to lose the tooth now or in 20 years time?
- What is the status of the pulp?
- Are the root apices fully formed?
- Are the third molars present?

General considerations
- The decision to extract is often best made in conjunction with an orthodontist.
- If the tooth is unrestorable no matter what the occlusion, then it should be removed. Even if successful root-canal therapy can be completed, the status of the crown is most important. Commonly, these teeth have extensive loss of tooth structure with only an enamel shell remaining.
- Non-vital, immature teeth have a poor prognosis. It is usually not indicated to perform a root-canal therapy on these teeth, especially as they would need an apexification procedure.
- If the upper molars are retained, a removable appliance such as a Hawley should be used to prevent over-eruption of these teeth before the eruption of the lower second molars.
- The ideal time for lower first permanent molar extraction is about the time of furcation calcification or before alveolar eruption of the second molar. These

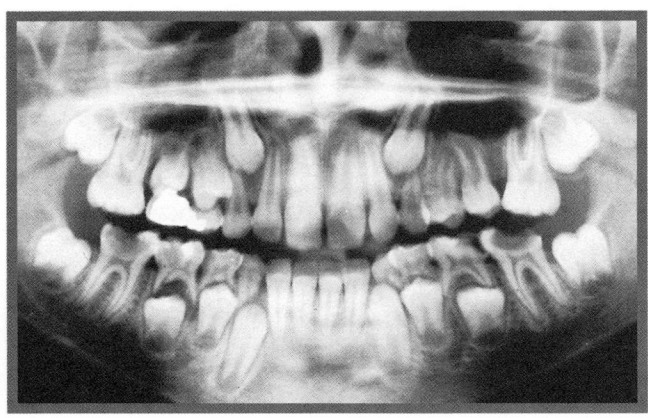

Figure 9.5 Gross caries affecting the lower first permanent molar teeth. Both teeth are necrotic and should be removed. This is a perfect time for extraction as the second molars will migrate mesially. The upper molars should be retained with a night-time removable appliance to prevent overeruption.

teeth will migrate mesially and assume the position of the first molar (Figure 9.6).
- If three molars are grossly carious and require removal it is probably better to keep the extractions symmetrical and extract all four teeth.

Timing of extractions

Although the timing of extractions will be determined in individual cases, some general rules should be followed if possible.

Class I (with no crowding)
- Extract all hopeless teeth as soon as possible.

Class I (crowding) or class II
- Extract lower teeth early.
- Retain upper molars until the second molars begin to erupt. The extraction space will close rapidly in the upper arch and this space will be required for anterior tooth retraction.

Class III
- Extract all hopeless teeth as soon as possible.

Extraction of over-retained primary teeth

The earlier one can recognize and remove over-retained primary teeth that may be causing ectopic eruption of a succedaneous tooth, the better the chance that a permanent tooth will erupt in a satisfactory position. The greatest damage that may result from over-retained primary teeth comes in the wake of ankylosed primary molars (Figure 9.6).

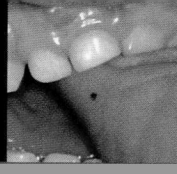

Diagnosis

The ankylosed primary molar may not be recognized in the very early stage. Its condition can readily be diagnosed a short time later because the vertical level of the occlusal surface of the ankylosed tooth becomes noticeably lower than the level of adjacent teeth, and as time progresses this difference in vertical level becomes more extreme.

Because ankylosed teeth seem to be submerging, they have been called 'submerged' teeth, but the term cannot be applied accurately to ankylosed teeth. It is more appropriate to call them 'engulfed' teeth. The continued vertical eruption of the uninvolved adjacent teeth and the vertical growth of the alveolar process and periodontium creates the illusion that the ankylosed tooth is submerging. The primary ankylosed molar may be totally engulfed by the continuing vertical growth of the jaw.

Management

- Ankylosed primary molars may be retained as long as they are maintaining arch length (i.e. preventing mesial shifting of the first permanent molars) or as long as they do not prevent the eruption of the succedaneous teeth (Figure 9.7).
- If there is evidence of root resorption these teeth will eventually be lost normally and there is no indication for early removal.
- The union between the cementum and dentine of the tooth and the bone of the alveolar process is physically strong and removal may require a surgical procedure, depending on how far the tooth has been submerged.
- A space-maintaining appliance must be used if the primary tooth is removed before the imminent eruption of the succedaneous tooth.

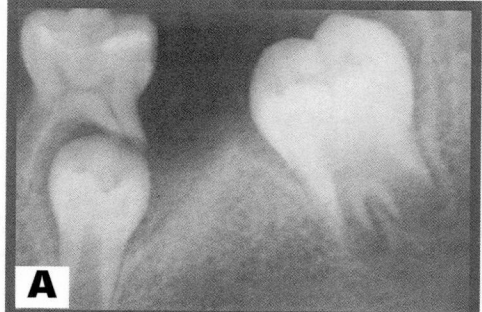
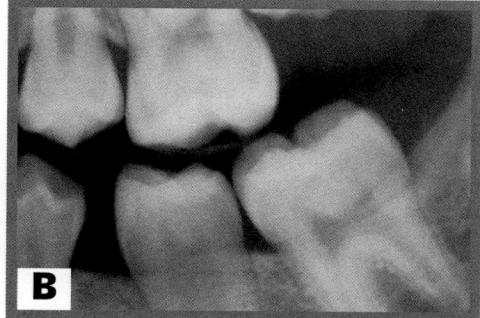

Figure 9.6 **A** The lower-left first permanent molar was extracted because of caries. **B** The second molar has migrated mesially into a good relationship without tipping. Note that there has been a degree of over-eruption of the opposing first permanent molar and some distal movement and rotation of the lower second premolar.

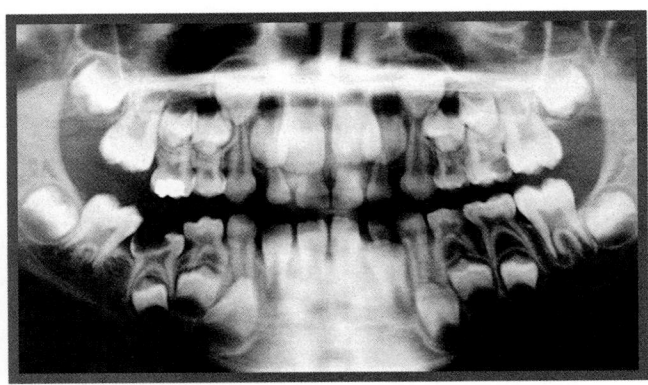

Figure 9.7 An ankylosed lower second primary molar in infra-occlusion. The tooth is subgingival and grossly carious. Surgical removal is indicated and a space maintainer should be inserted to prevent tipping of the first permanent molar.

- An over-retained tooth often accounts for the ectopic eruption, or impaction, of its succedaneous tooth; and because the ankylosed tooth is ultimately unable to withstand the mesial shifting of the first molar and the loss of arch length, the extraction of an ankylosed primary tooth is an effective means of practising interceptive–preventive orthodontics.

Basic requirements of orthodontic appliances

Appliance design
- Permit control of the degree, distribution, duration and direction of the force they exert.
- Be harmless to the oral tissues and not be adversely affected by oral secretions.
- Allow teeth and soft oral tissues to function normally.
- Allow wearer to maintain oral hygiene.
- Exert sufficient force or offer sufficient anchorage resistance to induce histological bone changes necessary for desired orthodontic tooth movement.
- Respond to the control of the operator.
- Allow movement of individual teeth or of groups of teeth in desirable directions.

Safety measures in appliance therapy
Appliances should be examined to see whether the bands are properly soldered, aligned and cemented in correct position to avoid undesirable movement of teeth, excessive plaque accumulation and unnecessary interruption of treatment. Arch wires should be examined for brittleness and unwanted crimping. Irritation of the mucous membranes can result from rough ends or arch wires. Small, smooth wires soldered to the lingual surface of bands afford a grip for the band remover and facilitate removal.

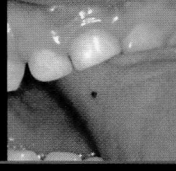

Removable appliances
Biteplanes

- Biteplanes used for tooth movement produce tipping. The tipping can be minimized, and in some cases the root will tend to follow the crown if the force in tooth movement is light. In some instances, by moving the crown of one tooth against that of the adjacent tooth and by applying spring force gingivally, an inclined tooth can be uprighted. Control of the axial inclination of teeth to be moved is an important consideration when they are moved by means of biteplanes.
- When incisor teeth are in protrusion a change of the position of the root is not required. The biteplane can be used with a flat plane to open the bite sufficiently to free interlocking cusps. Additionally, removal of the palatal acrylic and the placement of 3/8" labial elastics will effect the retraction of the incisors.

Springs

- Wire springs attached to plates should be cut to size when fitting the appliances in the mouth. The ends of the wire can then be rounded by adding a drop of solder or by turning the end of the spring on itself.
- Activation of springs for moving teeth should be a little less than half the width of the tooth to be moved.
- If the appliance is to be used for closing spaces in extraction cases, impressions should be taken and the appliance constructed before the extractions are performed.
- Distal movement of premolars can best be obtained by freeing the occlusal surfaces and by opening the bite so that the maxillary and mandibular teeth are slightly out of occlusion.
- Distal movement of molars can be performed with finger springs attached to a plate. Space closure in the mandible is not easily accomplished with a removable appliance, especially if there is a need for bodily movement of the mandibular incisors.

Retention While the use of biteplanes for tooth movement appears to be a simple form of treatment, retention is important, as is control of the axial position of the teeth. Removable appliances require exact knowledge of appliance manipulation, as do the fixed appliances. The use of a biteplane to correct excessive overbite frequently meets with failure when the correction of excessive overbite requires changes in the axial relations of the maxillary to the mandibular incisors. This cannot be accomplished easily with biteplanes.

Use of biteplane appliances

- Forward positioning of the head of the condyle of the mandible; repositioning the mandible, especially in young children when growth is active.
- Opening the bite and diminishing overjet of the anterior teeth.

- Elevation of the posterior teeth; the anterior teeth may be slightly depressed or both changes may occur.
- A more normal anteroposterior relationship of the occlusion.
- Retention after correction of disto-occlusion.
- As an aid in myofunctional therapy.
- Relieve locking of individual teeth or groups of teeth.
- Eliminate tongue habits, lip biting, thumb sucking and other deleterious habits.
- In class II, division 2 (angle) malocclusion the interference of the anterior and other teeth should be removed before the biteplane is used. Biteplanes should not be used where there is a tendency towards an open bite.
- To retain space when teeth are lost prematurely.
- With additional spring attachments, to move groups or individual teeth.
- For correcting the mesial position of the mandibular teeth in the primary dentition.

Most of the increase in face height following the use of Hawley-type biteplanes is caused by vertical increase in the posterior dental region, mostly in the maxillary posterior teeth. Increase in vertical dimension is also accompanied by change in the mandibular position.

Treatment of anterior and posterior crossbites

Anterior cross-bites (Figure 9.8)

Up to 10% of children present with cross-bites; there is a strong genetic component. There are three types of anterior cross-bites which may present in the mixed dentition.

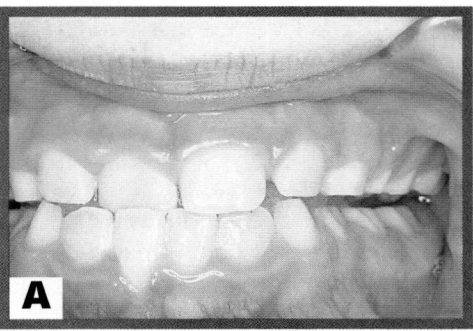
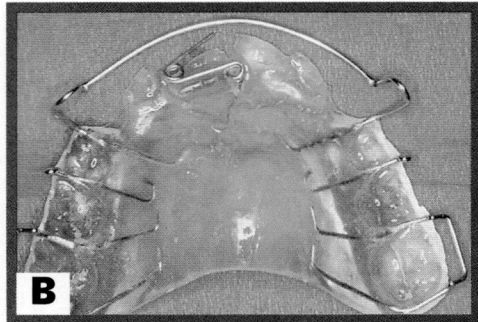

Figure 9.8 **A** Anterior dental cross-bite involving tooth 11. **B** Hawley appliance used to correct the malocclusion with Adams' cribs on the first permanent molars, ball retainers between the primary molars, posterior-bite planes and a labial bow. A Z-spring is activated approximately 2 mm to procline the incisor. The cross-bite was corrected within 4 weeks and was self-retaining because of the amount of overbite.

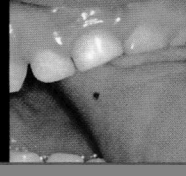

Ectopic incisors An incisor may erupt ectopically either palatally in the maxilla or labially in the mandible to a cross-bite relationship in centric occlusion. This may occur in a child with a balanced skeletal relationship.
- Early treatment is only necessary if there is a deviation on opening and or closing or if there is a traumatic occlusion or periodontal concern. Otherwise treatment can be delayed until the full permanent dentition erupts.

Skeletal class-III malocclusion An anterior cross-bite may be associated with a skeletal class-III discrepancy such that, although the incisors are positioned correctly within the alveolar ridges, they are in negative overjet on closing into centric occlusion with no deviation of mandibular closure.

Pseudo class-III malocclusion This pattern occurs where there is an habitual mandibular closure pattern such that the mandible goes into a protrusive bite and thus cross-bite of incisors avoiding traumatic occlusion with lingual position of one or more maxillary incisors. Thus anterior shift of the mandible can affect the growth of both the maxilla and the mandible with undesirable muscle adaptation.

Management
Incline planes
- Where there is a functional shift of the mandible into an anterior cross-bite, an acrylic inclined plane can be fitted to the lower incisors to restrict the forward posturing and place pressure on the palatal of the maxillary incisors to push them labially.
- Treatment is usually complete within 1 month. This appliance works best where there is a slight increase in overbite, which helps to retain the incisors in positive overjet once the appliance is removed.

Tongue blade technique Where the cross-bite is minimal and retention favourable, this technique may be used. Good patient cooperation is required but this technique can be an effective and cheap method of cross-bite correction.
- A disposable tongue depressor or ice-cream stick is placed lingual to the upper incisor tooth in cross-bite, and the patient is instructed to close the lower incisor teeth firmly against the blade.
- The blade is guided downwards and backwards against the lower lip and the chin, making sure that firm biting pressure is maintained.
- Holding the tongue depressor blade in this position and biting firmly against it, the patient is instructed to count slowly to 30. As with all removable appliances the more frequent the activation, the more effective the movement of the teeth.
- Both the patient and the parents are advised that if the tongue blade is used in the proper fashion the teeth will become tender after the first day of use, but that in spite of this it needs to be carried out daily. If the exercise is

discontinued for a day or two until the teeth are more comfortable, all prior progress will be lost.
- Correction of a simple incisor cross-bite is often complete within a few days but the patient should be reviewed every week.

Removable appliances
- A modified Hawley appliance can be used in the maxilla to correct one or two teeth in cross-bite.
- Occlusal surfaces of both the primary and permanent molars should be covered to open the bite and allow free labial movement of the teeth in cross-bite.
- Adam clasps are placed on the first permanent molars with a labial arch wire.
- If the primary molars are present, ball-ended clasps can be fabricated to engage the interproximal areas of these teeth.
- Where a single tooth is in cross-bite, a Z-spring placed palatally to the malposed tooth can be used, or if both central incisors are in cross-bite, two springs can be used to provide sweep arms on the palatal surface. Initially, the appliance should be fitted and checked for comfort with the springs passive. The springs are then activated one-half of the distance to be moved. The patient is reviewed after 4 weeks to reactivate the springs as required and to check the retention of the appliance.
- As with all removable appliances the success of treatment is reliant on cooperation and compliance. If these qualities can be encouraged and the patient takes responsibility for the wearing of the appliance, treatment will progress satisfactorily.

Fixed appliances Fixed appliances can be used when two or more incisors are in cross-bite.
- Brackets are bonded to the incisors with bands cemented to the first permanent molars.
- A labial arch of 0.016 round wire is used with vertical loop stops mesial to the molar tubes. These loops are expanded to procline the incisors, and the round wire permits labial tilting of the incisors to correct the cross-bite.
- Where the incisor cross-bite is a combination of palatal inclination of maxillary incisors and labial inclination of the lower incisors, fixed appliances can be used in both upper and lower arches on the incisors and first permanent molars.
- Class-III elastics (from maxillary molars to mandibular canines) can be used. The elastics need to be worn 24 hours per day, except for tooth brushing, and replaced every 3–4 days. This appliance will provide rapid correction of the cross-bite within 6 months.
- Retention with a removable appliance should follow for at least 6 months.

Posterior cross-bites
A posterior cross-bite is an abnormal, buccolingual relationship of a tooth or teeth when the two dental arches are brought into centre occlusion. There are three types of posterior cross-bites.

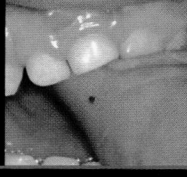

Dental cross-bite A dental cross-bite involves only the tilting of teeth.

Muscular cross-bite A muscular cross-bite involves a mandibular shift with muscle adaptations as a result of the tooth interferences.

Osseous cross-bite An osseous cross-bite is related to skeletal discrepancies between maxilla and mandible.

Insufficient arch length or prolonged retention of primary teeth can deflect teeth during eruption and produce a cross-bite. Prolonged thumb and finger sucking has also been implicated in the narrowing of the maxillary arch with molar cross-bites. This is also a regular presentation in patients with cerebral palsy.

Management

Posterior cross-bites should be treated as early as possible to allow normal growth and development of the dental arches and temperomandibular joints. When planning treatment it is important to determine whether the cross-bite is unilateral or bilateral.

The majority of cross-bites are bilateral but often present as unilateral when the teeth are in full intercuspal position. In these cases the dental midlines will not be coincident on closing and there will be a deviation of the mandible towards one side at the end on closing.

When the teeth are closed with the dental midlines coincident, the posterior segments will be in an edge-to-edge, buccolingual position, reflecting the overall constriction of the maxillary dental arch, and bilateral maxillary expansion is indicated.

Cross-elastics When only a single molar is in cross-bite, this can often be corrected with a bonded attachment, button or hook, to the palatal of the maxillary and buccal of the lower molar.
- An elastic is stretched between these teeth; it is worn 24 hours per day and changed every time it breaks (which is often).
- Cross-bites will normally correct within 3–4 months with continuous wearing of the elastic. The major change will be reflected in the position of the maxillary molar because of the cancellous nature of the maxillary alveolar bone as against the denser bone around the mandibular molar.

Removable appliances A true unilateral posterior cross-bite to two teeth can be corrected with a removable appliance with a jackscrew offset in the palate.
- This appliance relies on good retention using Adam cribs.
- The screw is activated one-quarter turn each week.
- Where the jackscrew is central over the midpalatal suture, such an appliance can also be used for bilateral expansion of dental arches. With both these appliances the correction is dental only, the major component of tooth movement being a tipping only.

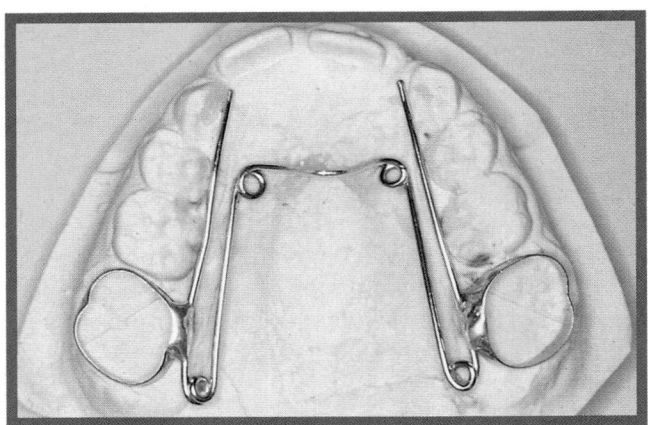

Figure 9.9 Quad helix used to correct posterior cross-bites in the mixed dentition. These appliances are simple to construct, are well tolerated by the patient and are efficient. They have the advantage that they are fixed and will also act as retainers once the malocclusion is corrected.

Fixed appliances (Figure 9.9) Fixed appliances may be directed at dental or orthopaedic correction, involving splitting of the midpalatal suture.
- A quad helix appliance soldered to molar bands cemented to the first permanent molar provides predictable dental correction.
- This appliance requires little cooperation from the parents or patients (apart from avoiding sticky foods) in that activation is controlled by the dentist.
- After activation, the patient is seen each 4 weeks with the appliance removed, expanded and recemented at alternate appointments.
- The expansion should continue until the molars are overcorrected, then retained with the same appliance for a further 3 months. The cross-bite is usually corrected within 4–6 months, with a further 3 months for retention.

Rapid maxillary expansion This involves the splitting of the midpalatal suture and produces an orthopaedic increase in maxillary width.
- The appliance uses a midpalatal screw (Hyrax) soldered to bands on the first permanent molars, primary molars or premolars. In contrast to the removable appliance, the screw is activated a quarter turn twice each day and the patient should be monitored once a week.
- As the expansion proceeds, a diastema will show between the central incisors, reflecting the splitting of the midpalatal suture. This will close as the bone remodels and the parents and patients should be warned of this. As with a quad helix, the cross should be overcorrected and retained in this position for at least 3 months with the same appliance.

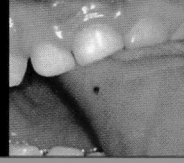

References

Crowding

BECKER A, KURNEI-R'EM RM. The effects of infra occlusion: Part I. Tilting of the adjacent teeth and local space loss. *Am J Orthod Dentofac Orthop* 1992, **102**:256–264.

IRWIN RD, HEROLD JS, RICHARDSON A. Mixed dentition analysis: a review of methods and their accuracy. *Int J Paediatr Dent* 1995, **5**:137–142.

MOORRES CFA, CHADHA JM. Available space for the incisors during dental development: a growth study based on physiological age. *Angle Orthod* 1965, **35**:12–22.

PAPANDREAS SG, BUSCHANG PH. Physiologic drift of the mandibular dentition following first pre-molar extractions. *Angle Orthod* 1993, **63**:127–134.

Digit sucking

LARSEN E. The effect of dummy sucking on the occlusion: a review. *Eur J Orthod* 1987, **8**:127–130.

MITCHELL EA, TAYLOR BJ, FORD RP, STEWART AW, BECROFT DM, THOMPSON JM, SCRAGG R. Dummies and the Sudden Infant Death Syndrome. *Arch Dis Child* 1993, **68**:501–504.

OULIS CJ, VADIAKAS GP, EKONOMIDES J, DRATSA J. The effect of hypertrophic adenoids and tonsils on the development of posterior cross-bite and oral habits. *J Clin Pediatr* Dent 1994, **18**:197–201.

Timed extraction

GIANELLY AA. Crowding: timing of treatment. *Angle Orthod* 1994, **64**:415–418.

JACOBS S. A reassessment of serial extraction. *Aust Orthod J* 1987, 10:90–96.

JACOBS SG. Reducing the incidence of palatally impacted maxillary canines by extraction of deciduous canines. A useful preventive/interceptive orthodontic procedure. *Aust Dent J* 1992, **37**:6–11.

LITTLE RM. The effects of eruption guidance and serial extraction on the developing dentition. *Pediatr Dent* 1987, **9**:65–70.

MACKIE IC, BLINKHORN AS, DAVIES PHJ. The extraction of permanent molars during the mixed-dentition period—a guide to treatment planning. *J Paediatr Dent* 1989, **5**:85–92.

Treatment timing

COUTINHO S, BUSCHANG PH, MIRANDA F. Relationship between mandibular canine calcification stages and skeletal maturity. *Am J Orthod Dentofac Orthop* 1993, **104**:262–268.

BOLTON WA. The clinical application of a tooth–size analysis. *Am J Orthod* 1962, **48**:504–529.

Ectopic eruption

BREARLEY LJ, MCKIBBEN DH. Ankylosis of primary molar teeth. I Prevalence and characteristics. *J Dent Child* 1973, **40**:54–63.

ERICSON S, KUROL J. Early treatment of palatally impacted maxillary canines by extraction of the primary canines. *Eur J Orthod* 1989, **10**:283–295.

PROFFIT WR, VIG KWL. Primary failure of eruption. *Am J Orthod* 1981, **80**:173–190.

Appliances
BISHARA SE, ZIAJA RR. Functional appliances: a review. *Am J Orthod* Dentofac Orthop 1989, **95**:250–258.

Maxillary expansion
BISHARA SE, STALEY RN. Maxillary expansion: clinical implications. *Am J Orthod Dentofac Orthop* 1987, **91**:3–14.
HENRY RJ. Slow maxillary expansion: A review of quad helix therapy during the transitional dentition. *J Dent Child* 1993, **606**:408–413.
THILANDER B, WAHLUND S, LENNARTSON B. The effect of early interceptive treatment in children with posterior x-bite. *Eur J Orthod* 1984, **6**:25–34.

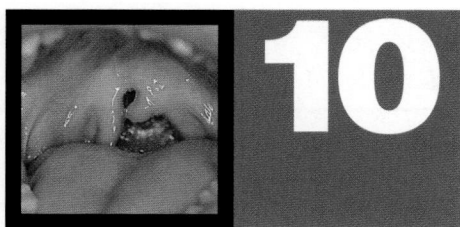

10 Management of cleft lip and palate

Contributors

Tissa Jayasekera, Roger Hall, Sandy Lopacki

Introduction

Cleft palate, with or without cleft lip, is one of the more common congenital malformations in humans. Although many factors have been associated with this condition, from a practical preventive aspect, the aetiology remains undetermined. Reported incidence has varied from 1 out of 600 to 1 out of 800 live births in Caucasians, with a relatively higher incidence in orientals and lower incidence in blacks. The offspring of patients with a cleft lip have an increased risk, of 1 in 20, of having a clefting condition. If other siblings or close relatives also have clefts the frequency is 1 in 6 (Bixler, 1981).

More recent Scandinavian studies have claimed to show a rise in incidence of the cleft condition. The authors have proposed several contributory factors such as decreased neonatal mortality, the use of some medications during pregnancy (e.g. retinoic acids) and an increase in intermarriage and childbirth in people with cleft conditions.

Children with clefting conditions will require extensive interdisciplinary medical care throughout early life, involving plastic surgery, maxillofacial or craniofacial surgery, dentistry (paediatric dental, orthodontic and oral surgical care, etc.), ear nose and throat surgery, audiology, speech therapy, psychology and in some cases ophthalmology and neurosurgery. The highest standards of oral health must be maintained for these patients. Intact primary and permanent dentitions will permit optimal orthodontic and surgical treatment, maximising long-term results.

The anatomy of the facial skeleton in cleft lip and palate

The presentation of clefting conditions can be categorized into the following groups:

Clefts of the lip and alveolus (primary palate)

These may vary from a minimal defect involving just the vermilion border to a complete defect extending from the vermilion border to the floor of the nose and clefting the alveolus. The primary palate forms anterior to the incisive foramen. The defect may also exist as a submucous cleft in the muscle band of the upper lip bridged only by mucosa, skin and fibrous connective tissue (Figure 10.1A).

The nasal alar cartilage on the side of the cleft is displaced and flattened to a greater or lesser degree, depending on the extent and width of the cleft. The tip of the nose tends to deviate to the non-cleft side.

The cleft may be unilateral or bilateral, and the latter may be symmetrical or asymmetrical in extent. In bilateral clefts the median portion of the lip contains the philtrum and is attached to the columella and the premaxilla. In humans, except for a brief period in the early embryo, the premaxilla does not exist as a separate entity. The term is retained with reference to cleft lip and palate conditions, however, because of its descriptive convenience and homology with experimental animals. The term 'premaxilla', therefore, refers to that portion of the maxilla anterior to the incisive foramen and mesial to the canine teeth. In bilateral complete clefts of the lip and alveolus, the premaxilla protrudes considerably forward of the facial profile. It is attached to a stalk-like vomer and the nasal septum. The columella appears deficient and the alar cartilages are flattened on both sides.

Cleft lip and cleft palate

Clefts of the lip and palate may be unilateral or bilateral, complete or incomplete.

Unilateral cleft lip and palate Varying degrees of clefting in the lip and palate can exist, in a wide range of combinations. In complete clefts a direct communication exists between the oral and nasal cavities on the cleft side (Figure 10.1A). There can be substantial variation in the degree of palatal shelf separation.

Premaxillary segment and nasal septum The premaxillary segment in the frontal view tilts upwards into the cleft. The cartilaginous nasal septum is also bent in the same direction. The nostril on the non-cleft side is constricted and may be functionally occluded. This constriction is caused by a combination of deviation of the nasal septum and approximation of the alar base and columella. The alar of the cleft side is usually stretched and flattened.

The lip and columella The anatomy of the orbicularis oris muscle is disrupted. The muscle fibres proceed horizontally from the corner of the mouth towards the midline and turn upwards along the margins of the cleft. The muscle fibres terminate beneath the alar base in the lateral segment and beneath the columella in the medial segment. Most fibres attach to the periosteum of the maxilla, but a few blend into the subepithelium. Where the cleft is less than two-thirds of the lip height, the muscle fibres above the level of the cleft remain intact. A protrusion of excess muscle may be seen and palpated on the lateral aspect of the cleft, due to heaping up of the disrupted fibres. The medial segment tends to be underdeveloped.

Vomer and palatal process The palatal segment on the cleft side is often tilted medially and superiorly into the cleft. The vomer is deviated laterally at its line of

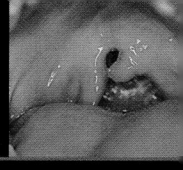

attachment to the palatal process of the non-cleft side. This deviation may be so severe in some cases that the vomer assumes a nearly horizontal position at its inferior margin.

Bilateral cleft lip and palate

Clefting can be either symmetrical or asymmetrical. In the bilateral complete cleft lip and palate both nasal chambers are in direct communication with the oral cavity. The palatal processes are divided into two equal parts and the turbinates are clearly visible within both nasal cavities. The nasal septum forms a midline structure that is firmly attached to the base of the skull but is fairly mobile anteriorly, where it supports the premaxilla and columella (Figure 10.1B).

Premaxilla There is a malformation of the premaxilla characterized by its protrusion relative to the nasal septum. The columella is usually non-existent, the lip attaching directly to the nasal tip. The basal bone of the premaxilla articulates with the cartilaginous nasal septum superiorly and the vomer posteriorly. In normal structure the alveolar process of the premaxilla is inferior to the basal component. However, in the bilateral cleft condition the alveolar component is anterior to the basal component, in horizontal arrangement.

The lip and columella The lip moiety in the medial segment contains only collagenous connective tissue. It is, therefore, grossly deficient in bulk and lacks the features normally produced by muscle (Figure 10.1C).

Although the columella would appear to be absent clinically, in anatomical terms it may be present in that the medial crura of the alar cartilages appear to occupy a normal position relative to the tip of the nose and the nasal septum. There is a deficiency of columellar skin, however, which complicates the re-establishment of normal anatomical relations during treatment.

The maxillary arch form generally appears normal at birth, but medial collapse of the maxillary segments occurs soon afterwards. The medial aspect of the palatal processes is often tilted superiorly into the cleft.

Cleft palate

The cleft may involve only the soft palate or both soft and hard palates, but almost never the hard palate alone. The cleft may extend forward from the uvula to varying degrees, from a bifid uvula (Figure 10.3) to a 'V'-shaped cleft extending through the hard palate to the incisive foramen. Deficiency of mucosa and bone is the main feature of clefts of the hard palate (Figure 10.2).

In the soft palate, deficiency of mucosa is combined with shortening of the velar musculature, which has abnormal sites of insertion. Submucous clefts of both soft and hard palate can also occur to varying degrees. In these cases the mucosa is intact, but deficiency of bone or muscle exists (Figure 10.3).

291

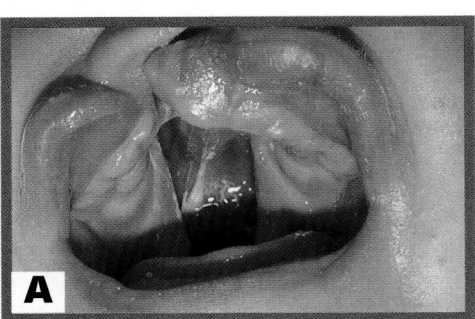
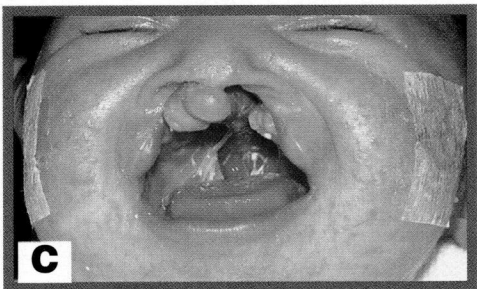
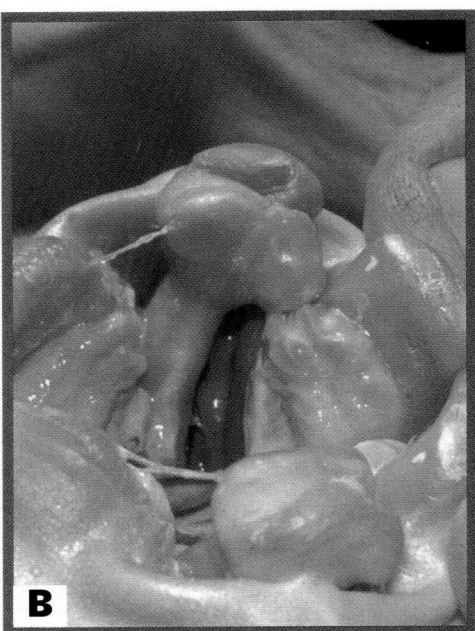

Figure 10.1 **A** Unilateral complete cleft lip and palate, showing the extent of the malformation in the palate. **B** Bilateral complete cleft lip and palate. The premaxillary segment is clearly visible as an extension of the nasal septum. The central incisors are contained within this process. **C** Anterior view of a child with a bilateral complete cleft of the lip and palate. The columella and philtrum are extremely short and there is a wide defect between the segments.

Dental anomalies

Dental anomalies are extremely common in children with orofacial clefting. The most commonly affected tooth is the maxillary lateral incisor on the cleft side. This is caused, in part, by disruption of the dental lamina. Anomalies may include:
- Agenesis of teeth.
- Supernumerary teeth.
- Concurrent agenesis and supernumerary teeth within or adjacent the cleft.
- Disorders of morphogenesis (size and shape).

Supernumeraries are customarily termed 'fissural teeth'. They may occur in either the medial or distal segment and much less frequently in both segments (Figure 10.4).

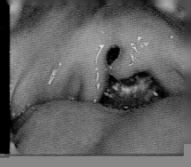

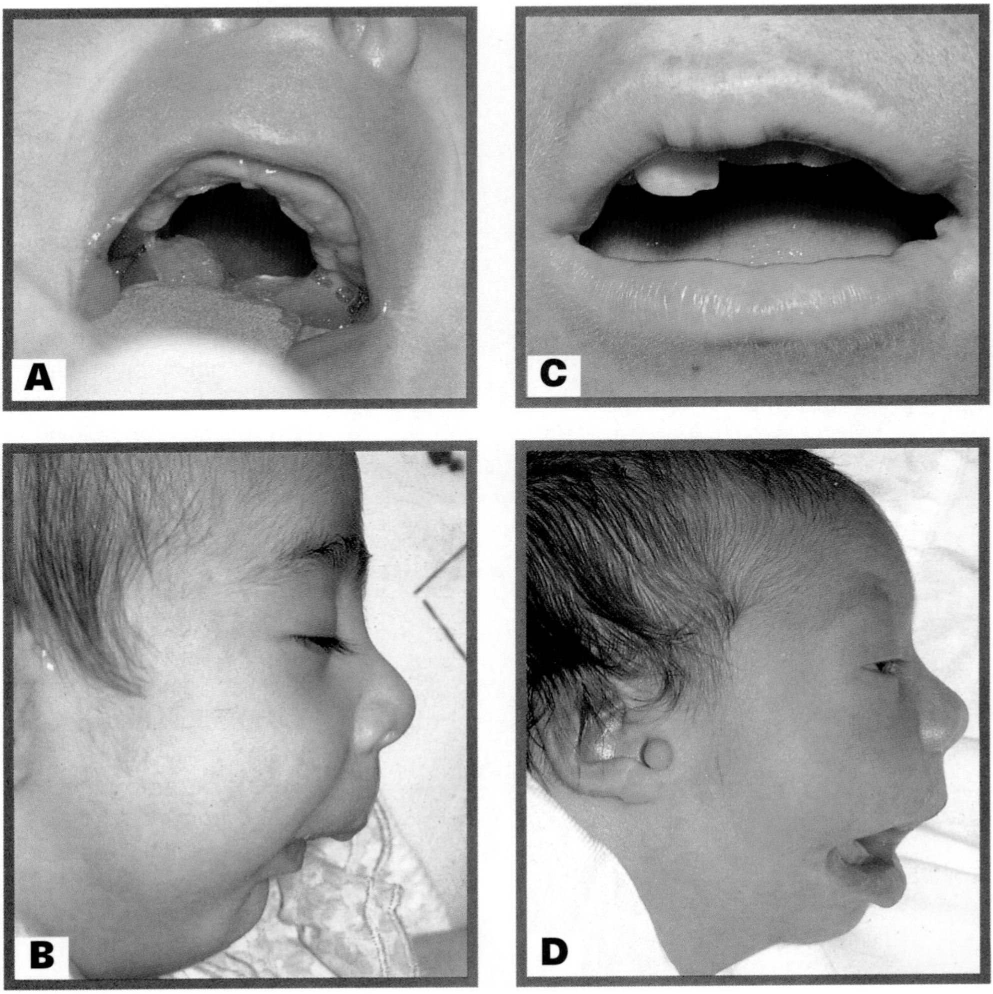

Figure 10.2 **A** Cleft of the palate with an intact lip and alveolus. This U-shaped cleft was associated with the Pierre Robin sequence and resulted from a failure of embryonic head rotation. This maintained the tongue in the oral cavity and the palatal shelves subsequently formed around the tongue giving rise to the characteristic cleft shape. **B** Another manifestation of this condition is extreme micrognathia. The Robin sequence may also be associated with transverse clefts of the face. These transverse clefts may be rather subtle as demonstrated in patient **C**, or severe as in **D**. This latter patient has a first and second branchial-arch deformity associated with Goldenhar syndrome. Note the pre-auricular skin tag.

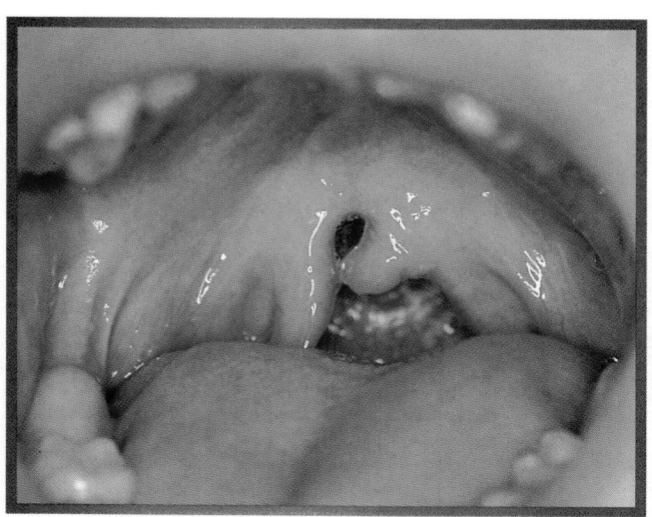

Figure 10.3 A bifid uvula associated with a submucous cleft palate. The fibres of tensor palati are not joined although the epithelium is intact. These children may present with nasal air escape caused by a shortened palate and velopharyngeal incompetence. There is often a notch felt at the posterior border of the hard palate and a bluish median line extends to the uvula.

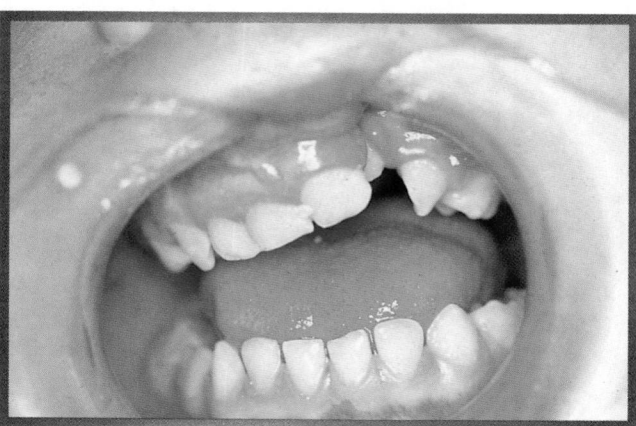

Figure 10.4 A supernumerary tooth erupting in the cleft. Such teeth often become carious, but should be retained until bone grafting is performed. Where permanent teeth are congenitally absent, especially the lateral incisor, the supernumerary may be used if of adequate size.

Current concepts of cleft management

The need for treatment
- Facial aesthetic appeal.
- Feeding difficulties caused by poor oral seal and nasal reflux.
- Severe speech problems associated with poor pharyngeal seal or oronasal communication.
- Chronic middle ear problems caused by poor Eustachian tube function.

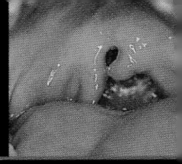

It is of interest that general growth of the maxilla and midface does not appear to be adversely affected in cleft patients left untreated until physical maturity.

The cleft palate team Treatment is generally undertaken in a coordinated 'team' environment. Cleft palate teams are located in the major paediatric hospitals throughout the world. The cleft palate team comprises:

- Plastic surgeons.
- Paediatric dentists.
- Orthodontists.
- Speech pathologists.
- Maxillofacial surgeons.
- Ear, nose and throat surgeons.
- Social workers.
- Other specialists, such as geneticists, who are consulted as required in individual cases.

There appear to be as many variations in technique, sequencing and timing of treatment as there are cleft palate teams. There are, however, some commonly accepted aims and principles of treatment.

Aims of cleft treatment

The ultimate goal is to attain normal form and function (especially speech and mastication) with the least possible damage to growth and development through surgical intervention.

Specific treatment objectives are:

- Provide a long mobile palate capable of completely closing off the oropharynx from the nasopharynx.
- Produce a full upper lip with a symmetrical cupid's bow and reconstruction of the columella and the alar architecture of the nose.
- Achieve an intact, well-aligned dental arch with a stable inter-arch occlusion.

Importance of dental care in overall management

Children with clefting conditions will require extensive interdisciplinary medical care throughout early life and the highest standard of oral health must be maintained for these patients. The presence of dental disease severely compromises both surgical and orthodontic success.

Patient referral

All patients with facial and jaw anomalies should be referred to a cleft palate clinic for multidisciplinary care. Although definitive care may not be provided by this particular team (depending on how close the child lives to the cleft centre), advice can be given on coordinated treatment through childhood and adolescence.

Initial consultation

Examination of baby The baby is examined and a record made of the type of cleft or other deformity present and the relation of the lip, alveolar and palatal clefts (i.e. arch form etc.), with a note of any overriding of segments, distortion of premaxilla, etc. Any erupted teeth are charted and a note made of any natal or neonatal teeth in the cleft or other regions.

The parent interview If the parents are not present when the baby is examined, a separate appointment must be made with them. The parent interview is one of the most important aspect of the initial consultation.

The approach in speaking to parents at this consultation should be relaxed and informative—a mostly 'getting to know you' introduction of the dental team as a preparation for later visits. It must be remembered that because of the emotional impact of the facial abnormality on the mother, father and family, they may not be fully receptive to advice at this early visit or remember much of what is said. At this interview it is important to explain:

- The dental aspects of the clefting process.
- The likely course of dental management. The involvement of different specialties, including restorative, radiological, orthodontic and possible later oral surgical care.
- The probability of the absence of the normal tooth in the region of the cleft, and the presence of one or more supernumerary teeth instead in the cleft region should be mentioned.
- The likelihood of the presence of crown and root morphological abnormalities

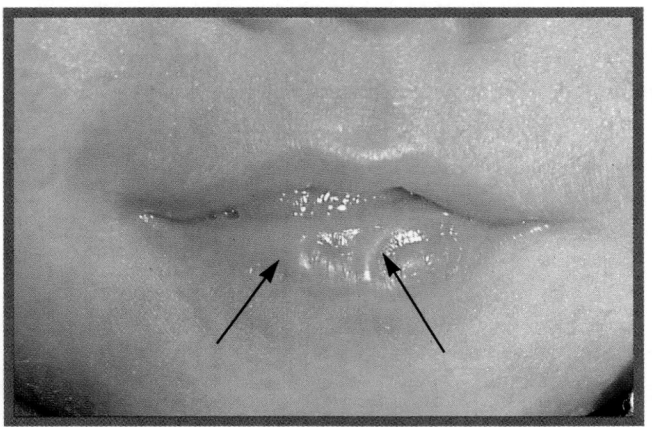

Figure 10.5 There are over 50 syndromes of the head and neck which manifest clefting. Congenital lip pits (arrowed) although uncommon are an important malformation associated with clefting of the palate.

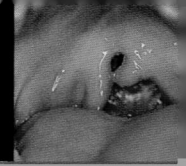

and enamel hypoplasia of the incisor and canine teeth adjacent to the cleft should be indicated with the positive reassurance that these can be treated relatively simply soon after they appear.
- The absolute importance of sound preventive care and regular dental visits should be emphasized.

It will almost certainly be necessary to reinforce the introductory information and advice given at this visit at many subsequent outpatient visits over the years of treatment. Many cleft palate clinics produce parent handbooks which are particularly useful.

Medical history A full medical history must be conducted at this time. Many clefts are merely one component in one of the 50 clefting syndromes—and it is common for other congenital abnormalities to be present in addition to the cleft (e.g. congenital heart disease).

Dental records
- Photographs should be taken at all major review visits.
- Dental impressions should be taken by the paediatric dentist, or the plastic surgeon under general anaesthesia before the lip repair.
- An initial screening panoramic radiograph is useful at 5–6 years of age (or earlier if pathology is present or suspected).
- All children should have study models and panoramic dental radiographs and lateral cephalometric radiographs at 8–9 years of age.

Role of the paediatric dentist
The role of the paediatric dentist is one of coordinator. Between the ages of 12 and 18 months the child should be seen by the paediatric dentist at regular intervals no greater than 12 months. In Australia the child is enrolled in the Cleft Palate Scheme at the first visit. This scheme provides government health benefits to pay for orthodontic, surgical and some general dental treatment. Parental support groups such as Cleft Pals are present in many countries and contact should be arranged as soon as possible with these organizations.

First follow-up visit
- Dental charting is carried out, including a record of the time of eruption of the first tooth.
- Body growth should be checked and height/weight entered on a growth chart. Details can be obtained from the child's Health Record Book.

These visits are essential for the general monitoring of growth and development and the control of dental disease. Updating of photographic, study model and radiological records will also be done. The paediatric dentist will generally coordinate all dental care aspects with those of other disciplines.

Preventive dental care

Preventive dental care is essential for these patients using all known techniques including:

- Toothbrushing.
- Home self-application of topical fluoride.
- Fissure sealing of both primary and permanent teeth.
- Oral hygiene technique instruction.
- Dietary advice to child and parents by paediatric dentist (or dietitian if necessary).

The prevention of dental caries and periodontal disease will help with cooperation for ultimate definitive orthodontic treatment, by reducing unpleasant visits for treatment in early childhood. Motivation is especially important for later orthodontic treatment in these patients. This should be assessed early, and enhanced during preventive visits during childhood.

General dental practitioner care

The role of the general practitioner is paramount. Children with craniofacial anomalies have significantly greater rates of dental disease, all of which is preventable and will affect the prognosis and course of future treatment. The child should if possible attend a general dental practitioner at 6-monthly intervals for preventive care, dietary advice and oral hygiene technique follow-up, together with routine restorative care if necessary. The parents should agree to attend the local dentist regularly. One of the most important duties is to establish early contact with the cleft palate team or surgeon and maintain a frequent dialogue.

Dental extractions and minor oral surgery

- Except in an emergency, dental extractions should not be done for these children by the general dentist without first checking and clearing this with the supervising paediatric dentist or orthodontist.
- Primary molars should be retained by pulpotomy, or the space maintained after extraction as advised by the paediatric dentist.
- Erupted supernumerary teeth should be retained until 6 or 7 years of age, unless impossible to clean, resulting in progressive dental caries, gingival or mucosal inflammation.

Extraction of such teeth should then, in most cases, be carried out in the supervising hospital either under local or general anaesthesia. If general anaesthesia is required superficial or obstructing unerupted supernumerary teeth may be removed at the same time, but only after discussion with the coordinating paediatric dentist. If a bone graft is planned for the alveolar cleft, the paediatric dentist coordinator may advise retaining unerupted supernumerary teeth, especially if it is one of the permanent tooth series. This tooth is removed by the maxillofacial or plastic surgeon at the time of bone grafting.

 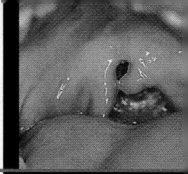
Cosmetic restoration of malformed anterior teeth and alveolar cleft

The appearance of the teeth should be improved early for affected children, who may have a poor self-image.

- Enamel-bond crowning or veneering should be carried out for hypoplastic or morphologically abnormal permanent incisor teeth adjacent to the cleft(s) as soon as they are sufficiently erupted.
- Even though a temporary measure, in suitable cases an acid-etch bridge may be constructed to temporarily fill the cleft space in the dental arch, until the primary teeth retaining it are shed or until orthodontic treatment of permanent teeth commences. This fixed bridge should now be used whenever possible in preference to a removable partial denture. Speech may also be helped by the use of fixed prosthodontics.

Surgical management

Surgical management can be divided into four steps:

Primary lip repair

Generally undertaken at 10–12 weeks of life, provided the infant is otherwise developing well (Figure 10.6).

Closure of soft and hard palate defect

The extent and timing of palatal surgery is one of the major and continuing controversies in cleft management; they relate to the perceived balance between the benefits of good speech development versus the deleterious effects on mid-facial growth through surgical trauma and associated scarring. 'Early' closure is generally carried out between 6 and 18 months of age, depending on the institution, before the development of speech. Some centres carry out soft palate closure

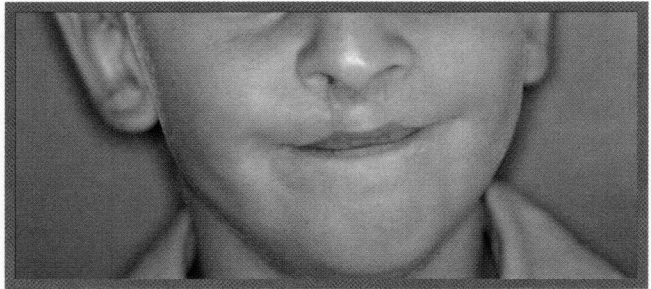

Figure 10.6 Surgical repair of a bilateral complete cleft lip with columella lengthening. The alar base is symmetrical although there is an accentuation of the cupid's bow and a eversion of the vermilion border.

'early' or even at the time of primary lip repair, but delay closure of the hard palate until age 4–5 years. An obturator is used in the interim period for these cases.

Alveolar bone grafting

The aim of bone grafting is to restore the bony contour of the alveolus and stabilize the maxillary expansion. It also provides a matrix through which teeth (especially the canine) may erupt. The grafting material of choice is autologous iliac crest cortico-cancellous bone. Cortico-cancellous bone from the calvarium and chin is also frequently used. The procedure may include revision of lip and/or palate repair if necessary, and will definitively close any remaining fistulae.

Although some centres advocate bone grafting of the maxillary alveolar defect at the time of primary lip repair, the majority of teams do this as a secondary procedure, either 'early', before the eruption of the permanent lateral incisor, or later, before eruption of the permanent canine tooth. The object here is to have these teeth erupting through and consolidating the bone graft (Figure 10.7).

Orthognathic surgery

If a maxillary/mandibular skeletal discrepancy exists at physical maturity an osteotomy may be required along with any further soft tissue revision that is also undertaken at the same time if needed.

Between these surgical 'milestones', other ancillary procedures such as pharyngoplasty and ear, nose and throat surgery may be required in individual cases.

Orthodontic management

Isolated clefts of the lip and soft palate do not generally involve any dental deformity, although in the latter case growth retardation of the maxilla and consequent skeletal class-III jaw relation may occur as a result of postsurgical scarring. Where the hard palate is also involved, there is a greater likelihood of growth retardation and maxillary constriction in the buccal segments with an associated buccal cross-bite.

Complete clefts of the lip and palate require extensive orthodontic treatment, from shortly after birth in some cases, until physical maturity. The first orthodontic referral is made routinely at 8 years of age, unless the child has been seen as a baby for presurgical orthopaedics. In such cases the child is reviewed with the paediatric dental appointments. In certain circumstances of incisor cross-bite or other incisor relationship problems, it may be necessary to request an earlier orthodontic referral, at around 7 years of age, for correction of this problem. However, in most instances the simple treatment involved comes within the province of normal paediatric dental care (i.e. palatal expansion). Orthodontic management in this instance can be divided into three stages—presurgical orthopaedics, mixed dentition treatment and full permanent dentition correction.

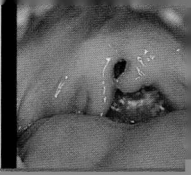

Presurgical orthopaedics

An alginate impression of the maxillary arch is taken as early as 24 hours after birth. A passive acrylic appliance is constructed as in Figure 10.8, with the aim of:
- Normalizing oral function in regard to feeding, swallowing and tongue posture.
- Re-approximating grossly divergent maxillary segments to facilitate primary repair.

Mixed dentition treatment

Treatment is commenced approximately 12 months before alveolar bone grafting,

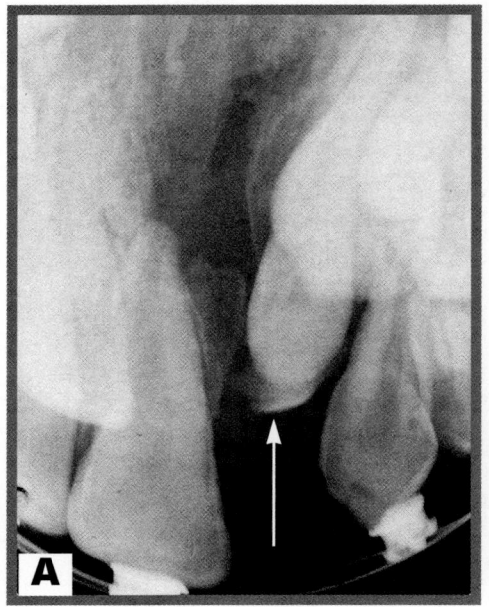
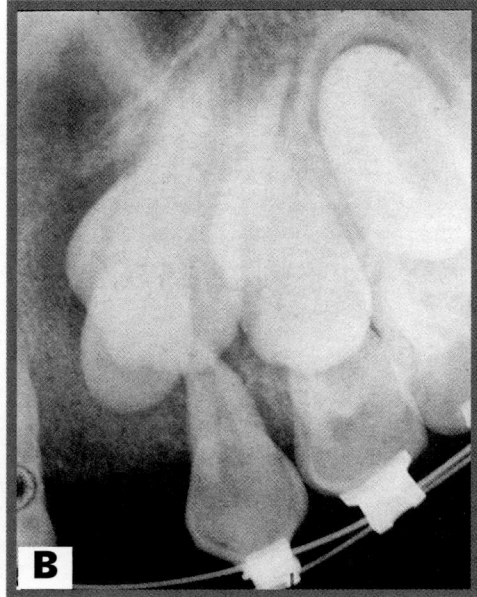

Figure 10.7 A Periapical radiograph of a cleft before bone grafting. The lateral incisor is present on the palatal aspect of the canine tooth. A small supernumerary tooth (arrowed) is also present, and was removed at the time of surgery. **B** The cleft has been filled with cancellous bone, harvested from the iliac crest. After 3 months there is already movement of the lateral and canine and both these teeth erupted through the graft to the mouth where they were aligned orthodontically.

which is undertaken when the cleft-side permanent canine tooth shows between one-half and two-thirds root development. The sequence of treatment is as follows:
- Initial expansion of collapsed maxillary arch segments with a quad (Figure 10.9).
- Limited fixed appliances are placed to align the maxillary incisors before bone grafting of the alveolar cleft defect. The appliance is maintained for 4–6 months after the graft for stability, at which time it may be replaced with a passive retainer.

Full permanent dentition correction

Once the full permanent dentition is established, final tooth alignment and interdigitation is undertaken. In the mixed dentition only the minimum of active orthodontic treatment, if any, is done, leaving the bulk of the orthodontic treatment to be carried out in the shortest possible time when the full permanent dentition is present.

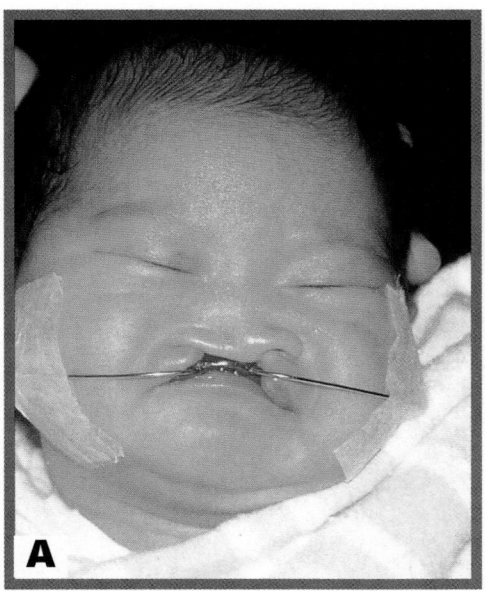
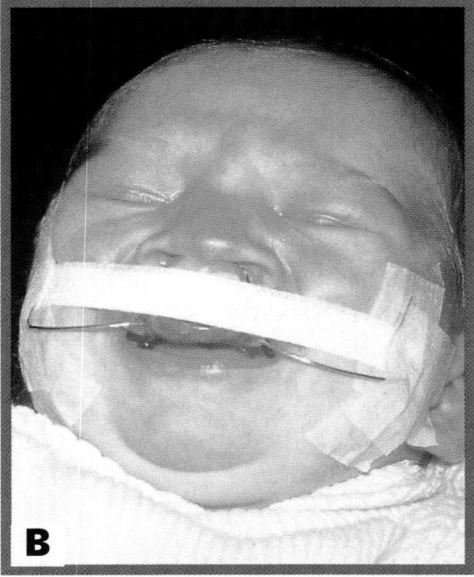

Figure 10.8 A Presurgical orthopaedic appliance. The plate is held by Micropore tape to the cheeks. **B** Strapping aids in the positioning of the labial segments, especially in cases of bilateral complete clefts. Depending on the institution, these appliances are used in cases of bilateral cleft lip and those with very wide unilateral clefts as shown in **A**.

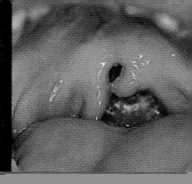

At 12–16 years dental suitability and motivation to cooperate with orthodontic treatment are assessed before the commencement of full fixed appliance therapy. Rapid palatal expansion and/or fixed appliance orthodontic treatment is undertaken at optimum timing; sometimes elective extraction of teeth for orthodontic reasons is indicated.

Further orthodontics in conjunction with orthognathic surgery may be required in the event of significant skeletal dysplasia.

Speech therapy

Speech pathologists are actively involved in the management of children with craniofacial clefts from birth. They play an important role in the following areas:

Feeding

An infant with a cleft of any kind may experience feeding difficulties. Babies with clefts of the lip only may be breast-fed, but clefts of the palate typically preclude this option. The infant is unable to achieve the requisite negative air pressure for its sucking efforts to be successful. The speech pathologist offers advice regarding appropriate feeding techniques and equipment. A soft-squeeze bottle and adapted teat to enhance the liquid flow is usually recommended in addition to an upright positioning of the baby to reduce the likelihood of nasal regurgitation. In wide palatal clefts a specialized feeding plate may be required.

Speech and language development (see Chapter 11)

Children with clefts and other craniofacial malformations are at increased risk of speech and language difficulties. Frequent assessments are required to monitor the language acquisition process, to assist in making surgical decisions and to provide therapy interventions.

Velopalatal competence

Children with clefts are at increased risk of hypernasality and nasal air escape during speech. The speech pathologist's assessment of speech production is critical in the identification and management of this problem. This may involve measurements of velopharyngeal competence such as naso-endoscopy and videofluoroscopic evaluation of soft palate function during speech. These procedures document the presence of the problem and assist the cleft palate team in planning palate surgery or pharyngoplasty.

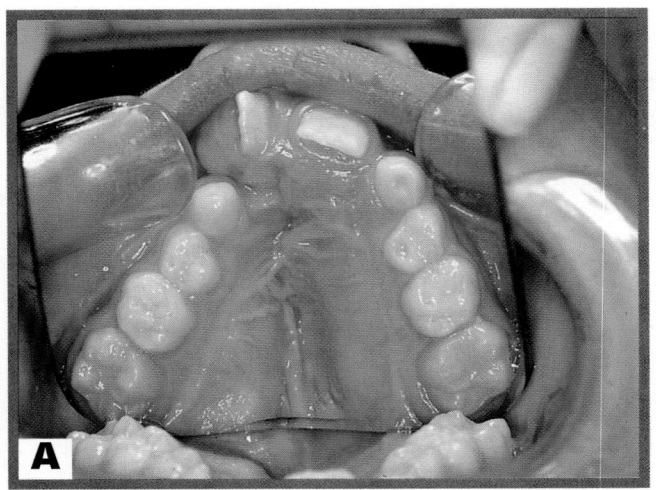

Figure 10.9 **A** One of the effects of early surgery and scarring is collapse of the palatal segments because of an inhibition of growth. Rotation of the central incisor adjacent to the cleft can also be seen. **B** Palatal expansion with a quad-helix appliance to correct the posterior cross-bite and open space for the bone graft.

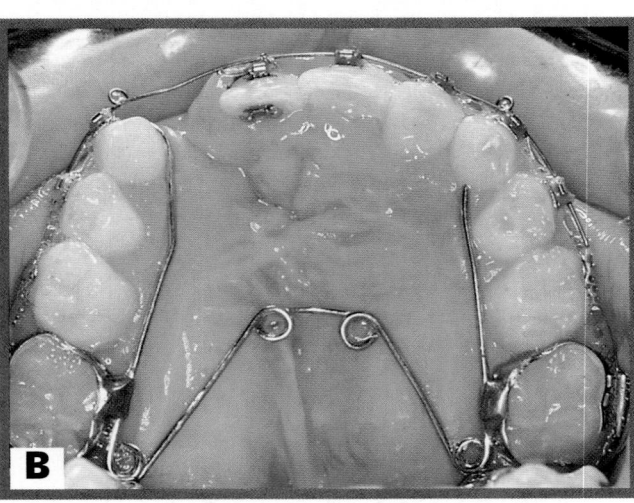

References

ABYHOLM FE, BERGLAND O, SEMB G. Secondary bone grafting of alveolar clefts. *Scand J Plast Recon Surg* 1981, **15**:127–140.

BERGLAND O, SEMB G, ABYHOLM FE. Elimination of the residual alveolar cleft by secondary bone grafting and subsequent orthodontic treatment. *Cleft Pal J* 1986, **23**:175–205.

BIXLER D. Genetics and clefting. *Cleft Pal J* 1981, **18**:10–18

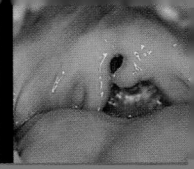

Table 10.1 Protocols for total dental management of children with cleft lip and palate

Age	Paediatric dental	Orthodontic	General practitioner	Surgical
Birth	Initial contact and interview with parents. Registration with cleft palate scheme. Arrange contact with parental support groups.	Construction of presurgical orthopaedic appliance if required.		Initial assessment.
3–5 months	Initial contact, if not at birth. Introduce dental care plan. Study models at time of lip repair.			Primary surgical repair of lip.
12 months	Review.			Surgical repair of palate.
2–6 years	12-monthly reviews for assessment of growth and development, caries and preventive advice.		Initial visit, then 6-monthly for preventive advice, topical fluoride applications and fissure sealing.	Possible revision of lip repair. Pharyngoplasty if required. Myringotomy and grommets by ENT.
6–7 years	Fissure sealing of first permanent molars. Composite resin restoration of hypoplastic teeth adjacent cleft. Preventive advice.		Fissure sealing of first permanent molars. Composite resin restoration of hypoplastic teeth adjacent cleft. Preventive advice.	Myringotomy and grommets by ENT as required.
8–10 years	Case conference with surgical and orthodontic teams for bone grafting.	Assessment for maxillary expansion prior to bone grafting Skeletal age assessments.	6-monthly reviews. Possible extractions of erupted super-numerary teeth. Interim bridge or partial denture.	Bone grafting at one-half to two-thirds root development of canine.
11–12 years	Retention of palatal expansion.		6-monthly reviews.	
12–15 years	12-monthly review.	Full fixed-appliance therapy.	Fissure-sealing of bicuspids and second molars.	Review and possible surgical revision if required.
16–17 years	Restoration of teeth adjacent cleft. Referral to general practitioner.	Retention post orthodontic therapy.	Restoration of teeth in the cleft, including crowns, bridges, implants, dentures.	Assessment of the need for orthognathic surgery.

Source: adapted from Hall RK. *Int J Dent* 1986.

BOHN A. Dental anomalies in hare lip and cleft palate. *Acta Odont Scand* 1963, **21**(suppl.):38.

EL DEEB M, MESSER LB, LEHNERT MW, HEBDA TW, WAITE DE. Canine eruption into grafted bone in maxillary alveolar cleft defects. *Cleft Pal J* 1982, **19**:9–16.

EL DEEB M, HINRICHS JE, WAITE DE, BANDT CL, BEVIS R. Repair of alveolar clefts with autogenous bone grafting: periodontal evaluation. *Cleft Pal J* 1986, **23**:126–136.

ENEMARK H, PEDERSON S. Surgical-orthodontic treatment of severe lateral open bite and cross bite in unilateral cleft lip and palate patients. *Int J Oral Surg* 1983, **12**:277.

HALL HD, POSNICK JC. Early results of secondary bone grafts in 106 alveolar clefts. *J Oral Maxillofac Surg* 1983, **41**:289–294.

HALL RK. Care of adolescents with cleft lip and palate: the role of the general practitioner. *Int J Dent* 1986, **36**:120–130.

HEGGIE AC, WEST RA. Co-ordinated treatment of secondary cleft deformities. *Aust Dent J* 1988, **33**:116–128.

HELLQUIST R, SVARDSTROM K, PORTER B. A longitudinal study of delayed eruption due to the cleft alveolus. *Cleft Pal J* 1983, **20**:277–288.

KINNEBREW MC, MCTIGUE DJ. Submucous cleft palate: review and two clinical reports. *Pediatr Dent* 1984, **6**:252–258.

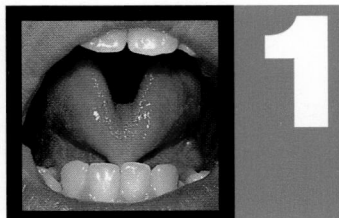

11 Speech and language development

Contributors

Sandy Lopacki, Sarah Starr, Linda Kingston, Justine Hemmings

Introduction

The ability to communicate effectively is vital to a person's functioning in society. Speech and language acquisition is a developmental process occurring most dramatically in the first years of life but one that proceeds throughout a person's lifetime. Difficulties may be encountered at any point during the language acquisition process. Children may experience problems acquiring the sounds of the language, learning how to combine words meaningfully or comprehending others' questions and instructions. Communication problems in adults may arise from loss of language functioning associated with stroke or head injury. In all these cases, a speech pathologist is the primary health-care professional responsible for the identification and treatment of individuals with communication problems. Paediatric dentists should be aware of the symptoms and problems associated with communication difficulties and should know how to refer children and their families to speech pathologists.

Communication disorders

There are five main areas to be considered when assessing a child's communication:
- Oral motor and feeding problems.
- Articulation.
- Language.
- Voice.
- Fluency.

Oral motor and feeding problems
Problems in this area constitute the earliest at which children are referred to a speech pathologist. Significant problems can result when an infant does not develop control of the oral mechanism sufficient for successful feeding. Early reflex development typically facilitates feeding behaviour, but neuromotor factors, prematurity, cleft lip and palate, long-term non-oral feeding and other reasons may interfere with a child's development of the movement patterns essential for sucking,

swallowing and feeding. Because these patterns form the scaffolding of movement for early speech sound development, it is not uncommon for children with a history of feeding difficulties to have subsequent difficulties in producing sounds for speech.

Referral

- Sucking, swallowing or chewing difficulties.
- Coughing or choking with feeds.
- Moist vocal quality.
- Poor cough or gag reflex.
- Persistent drooling (not coincident with teething).
- Recurrent chest infections.
- Presence of a craniofacial malformation.
- Parental report of feeding difficulty or refusal.

Articulation

Articulation refers to the production of speech sounds by modification of the breath stream by using the various valves along the vocal tract: lips, tongue, teeth and palate. Problems in these areas can vary from a fairly mild distortion of sounds, such as a lisp, where the child's speech is still easy to understand, through to a more severe speech production problem in which all speech attempts are unintelligible or the child makes very few speech attempts. Errors are classified in the following ways:

- **Speech sound omissions**
  'cu' for 'cup'.
  'te-y' for 'teddy'.
- **Substitutions of sounds**
  'wed' for 'red'.
  'tun' for 'sun'.
- **Distortions**
  lateral lisp—'s' that sounds slushy.

Children learn to produce sounds in a developmental sequence, with adult-like sound systems expected by 8 years of age (Table 11.1). For example, it is acceptable for a 2-year-old to mispronounce an 's' sound but it would be considered a problem if a similar error were made by a 5-year-old child.

Language

In contrast to the fairly straightforward examples listed above to illustrate speech sound learning, language development is much more complex. Skills emerge on two parallel levels.

Receptive language This is the ability to understand language.

Expressive language This refers to the ability to initiate communication.

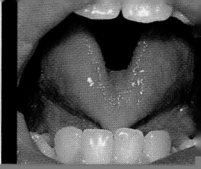

Table 11.1 Development of sounds with age		
Age	**Sounds correctly produced**	**Comments**
2	m, n, h	Speech is sometimes difficult to understand, especially for unfamiliar people.
2½	p, b, ing, w, d, g	
3	y, k, f, sh	By 3 years of age, 80–90% of a child's speech should be easily understood.
3½	t, ch, dge	
4	l, s zh (measure)	Blends of sounds (e.g. st, cl, dr) are acquired later than individual sounds but are usually mastered by 5 years.
5	r	
5½	z	The ages quoted here are only a guideline as to when the average child acquires the sound, but by 8 years of age all sounds should be mastered.
7½	th	
8		

A child with a language disorder may present with difficulties in both comprehension and expression of language, or in only one area of language learning.

Language learning proceeds in a predictable order but there is more variability in the emergence of these skills than the acquisition of speech sounds. Vocabulary grows, as does a child's ability to progressively understand more complex language. Words are combined into phrases and eventually sentences, and comprehension becomes more adult-like over time. Eventually, language that is heard and said becomes the language of literacy, reading and writing. School success is highly correlated with language learning, especially in the early years.

Children may experience language learning problems at any stage of the acquisition process. There may be:

- Difficulties interpreting the meaning of words and gestures.
- Excessive delay in the production of first words and phrases.
- Lack of understanding of questions and instructions.
- Inability to produce sentences that are grammatically correct.
- Inability to participate in conversations.

A delay at any single stage may not necessarily constitute a long-standing problem, although it should be investigated further. Problems with language acquisition are the most subtle indicators of difficulties with childhood development, and therefore should never be ignored.

Voice

The voice is produced when the vocal cords in the larynx are vibrated. Changes in air flow and the shape of the vocal folds can affect the loudness, pitch and quality of the voice. Once the voice is produced, its tone (resonance) and quality are modified by the throat, oral and nasal cavities. A child with a voice problem may present with:

Abnormal voice quality Harsh, breathy or hoarse in the absence of upper respiratory tract infection.

Abnormal resonance or tone Hypernasal (excessive nasal resonance). Hyponasal (lack of nasal resonance, due to some type of nasopharyngeal obstruction).

Inappropriate loudness levels Voice too soft to be heard or so loud that it distracts from the message of the speaker.

Problems with pitch Pitch too high or low for age or sex. Causes of voice problems include:
- Vocal abuse and misuse (in some cases producing vocal nodules).
- Neurological problems.
- Vocal polyps.
- Muscular pathology.
- Vocal cord paralysis.
- Irritants caused by exposure to smoking or aerosol sprays.
- Physical conditions including cleft palate, laryngectomy and hearing loss.

Fluency

Fluency refers to the smooth flow of speech. Where there are interruptions in the flow of speech, stuttering occurs. Many children experience brief periods of stuttering as they learn to speak in longer sentences. The phenomenon is not a disordered pattern that will persist, and is best resolved by reacting to the message the child is attempting to convey. When stuttering outlasts this normal period and when it is becoming stressful for the child, referral is indicated.

A child or an adult with a stutter experiences involuntary repetition of words, prolongations of sounds in words and blocks where no sound is produced at all. Some speakers with a stutter will use words like 'um' to help them initiate speaking. Often secondary features such as a facial grimace will occur with the stutter.

Recent research suggests that the problem is not psychological in origin The majority of people who stutter have been born with an inherited predisposition to disfluency (e.g. it is usually a familial trait). Stutterers do not have more emotional or psychological problems when compared with the general population, nor is there evidence of decreased mental aptitude. Approximately 3% of the population

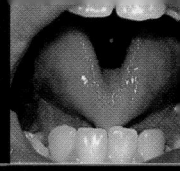

stutter, with a predominance of males (3:1). The disorder usually has its onset in the early years of life with an improved prognosis when treatment is undertaken early. Hence the importance of prompt referral.

Structural anomalies and their relationship to speech

The speech pathologist is actively involved in the assessment of the structural and functional status of the orofacial, pharyngeal and laryngeal areas. These structures, as well as the nasal and respiratory areas, are often objectively assessed by video-fluoroscopic X-ray studies or by naso-endoscopy during both speech production and swallowing. These important diagnostic procedures are often critical in the diagnosis of structural and functional problems affecting feeding skills and speech production.

Dental anomalies

Severe class-III malocclusion Tongue tip elevation to the alveolar ridge may be restricted, resulting in speech sound distortions and an interdental tongue position for sounds such as 's', 'z', 't', 'd,' 'l' and 'n'.

Severe class-II malocclusion Lip closure may be poor during eating and drinking. Distortion or substitution of the lip sounds 'p', 'b' and 'm' may occur with the child compensating by placing the lower lip and upper teeth together.

Maxillary collapse This condition may occur after cleft palate surgery. Distortion of sounds requiring tongue and palatal contact—'s', 'z', 'sh', 'ch' and 'dge'—may result.

Absence of teeth Chewing difficulties may result. Lateral or forward displacement of the tongue during speech may occur, resulting in distortion of sounds.

It is important to note that speech and feeding difficulties are not always associated with these dental conditions. Each patient must be considered individually in the light of his or her ability to compensate for these conditions. In cases where problems are identified, treatment is coordinated with dental and orthodontic management, as some individuals may not be able to improve their speech or feeding until the dental anomaly is remedied.

Palatal anomalies

The soft palate and pharyngeal walls work simultaneously to close off the nasopharynx during speech production and while swallowing. This action prevents excessive airflow into the nasal cavity during speech and prevents nasal regurgitation during the swallow. If there is a palatal abnormality, this action cannot take place efficiently and there is often escape of food and liquid into the nose. Speech is nasal and breathy, sounds are unclear and volume may be reduced.

Palatal anomalies:

- Cleft palate (with or without cleft lip).
- Submucous cleft palate, characterized by a bifid uvula, separation of the palatal muscles, which results in a midline furrow on the soft palate, and a notching of the posterior margin of the hard palate.
- Congenital palatal abnormalities: short palate, deep nasopharynx, uncoordinated or inefficient velopharyngeal movement.
- Acquired palatal abnormalities resulting from neurological damage, from surgery or from neoplasms.

Children with palatal anomalies are best referred to a specialist cleft palate clinic where they can receive multidisciplinary assessment and management (see Chapter 10).

Lingual anomalies

Abnormalities of the tongue may affect the precision, range and speed of tongue movement, resulting in speech or feeding difficulties. The most common expression of a lingual anomaly is the tongue tie.

Ankyloglossia— 'tongue tie' (Figure 11.1) This may occur with varying degrees of severity and does not always result in any functional problems. Some of the possible presenting speech problems of concern to the speech pathologist are:

- Substitutions and distortion of tongue tip sounds caused by restricted elevation of the tongue tip ('l', 't', 'd', 'n', 's', 'z').
- Slower than normal speech rate.
- Reduced speech precision during shouting (shouting requires the mouth to open more widely and thereby may result in the tongue tie having a more negative effect on speech precision).
- Feeding difficulties, such as difficulty sucking in infancy and persistent 'messy' eating.

If a child's speech or feeding appears to be affected by the presence of a tongue tie, comprehensive assessment by both a speech pathologist and a dentist is indicated to determine whether surgical release is required.

Maxillofacial surgery and its relation to speech production

When orthognathic surgery is being considered, consultation with a speech pathologist should be made to determine the possible consequences of the procedure for speech production.

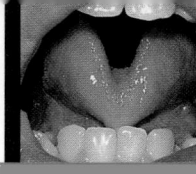

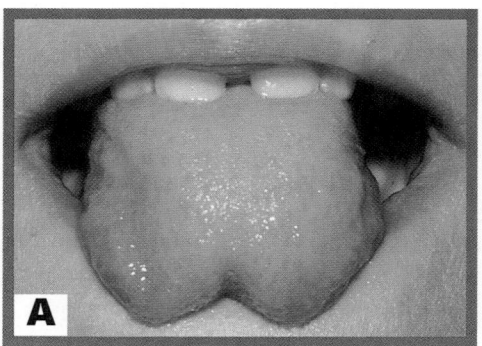
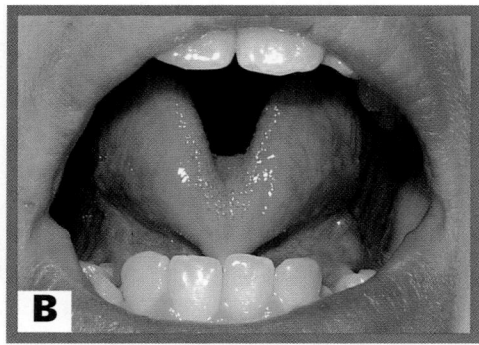

Figure 11.1 Ankyloglossia. Notice the tethering of the frenum to the anterior tip of the tongue restricting elevation and protrusion. It is important to assess the position of the frenum in the body of the tongue as well as any attachment into the gingival margin that may cause periodontal complications.

Maxillary advancement procedures

When the maxilla is advanced anteriorly, the hard and soft palatal structures are also displaced forwards, increasing the distance that the soft palate must move to achieve velopharyngeal closure. Most patients seem able to compensate for this alteration in the nasopharyngeal area, and their speech and swallowing are not affected. Some patients (e.g. those with cleft palate) are at risk of developing velopharyngeal incompetence and the consequent hypernasal and distorted speech production. Forward placement of the maxilla also means that tongue contact on the palate may be altered for some sounds. In patients with severe class-III malocclusions, tongue placement and sound production may be improved with this procedure.

Referral to a speech pathologist

When the presence of a communication or feeding problem is suspected, referral should be made as soon as possible.

Dentists should refer any child who experiences the dificulties outlined below.

Feeding and swallowing
- Has difficulty sucking, swallowing and chewing.
- Is coughing and choking during feeds.
- Is drooling excessively.

Articulation
- Is not babbling a wide variety of sounds by 8–10 months.

- Is not easily understood by caregivers by 2 years.
- Is not easily understood by familiar adults by 3 years.
- Is having difficulty in producing sounds accurately by 5 years.

Language
- Is not understanding a variety of questions/instructions by 18 months.
- Is not using single words by 18 months.
- Is not combining two words by 2 years (e.g. want drink).
- Has difficulty following instructions or answering questions.
- Gives inappropriate answers or frequently ignores language spoken to them.
- Is constructing sentences that are incorrect or immature by 3–4 years (e.g. 'me go to him house').
- Cannot maintain a topic of conversation by 4 years.

Voice
- Has a hoarse voice or often loses their voice.
- Has a nasal voice.
- Often sounds as though they have a cold.
- Has a voice that seems too high or low for their gender or age.
- Continually speaks abnormally loudly or softly.
- Has a sudden onset of any of these problems.

Fluency
- Shows evidence of stuttering at any age.

Referral procedures
It will be necessary to locate the most appropriate service to meet your patients' needs. Most often, access to a speech pathologist through a local community health centre or hospital will be all that is required. Some patients may require a more specialized service such as a developmental disability service or cleft palate clinic. Some patients may prefer the services of a private practitioner.

Referral is most efficient when the dentist provides a written referral outlining the areas of concern. Following an assessment, a treatment plan will be devised according to the individual needs of the patient. Treatment can be provided in individual or group sessions, and it may extend over a period of time depending on the nature and severity of the condition. Most speech, language and feeding problems are best treated with parental participation and a programme to facilitate carryover at home. Occasionally, it is useful to include a school component to fully integrate speech and language services into the child's daily life experiences.

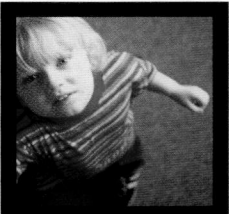
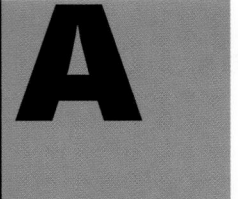

Appendices

Contributors
Angus Cameron, Richard Widmer, Neil Street, Christopher Olsen, Peter Cooper

Appendix A. Normal values in blood chemistry

Laboratory examination may be divided into two general categories: screening and diagnosis.

Screening studies are intended to identify individuals with disease in the early and asymptomatic stages. By definition, screening studies must be relatively simple and inexpensive, and are useful only when used to identify a disease that is relatively frequent (diabetes mellitus, haematocrit anaemia, syphilis, blood disorders).

Diagnostic examinations provide more specific information. The distinction between screening and diagnostic laboratory examination is not always rigid or absolute.

It must be remembered that laboratory examinations provide information that contributes to the diagnostic process; seldom is this information of value by itself. The results must be interpreted in conjunction with other information that is available about the patient. It should also be noted that a laboratory value outside the normal range does not necessarily indicate disease. That value may represent normal for that specific patient. Usually normal values are determined by testing supposedly healthy people, and these results are used to calculate the mean and normal range. Variables are not considered, and as a consequence normal ranges are not always valid for all patients. Conversely, if a clinical diagnosis appears valid, and is not substantiated by laboratory results, the tests should be repeated to rule out the possibility of laboratory error.

Haematology

Full-blood count
A full-blood count (FBC) usually includes a white blood cell count (WBC), red blood cell count (RBC), haemoglobin (Hb) haematocrit (Hct), red blood cell indices (mean corpuscular haemoglobin, mean corpuscular volume, mean corpuscular haemoglobin concentration and platelet count).

Platelet function tests are rarely ordered, usually only in consultation with a haematologist. If one asks for FBC and 'differential', one will also receive a breakdown of the RBC and WBC as listed on the form. If an FBC detects anaemia then

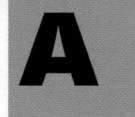
one should request serum ferritin, red cell folate and serum B_{12} analysis. However, interpretation of these results is difficult and advice should be sought.

White blood cells	Children		$4.0-15.0\times10^9$/L	
		Neutrophils	$1.5-7.5\times10^9$/L	50%
		Lymphocytes	$1.0-8.6\times10^9$/L	42%
		Monocytes	$0.5-1.5\times10^9$/L	5%
		Eosinophils	$0.3-0.8\times10^9$/L	
		Basophils	$<0.1-0.2\times10^9$/L	
	Adults		$4.0-11.0\times10^9$/L	
		Neutrophils	$2.0-8.0\times10^9$/L	60%
		Lymphocytes	$0.5-4.0\times10^9$/L	33%
		Monocytes	$0.2-1.0\times10^9$/L	4%
		Eosinophil	$0.04-0.5\times10^9$/L	
		Basophils	$<0.01-0.2\times10^9$/L	

Red blood cells	Children (3–12 years)		$4.0-5.5\times10^{12}$/L
	Adults	Male	$4.5-6.5\times10^{12}$/L
		Female	$3.8-5.8\times10^{12}$/L

Haemoglobin	Children (3–12 years)		115–145 g/L
	Adults	Male	130–180 g/L
		Female	115–165 g/L

| **Mean corpuscular volume MCV)** | Children | 70–90 fL |
| | Adults | 80–96 fL |

| **Mean corpuscular haemoglobin (MCH)** | Children | 23–31 pg |
| | Adults | 27–32 pg |

| **Platelets** | $150-450\times10^9$/L |

Erythrocyte sedimentation rate (ESR)	Children		0–10 mm
	Adults	Male	0–15 mm
		Female	0–20 mm

Reticulocytes	Children	$10-100\times10^9$/L
	Infants	2.0–6.0%
		or mean 150×10^9/L
	Adults	0.2–2.0%

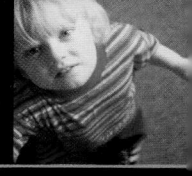

Red cell folate	340–2500 nmol/L
Serum folate	7–40 nmol/L
Vitamin B$_{12}$	150–700 pmol/L

Coagulation and bleeding tests

Problems relating to bleeding are relatively infrequent in dental practice. Most inherited defects will usually have been identified early in life, and so it is usually acquired bleeding problems about which the dentist must be aware. Screening studies will identify whether there is a bleeding problem, and in which of the three systems it is, namely: platelets, coagulation, or vascular abnormalities.

Activated partial thromboplastin time (APTT)		24–38 sec
Prothrombin time		11–17 sec
Factor-VIII assay		50–200%
	Mild haemophilia	20–25%
	Moderate	2–5%
	Severe	<1%
Skin bleeding time		< 9 min

Clinical chemistry

It is not appropriate to simply request an MBA12 (12 tests for multiblood analysis). The following abbreviations are used when ordering tests:

EUC (electrolytes, urea, creatinine)
LFTs (liver profile, including serum proteins)
CA (calcium)
PHOS (inorganic phosphate, alkaline phosphatase)

Blood chemistry		
	Sodium	136–146 mmol/L
	Potassium	3.4–5.5 mmol/L
	Chloride	94–107 mmol/L
	Total CO$_2$	24–31 mmol/L
	Urea	2.5–6.5 mmol/L
	Creatinine	60–125 mmol/L
	Glucose	
	fasting	3.9–6.1 mmol/L
	2 hours	

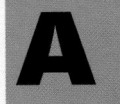

	postprandial	<7.8 mmol/L
	Calcium	2.13–2.63 mmol/L
	Phosphate	0.18–1.45 mmol/L
	Osmolality	275–295 mmol/L
	Lactate	0.63–2.44 mmol/L
	Alkaline phosphatase(ALP)	60–391 U/L
Liver function tests	Total bilirubin	2–21 mmol/L
	Total protein	63–79 g/L
	Albumin	35–53 g/L
	ALP	30–115 U/L
	γ-Glutamyl transpeptidase (γGT)	
	Male	8–43 U/L
	Female	5–30 U/L
	Alanine amino-transferase (ALT)	7–47 U/L

Iron studies These tests are used when there is suspicion of an underlying anaemia. The request for iron studies provides information regarding serum iron, total-iron binding capacity, and percentage iron saturation.

	Ferritin	
	Male	30–300 mg/L
	Premenstrual	15–150 mg/L
	Postmenstrual	25–200 mg/L
	Iron	7.0–29.0 mmol/L
	Transferrin	2.1–3.9 g/L
	Saturation	0.09–0.52
Urine chemistry	Sodium	40–220 mmol/L
	Potassium	25–120 mmol/L
	Creatinine	8.0–18.0 mmol/L
	Total protein	<0.15 g/d/L
Arterial blood gas	pH	7.35–7.45
	pCO_2	35–45 mmHg
	pO_2	75–100 mmHg
	HCO_3	22–26 mmol/L
	Base excess	–3+3 mmol/L
	SO_2	0.95–0.98

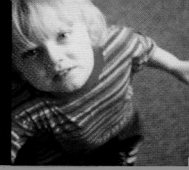

Appendix B. Fluid and electrolyte balance

Fluid and electrolyte replacement can be conveniently divided into:

Maintenance replacement
The fluid and electrolyte losses occur during a normal day. These values are modified by other factors such as patient and environmental temperatures, age weight and metabolic rate.

Deficit replacement
To replace any existing or ongoing abnormal losses such as dehydration from vomiting or diarrhoea and blood loss.

Maintenance replacement
The need for water and electrolytes is a function of the metabolic rate, as they are substrates for metabolism. Thus the younger the child, the higher the metabolic rate on a weight basis and the higher the turnover of water and electrolytes.

Water requirements

Infants		
	Day 1	60 mL/kg/day
	Day 2	80 mL/kg/day
	Day 3	100 mL/kg/day
	Day 4 to 1 year	120 mL/kg/day

Children	
	<10 kg 4 mL/kg/h
	10–20 kg 2 mL/kg/h + 40 mL/h
	>20 kg 1 mL/kg/hr + 60 mL/h

Modifying factors
Increased maintenance requirement
- Fever—add 12% per degree above 37.5°C.
- Hyperventilation.
- Extreme activity.
- High environmental temperature.

Decreased maintenance requirement
- Cardiac failure.
- Inactivity (patient sedated in intensive care unit [ICU])—decrease by 30%.
- Hypothermia—decrease 12% per degree less than 37.5°C.
- Head injury—decrease by 30%.
- Renal failure—decrease by 70% + urine output.

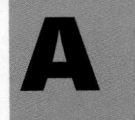
Electrolyte requirements

Normal electrolyte requirements are shown in Table A-1.

N/4 saline (0.225% normal saline + 3.75% dextrose) at normal maintenance rates will supply adequate sodium and chloride. Potassium should only be added to intravenous fluids if replacement is to continue for more than 24 hours and adequate urine output is present. Infants under 3 months of age will also require supplements of dextrose if they are to fast for longer than 4–6 hours.

Deficit replacement

Fluid deficit is usually expressed as a percentage of body weight. This allows for easy calculation of replacement fluids. Fluid imbalance may be as a result of any of the following:

Water loss
- Decreased intake.
- Increased respiratory loss
  (especially seen in children with high respiratory rates).
- Renal concentration impairment.

Water and salt loss
- Vomiting.
- Diarrhoea.
- Increased sweating.

Blood volume loss
- Haemorrhage.
- Septic shock.
- Anaphylaxis.
- Burns.

Table A-1 Electrolyte requirements			
	0–10 kg	**11–20 kg**	**>20 kg**
Fluids (mL/kg/day)	100	50	20
Ca (mmol/kg/day)	100	50	20
Na (mmol/kg/day)	3.0	1.5	0.6
K (mmol/kg/day)	2.0	1.0	0.4

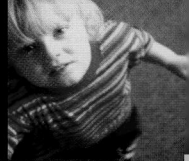

Assessment of deficit

Deficit assessment is difficult even for experienced paediatric workers. Some idea of the deficit can be gained from the history of the abnormal loss. For example:
- Has the vomiting persisted for more than 24 hours?
- Has the child passed urine in the past 12 hours?
- Is the child thirsty? Dehydration is generally assessed by estimating weight loss.

Mild dehydration (2–3% acute weight loss)
- Thirst.
- Mild oliguria.
- No physical signs.

Moderate dehydration (5% acute weight loss)
- Slight decrease in skin tone.
- Sunken fontanelle in infants.
- Slight decrease in ocular tension.
- Tachycardia.

Severe dehydration (7–8% acute weight loss)
- Marked tachycardia.
- Loss of skin tone.
- Loss of ocular tension.
- Sunken eyes.
- Restlessness and apathy.

Profound dehydration (>10% acute weight loss)
- Circulatory collapse.
- Delirium and coma.
- Hyperpyrexia.
- Cyanosis.

Replacement of deficit

Usually the deficit is replaced with the fluid that most closely approximates the fluid that has been lost. Replacement therapy is aimed at restoring the fluid compartments in the order given below. If there is significant loss of blood volume, then this must be replaced as rapidly as is safely possible to preserve brain, heart and kidney perfusion.

Blood volume loss
- Blood-packed red cells or whole blood.
- Colloid 5% human serum albumin (HSA) or Haemaccel.
- Hartmann's solution or normal saline.
- Ionotropes if needed.

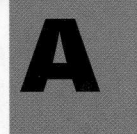

Salt and water loss
- Hartmann's solution or normal saline.
- 0.45% normal saline + 2.5% dextrose (N/2 saline).

Water loss
- 0.255% normal saline + 3.75% dextrose (N/4 saline).
- Maintenance fluids should be added to the deficit losses and given over the normal period.

Calculation of deficit Deficit (mL) = % dehydration × weight (kg) × 10.

Examples
Mild dehydration Where there is no circulatory compromise the loss will be water and electrolytes from all body compartments. This can be replaced with dextrose saline solutions over many hours.

Severe dehydration There is loss of intracellular, interstitial and most importantly blood volume. The priority is to rapidly restore blood volume, and consequently cardiac output, with colloid or blood (10–20 mL/kg over 20–30 minutes) or saline solutions (20–40 mL/kg) to allow adequate vital organ perfusion. After this is achieved, electrolyte and water deficits should be replaced, as calculated, with dextrose/saline solutions over a longer period of time (several hours to 24 hours).

Severe blood loss In cases of trauma or bleeding there will initially be loss of blood volume. This is treated in the same way as above, i.e. restoring circulating blood volume with colloids or blood and reassessment of losses. If the blood loss is unknown, initial therapy is to start with 20 mL/kg over 10–20 minutes and then reassess. If the blood pressure has returned to normal and fallen again, or has not responded to the initial bolus, a repeat of the initial bolus of fluid is indicated, followed by reassessment. The signs of adequate fluid replacement, without the aid of central-venous pressure or urine output measurement, are a return to normal blood pressure and heart rate values without the need for further boluses of fluid.

Notes on rehydration
The above guidelines apply to previously healthy children. Those children with cardiac disease or significant systemic disease require intensive intravascular monitoring in a paediatric intensive care unit.
- Constant reassessment of fluid therapy is essential throughout replacement.
- Measurement of electrolytes is essential in the replacement of greater than moderate deficits and applies especially to potassium.

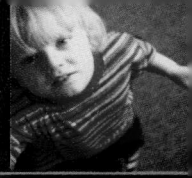

- Measurement of acid–base status with arterial blood gases is often necessary, as fluid deficit causes organ hypoperfusion and subsequent metabolic acidosis. This will usually correct itself with correction of blood volume and cardiac output over many hours.
- Fluid balance and acid–base disturbances are often very complex and life-threatening. If there is any doubt as to management, then specialist paediatric or anaesthetic advise should be sought.

Transfusion

Volume (mL) = weight (kg) × g% Hb rise required × 3.

Table A-2 Composition of intravenous crystalloid fluids

	Na^+ (mmol/L)	Cl^- (mmol/L)	Lactate (mmol/L)	Ca^{2+} (mmol/L)
Normal saline	150	150		
N/2 saline 5%	75	75		
N/4 saline 3.75%	37.5	37.5		
N/5 saline 4%	30	30		
Hartmann's solution	130	5	5	3

Table A-3 Composition of intravenous colloid fluids

	Na^+ (mmol/L)	K^+ (mmol/L)	Ca^{2+} (mmol/L)	Polygeline g/L	5% Solution of protein Globulin%	Albumin%
Haemaccel	145	5.1	6.25	35		
5% Human serum albumin	130–150	4–6	1.5–2.5		14	86

Appendix C. Management of anaphylaxis

Anaphylaxis is a symptom-complex accompanying the acute reaction to a foreign substance to which the patient has been previously sensitized.

Anaphylactoid

Same symptoms but the reaction is non-immunological or unknown.

Frequency	Anaesthesia	1:5000 to 1:30000
		(mortality 4% of reactions)
	X-ray contrast	2%
	Antibiotics	1:5000
	Local anaesthetics	rare
	Foods, insects, usually to preservatives	

Timing
98% occur within 5 minutes of drug administration, but may occur up to hours later.

Clinical presentation
Prodrome
- Metallic taste.
- Apprehension.
- Coughing.
- Choking sensation.
- Paraesthesia.
- Arthralgia.

Cutaneous
- Blushing.
- Urticaria.
- Angio-oedema.
- Pallor and cyanosis.

Cardiovascular
- Tachycardia.
- Hypotension.
- Shock.

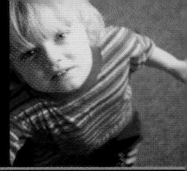

Respiratory
- Bronchospasm.
- Laryngeal obstruction.
- Pulmonary oedema.

Gastrointestinal tract
- Nausea, vomiting, diarrhoea.
- Abdominal cramps.

Others
- Disseminated coagulation disorders (DIC).
- Fitting.

Treatment
Adrenaline and colloid infusion are the mainstay of the treatment of anaphylaxis. Follow-up is essential. The patient must be transferred to an ICU, as symptoms may return up to hours later. A letter must be sent with the patient describing the event and all the drugs used until skin testing can identify the offending drug. Skin testing of all drugs used is performed 3 months after the reaction. A Medialert bracelet, identifying relevant drug reactions, should be worn.

Notes on management (see Figure A.1)
- Adrenaline is the main drug used in the treatment of anaphylaxis and anaphylactoid reactions. Adrenaline must be used if anaphylaxis is suspected.

Children (<12 years)

Dilute 1 ampoule into 9 mL of saline
1:1000 becomes 1:10 000   (1 mg/10 mL)
Inject 0.25 mL per year of age intramuscularly; this approximates 5 µg/kg

Adults

Inject 1:1000 intramuscularly
Small adults   (<50 kg) 0.25 mL
Average adults   (50–100 kg) 0.50 mL
Large adults   (>100 kg) 0.75 mL
IV-access lines must be large gauge, preferably 16 gauge or larger.
Colloid 10–20 mL/kg immediately

Note
- The doses of adrenaline and colloid must be repeated if the patient's vital signs have not improved.

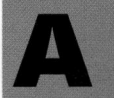
Anaphlyaxis

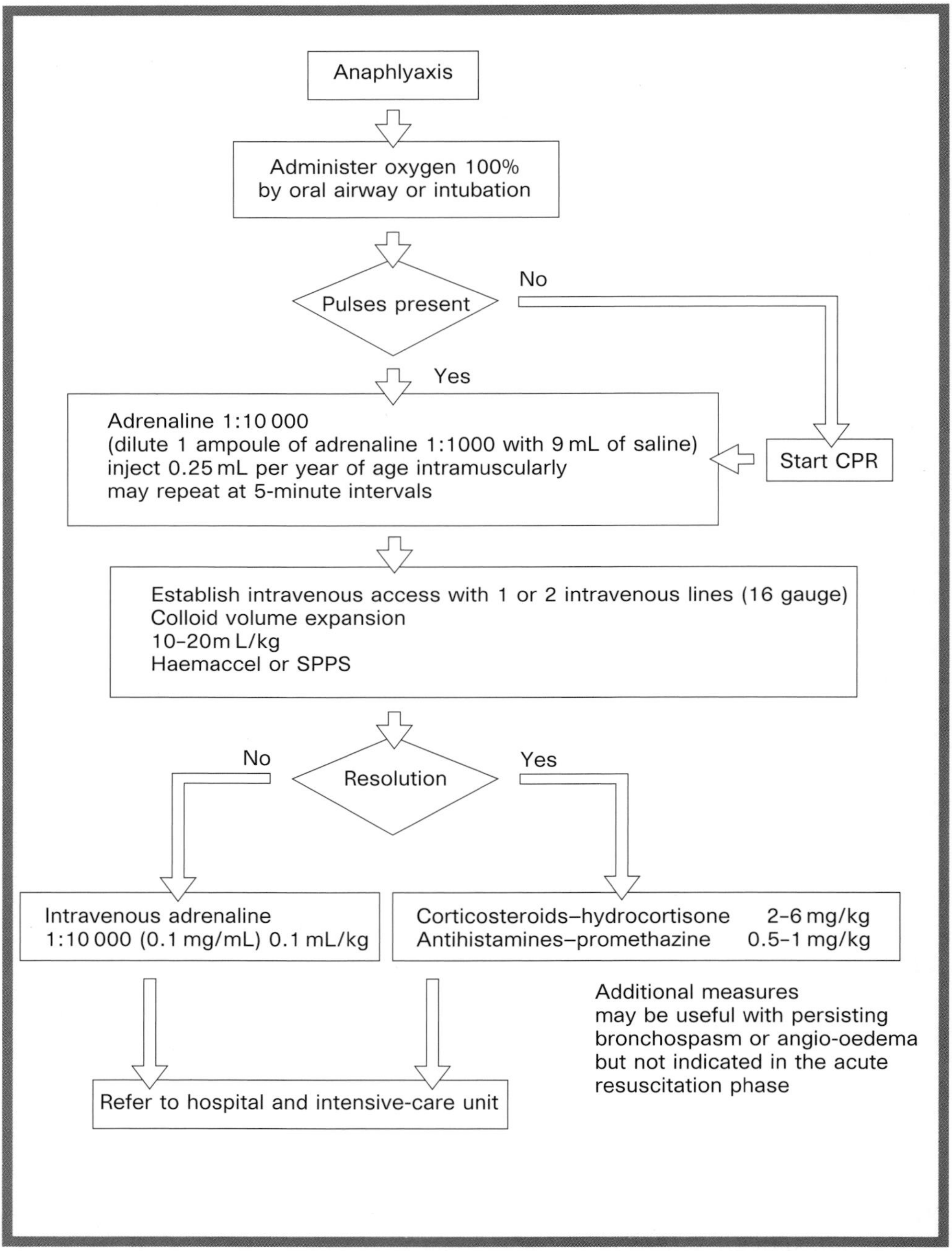

⇩

Administer oxygen 100%
by oral airway or intubation

⇩

Pulses present — No

Yes ⇩

Adrenaline 1:10 000
(dilute 1 ampoule of adrenaline 1:1000 with 9 mL of saline)
inject 0.25 mL per year of age intramuscularly
may repeat at 5-minute intervals

⇦ Start CPR

⇩

Establish intravenous access with 1 or 2 intravenous lines (16 gauge)
Colloid volume expansion
10–20m L/kg
Haemaccel or SPPS

⇩

No — Resolution — Yes

Intravenous adrenaline
1:10 000 (0.1 mg/mL) 0.1 mL/kg

Corticosteroids–hydrocortisone   2–6 mg/kg
Antihistamines–promethazine   0.5–1 mg/kg

Additional measures
may be useful with persisting
bronchospasm or angio-oedema
but not indicated in the acute
resuscitation phase

Refer to hospital and intensive-care unit

Figure A.1 Management of anaphylaxis.

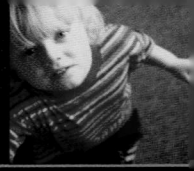

Appendix D. Management of acute asthma

Asthma is one of the most common childhood diseases in Australia and accounts for significant mortality and morbidity. The emphasis of treatment today is on prophylaxis rather than merely treating attacks.

Essential equipment for asthma kit (see also p. 329)

(see also p. 329)

- Ventolin inhaler.
- Bricanyl Turbohaler.
- Ventolin nebules (2.5 mg).
- Ventolin nebules (5 mg).
- Nebulizer unit and tubing for wall oxygen.
- Child mask for nebulizer.
- Aerochamber spacer.
- Volumatic spacer.
- Peak-flow meter.

Bronchodilators

Ventolin

Inhaler (blue)	100 µg/puff.
Dose	2–4 puffs by spacer.
Nebules	2.5 or 5 mg given by nebulizer.

Bricanyl Turbohaler 500 µg/inhalation.

Apparatus for administration of bronchodilators

Aerochamber Children 4 years and under:

- position aerochamber with mask over child's face.
- 4 puffs from Ventolin inhaler, patient inhales four to six times for each puff.

Volumatic spacer Children 4 years and over:

- position spacer between lips.
- 4 puffs from Ventolin inhaler, patient inhales four to six times for each puff.
- encourage child to breath deeply for 10–15 seconds.

Nebulizer For very young children or when not improved by inhaler, or with spacer, after 10 minutes:

- <5 years 2.5 mg Nebule.
- >5 years 5 mg Nebule.

Place contents of Nebule in bottom of Nebule bowl, fix to face mask and apply oxygen or air to mask at 6 L per minute flow rate. A fine mist will form which the child breathes deeply for about 10 minutes.

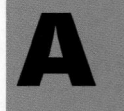

Management (see Figure A.2)

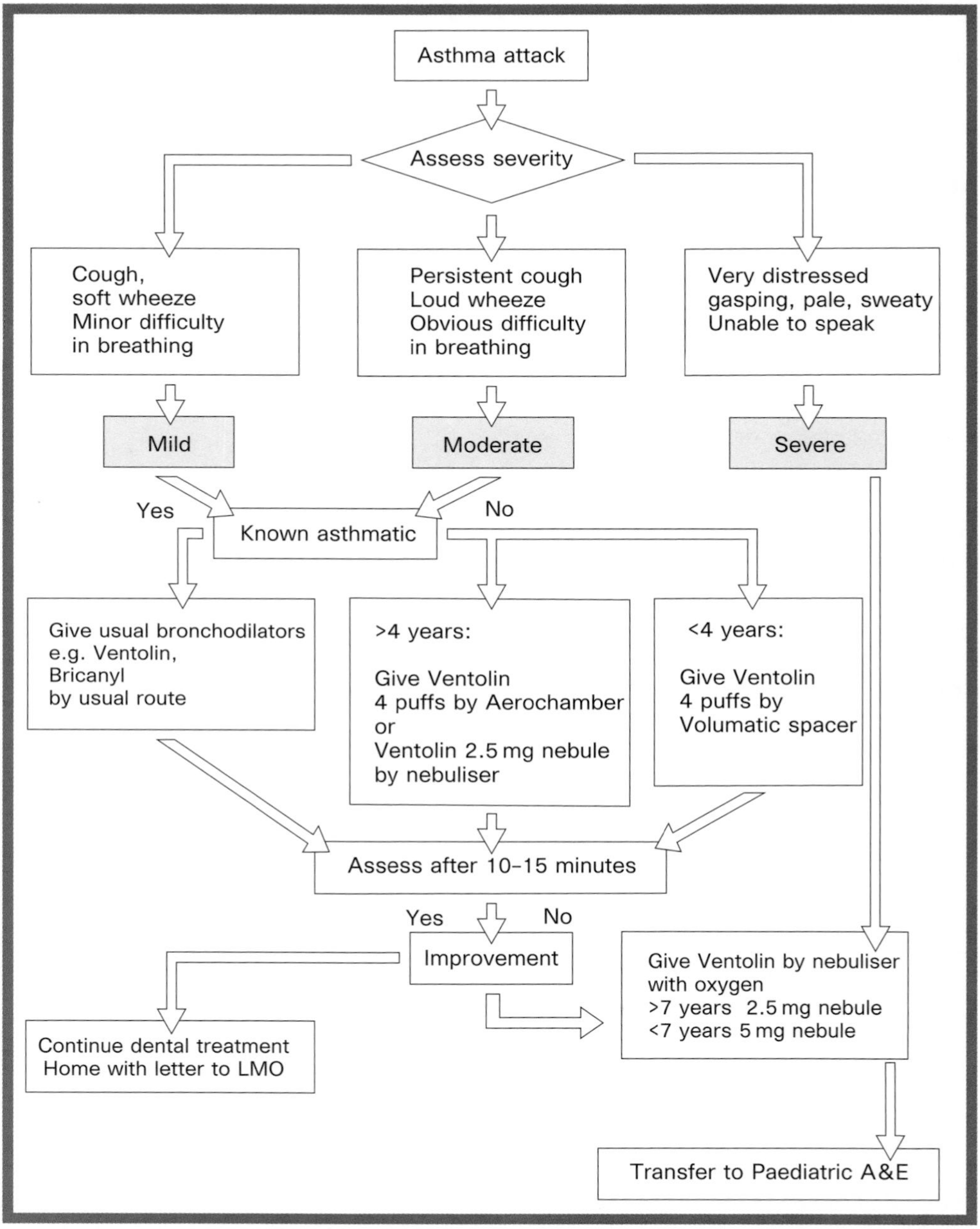

Asthma attack

Assess severity

Cough,
soft wheeze
Minor difficulty
in breathing

Persistent cough
Loud wheeze
Obvious difficulty
in breathing

Very distressed
gasping, pale, sweaty
Unable to speak

Mild

Moderate

Severe

Yes   No

Known asthmatic

Give usual bronchodilators
e.g. Ventolin,
Bricanyl
by usual route

>4 years:

Give Ventolin
4 puffs by Aerochamber
or
Ventolin 2.5 mg nebule
by nebuliser

<4 years:

Give Ventolin
4 puffs by
Volumatic spacer

Assess after 10–15 minutes

Yes   No

Improvement

Give Ventolin by nebuliser
with oxygen
>7 years 2.5 mg nebule
<7 years 5 mg nebule

Continue dental treatment
Home with letter to LMO

Transfer to Paediatric A&E

Figure A.2 Management of acute asthma.

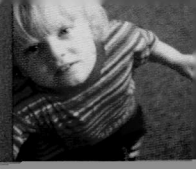

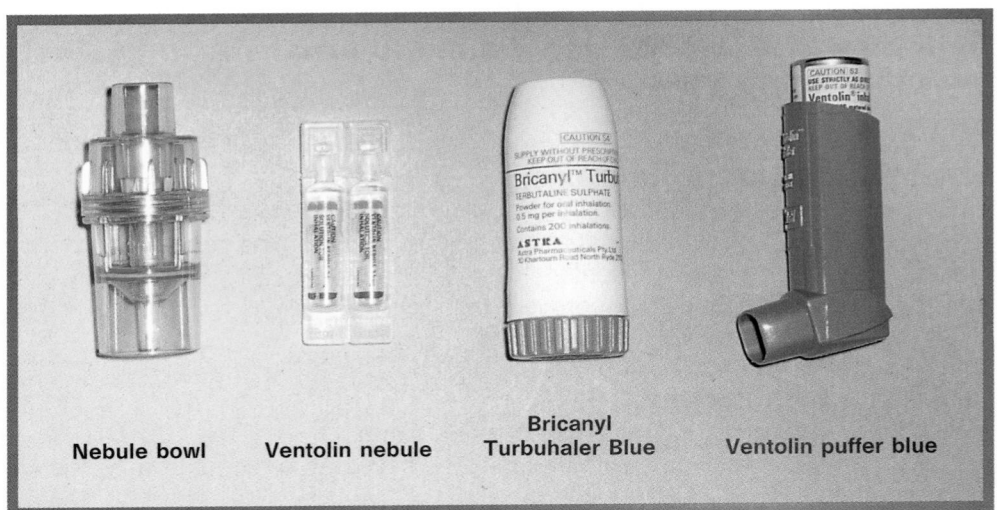

| Nebule bowl | Ventolin nebule | Bricanyl Turbuhaler Blue | Ventolin puffer blue |

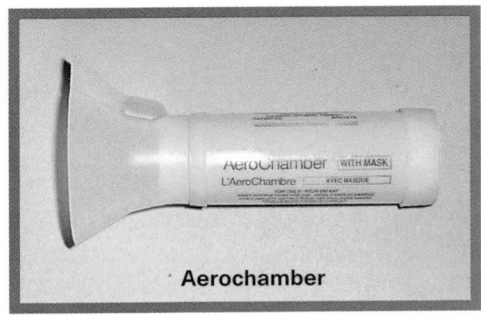

Aerochamber

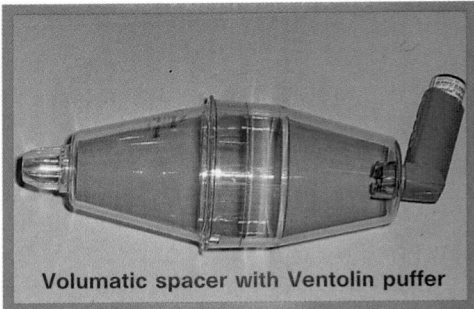

Volumatic spacer with Ventolin puffer

Appendix E. Protocols for antibiotic prophylaxis against infective endocarditis

The rationale for prophylaxis
- Bacterial endocarditis has a high mortality rate (10–15%).
- There is strong circumstantial evidence that endocarditis may follow dental treatment in susceptible patients.
- There is a need to provide approved antibiotic prophylaxis for potential at-risk patients receiving dental treatment.

Problems with prophylaxis
- No two sets of antibiotic guidelines are the same.
- Less than 15% of patients with endocarditis have had a recent invasive dental procedure.
- There is no direct evidence in humans that antibiotic prophylaxis works. Indeed, there have been many cases of endocarditis occurring in spite of 'appropriate' cover having been given.
- Disagreement over the efficacy of different protocols.
- Which patients to cover.
- Which dental procedures should be covered.

Protocols available
- American Heart Association adopted by the American Dental Association (1990).
- British Society for Antimicrobial Chemotherapy (1990).
- Victorian Drug Usage Advisory Committee, adopted by the Australian Dental Association (1992).

History
It is very important to accurately check a patient's history with respect to a cardiac problem. Always consult the local physician or cardiologist involved; ask for details of the complaint and whether antibiotic prophylaxis will be needed. If this information is not available a cardiac review should be sought.

Other considerations
- Is the patient on long-term antibiotics? Alternative drugs should be used.
- Does the patient have a convincing history of allergy to antibiotics?
- Anaphylaxis must always be considered when penicillin is used.
- Does the patient have impaired renal function which will necessitate dose modification?
- Is there a history of vomiting with oral antibiotics? If so consider parenteral medication.

The use of IV antibiotics, for patients undergoing general anaesthesia, has

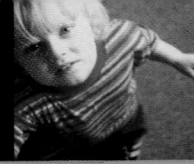

several advantages over oral and IM techniques. Blood levels are rapidly achieved, prophylaxis is more predictable and there are no problems with compliance.
- Is a general anaesthetic required?

Serious consideration should be given to arranging general anaesthesia and IV antibiotics for children who require multiple visits.
- In addition to antibiotic cover, it is considered routine in most paediatric dental departments to use a preoperative rinse of 0.2% chlorhexidine gluconate to reduce the risk of bacteraemia.

Classification of patients

Highly susceptible patients
- Prosthetic cardiac valves.
- Previous bacterial endocarditis.
- Recent surgical repair of cardiovascular defect within 6 months.
- Surgical systemic to pulmonary artery shunts or conduits.

Susceptible patients
- Renal dialysis with atrioventricular shunt appliance.
- Ventriculo-atrial or ventriculo-venous shunts for hydrocephalus.
- Hypertrophic cardiomyopathy.
- Indwelling vascular catheter.

Most congenital cardiac malformations
- Ventricular septal defect (unrepaired).
- Patent ductus arteriosus.
- Coarctation of the aorta.
- Tricuspid valve disease.
- Asymmetric septal hypertrophy.
- Tetralogy of Fallot.
- Aortic stenosis.
- Complex cyanotic heart disease.
- Bicuspid aortic valve.
- Idiopathic hypertrophic-subaortic stenosis.
- Mitral valve prolapse with mitral insufficiency and/or holosystolic murmur.

Patients with conditions not requiring prophylaxis
- History of rheumatic fever (more than 5 years previously) without clinical heart disease.
- Uncomplicated secundum atrial septal defect.
- Surgical repaired secundum atrial septal defect, ventricular septal defect, or patent ductus arteriosus beyond 6 months and without residua.
- Previous coronary artery bypass graft.
- Mitral valve prolapse without valvular regurgitation.

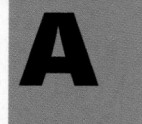
- Previous Kawasaki's disease without valvular dysfunction.
- Cardiac pacemakers and implanted defibrillators.
- Well-controlled diabetics.
- Atherosclerotic heart disease.
- Ventriculoperitoneal shunts for hydrocephalus.

There is great disagreement over the need to cover ventriculoperitoneal shunts. While theoretically there is no risk of a bacteraemia colonizing a shunt, which has no direct communication with the bloodstream, some neurosurgeons insist that their patients be covered. Dentists should be advised to check with the particular protocol of the neurosurgeon who is responsible for the patient.

Classification of procedures
Procedures that require prophylaxis
- All dental procedures likely to induce bleeding.
- First-visit endodontic procedures.
- Endotracheal intubation.

Procedures that do not require prophylaxis
- Simple adjustment of orthodontic appliances.
- Restorations above the gingival margin.
- Endodontic procedures confined to the root canal after pulp extirpation.
- Injection of local intra-oral anaesthetic (except intraligamentary injections).
- Exfoliation of primary teeth.

Relative risk of procedures It is considered that some procedures subject the patient to a higher level of risk of developing endocarditis than others. An open surgical procedure will produce a significantly greater bacteraemia than gingival scaling or placing a matrix band below the gingival margin.

If the procedure is determined to put a potentially susceptible patient at higher risk the use of parenteral antibiotics should be considered.

Protocols for antibiotic prophylaxis
These protocols are based on those published by the Victorian Drug Usage Advisory Committee (1992) and recommended by the Australian Dental Association.

Protocols for susceptible patients
Non-penicillin-allergic patients able to take oral medications
Amoxycillin

Children	50 mg/kg orally 1 hour before procedure
Adults	3.0 g

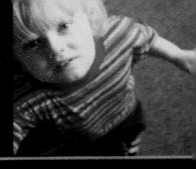

Penicillin-allergic patients   *Clindamycin*

    Children

10 mg/kg
orally or intravenously followed by 5 mg/kg
6 hours later

    Adults

600 mg orally 1 hour before procedure
followed by 300 mg 6 hours after initial
dose or
Vancomycin

    Children

20 mg/kg infused over 1 hour before
procedure

    Adults

1.0 g infused over 1 hour before procedure

**Susceptible patients under
general anaesthetic**   *Ampicillin* or *amoxycillin*

    Children

50 mg/kg intravenously just before procedure
followed by 25 mg/kg 6 hours later

    Adults

1.0 g intravenously just before procedure or
intramuscularly 30 min before procedure.
Then 500 mg intravenously, intramuscularly
or orally, 6 hours after initial dose

Protocol for highly susceptible patients or high-risk procedures
Non-penicillin-allergic patients
    Children

Ampicillin or *amoxycillin* 50 mg/kg intravenously + *gentamycin* 2.5 mg/kg (up to
80 mg maximum) followed by *amoxycillin*
25 mg/kg 6 hours later

    Adults

Ampicillin or *amoxycillin* 1.0 g intravenously +
gentamycin 1.5 mg/kg (up to 80 mg
maximum) intravenously just before
procedure 'or intramuscularly 30 minutes
before procedure followed by *amoxycillin*
500 mg 6 hours later

Penicillin-allergic patients

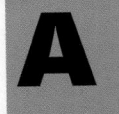

Children	*Vancomycin* 20 mg/kg infused over 1 hour before procedure followed by *gentamycin* 2.5 mg/kg intravenously (up to 80 mg maximum) before procedure commences
Adults	*Vancomycin* 1.0 g infused over 1 hour to end just prior to procedure, followed by *gentamycin* 1.5 mg/kg intravenously (up to 80 mg maximum) just before procedure commences

Further considerations
Paediatric dosage

Total paediatric dose should not exceed total adult dose.
- It is always preferable to prescribe on a dose per kilogram basis.
- Paediatric doses should be calculated up to the adult dose.
- It is expected that some cases of endocarditis will occur, despite the use of optimal prophylaxis protocols.
- Good history taking is essential.
- If in doubt, consult relevant medical authorities.

References

American Heart Association. Prevention of bacterial endocarditis. *JAMA* 1990, **2664**:2919–2922.
American Heart Association. Prevention of bacterial endocarditis. *JADA* 1991, **122**:87–92.
Recommendations from the Endocarditis Working Party of the British Society for Antimicrobial Chemotherapy. Antibiotic prophylaxis of infective endocarditis. *Lancet* 1990, **1**:88–89.
Antibiotic Guidelines Subcommittee of the Victorian Drug Usage Committee. Prevention of endocarditis or infection of prosthetic implants. In: *Antibiotic guidelines*, 7th ed.:Victorian Medical Postgraduate Foundation Inc, Melbourne, Australia; 1992:94–95.

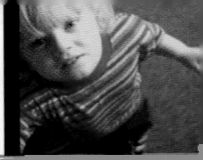

Appendix F. Vaccination schedules

2 months	DTP (Diphtheria, tetanus, pertussis) Sabin vaccine (Polio) Hib vaccine (a, b) (*Haemophilus influenzae* Type b)
4 months	DTP Sabin vaccine Hib vaccine (a,b)
6 months	DTP Sabin Hib vaccine (a)
12 months	MMR (Measles, mumps, rubella) Hib vaccine (b)
18 months	DTP Hib vaccine (a)
4–5 years (before school entry)	DTP Sabin vaccine
10–16 years	MMR Male and female
15 years (before leaving school)	ADT (Adult diphtheria and tetanus) Sabin
Every 10 years	Tetanus booster 0.5 mL IM
Hib vaccines	(a) HbOC (HibTITER) Lederle (b) PRP-OMP (PedvaxHIB) MSD

Source: National Health and Medical Research Council of Australia. *Australian Immunisation Procedures Handbook*, 5th ed. Canberra: AGPS, 1994.

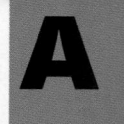
Appendix G. Isolation and exclusion from school for childhood infectious diseases

Condition	Isolation period/Incubation time
Acute conjunctivitis	Until all discharge has ceased.
Chickenpox	Until fully recovered. For at least 7 days after the first appearance of spots. No open sores should be present 10–21 days.
Diphtheria	Immediate isolation until certified by a medical practitioner. 3–6 days
Infectious mononucleosis	Until fully recovered or certified by a medical practitioner. 2–6 weeks
Infectious hepatitis	Until all symptoms have disappeared or until a medical practitioner certifies recovery. At least 7 days from the first signs of jaundice. 15–50 days.
Measles	At least 5 days from the appearance of the rash. 10–12 days.
Rubella	Until fully recovered. For at least 5 days after the appearance of the rash. 14–21 days.
Pertussis	Immediate isolation. Exclude from school for at least 3 weeks from the onset of the whoop, until full recovery or a medical certificate is obtained. 5–21 days.
Impetigo	Attendance at school is permitted if the sores are being treated and properly covered with a clean dressing. Exclusion from school is required, if the sores are not covered and are on exposed areas such as the scalp, hands or legs, until the sores have healed. 2–5 days.
Pediculosis (head lice)	Until treatment with antilice lotion or shampoo has been undertaken. Hair should be free of eggs.
Ringworm	Until appropriate treatment has begun.
Scabies	Until appropriate treatment has begun.

Source: NSW Department of Health, Australia, recommendations.

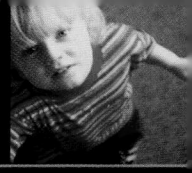

Appendix H. Somatic growth and maturity

Introduction
Assessment should begin as soon as the child enters the surgery. At the outset, the dentist should always look at children's size, development, appearance and behaviour in relation to their chronological age. Dental examination will initially include an assessment of dental age (based on time of exfoliation, eruption status and root development) in relation to the chronological age. Any marked discrepancies should then be investigated further.

Basic indicators of somatic growth and development
Height and weight
Height measurement Measure the child with shoes off, standing straight, with the Frankfort plane horizontal to the floor.

Measurement is taken on deep inspiration of the patient.

Sequential measurements are ideally taken at the same time of day.

Weight measurement Taken in light indoor clothing, with shoes off, ideally at the same time of day as height measurements.

Height Abnormalities
- Short stature <3rd percentile, tall stature >97th percentile over a 6-month period, or
- Rate of growth less than 3–5 cm/year consider referral to specialist growth unit at a paediatric hospital.
- Measurements must be considered in relation to height of parents and skeletal age.
- Height prediction possible using methods of Tanner–Whitehouse or Bayley–Pinneau.
- Prediction of adolescent growth spurt is achieved by serial measurements, and may influence the subsequent timing of myofunctional orthodontic treatment.

Weight abnormalities
- Children with an endomorphic appearance tend to mature early, while those who are ectomorphic (especially boys) tend to mature late.
- Underweight—consider anorexia/bulimia.
- Overweight—may indicate nutritional problems.
- When children are markedly outside norms for age, early referral to a paediatrician or dietitian is essential.
- Gross obesity may significantly alter drug metabolism and will affect the calculation of drug dosages.

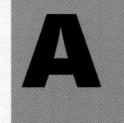
Skeletal assessment

- It has been consistently shown that bone age, as determined from hand-wrist radiographs using Greulich–Pyle, or Tanner–Whitehouse systems, has a high correlation with stature and general body development.
- Convention for anthropometric measurements uses the left hand.
- These methods assume bones of all patients consistently go through the same sequence of development, albeit at different rates. The Greulich and Pyle system is the most skeletally advanced for any age group, as it was derived in the USA from healthy children of a high socioeconomic group.

Greulich and Pyle Each bone is matched with a bone that appears similar in a series of standard radiographs of increasing age. Thus each bone has a bone age assigned to it and the modal (or most frequent) of these bone ages is taken as the bone age of the hand-wrist. Frequently, the step of assigning bone ages to each separate bone is omitted and instead the patient's hand-wrist radiograph is matched to the nearest standard radiograph, thereby determining the patient's skeletal age. Radiographic standards are provided at 6-monthly and 12-monthly intervals for both males and females.

Tanner–Whitehouse This method scores specified bones, according to their stage of development, using a written description and a radiographic standard of each stage of development. The total score for all bones is used to derive a skeletal age from tables provided. Generally, the Tanner–Whitehouse TW-2 (13 bone score) is used in preference to the Tanner–Whitehouse TW-20 bone method as it is about as accurate and quicker to use. The Tanner–Whitehouse TW-2 method is easier and more accurate than the Greulich–Pyle method for the occasional user.

Significance

- Used to calculate potential for further increase in height.
- Used to predict adolescent growth spurt for timing of orthodontic treatment.
- Used to monitor growth abnormalities.

Dental development

Eruption times

- The emergence of teeth in the primary and permanent dentitions is unreliable because of environmental influences (i.e. early extraction of primary teeth will delay eruption of the succedaneous tooth, while late extraction of a primary tooth will hasten the eruption of the permanent successor).
- Eruption is not a continuous event.
- Racial variations—published data on eruption times are generally of Northern European populations. Earlier eruption times may be the norm in Asian peoples, and later eruption times the norm in Eastern and Southern European groups.

Root development Using the scoring systems of Nolla, Moorees, Fanning, Demirjian and others. These quantify tooth development from initial calcification to final root closure as seen on radiographs.

Sexual development
Peak-height velocity (PHV)
- Hagg and Taranger observed that menarche occurred a mean 1.1 years after peak height velocity (PHV).
- Menarche is a highly reliable but not absolute indicator that PHV has been reached or passed.
- Menarche occurs at a bone age of 13.1 years.
- Boys attained a 'pubertal voice' (the pitch of the voice had changed noticeably but had not yet acquired adult characteristics) 0.2 years before PHV, and the 'male voice' (pitch of the voice had acquired adult characteristics) 0.9 years after PHV.
- Tanner found that in males, breaking of the voice happens relatively late in puberty and is caused by the increased length of the vocal cords which follows the growth of the larynx. Voice breaking is often a gradual process and is not reliable as a criterion of puberty. Facial hair appears in boys usually somewhat later than the PHV.

Correlation between dental development and other maturity indicators
Evidence so far indicates that the skeletal system, as well as height and the onset of puberty, develop largely independently of the dental system. Teeth are partly of epithelial origin, while bone is derived from mesoderm. Serious endocrinopathies, while severely retarding somatic growth and maturation, exert only a minor effect on the dentition. Demirjian found a very low correlation between dental age (root development) and skeletal age.

General observations on somatic growth
- Growth is nutrition-dependent and a well-fed infant gains length before weight.
- The pubertal-growth spurt is governed by growth hormone and anabolic steroids (testosterone and oestrogens).
- Girls enter the growth spurt about 2 years earlier than boys; however, they complete the growth spurt only about a year earlier than boys.
- The growth spurt is of greater magnitude and of shorter duration in boys than girls, as testosterone has a greater anabolic effect than oestrogen.
- Growth ceases from the feet up, so limb growth stops before spine growth.
- The pubertal-growth spurt adds 25–30 cm to final height over the childhood growth curve. Boys on average end up 12–13 cm taller than girls as their growth spurt occurs after an additional 2 years of childhood growth.

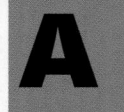

Appendix I. Growth charts

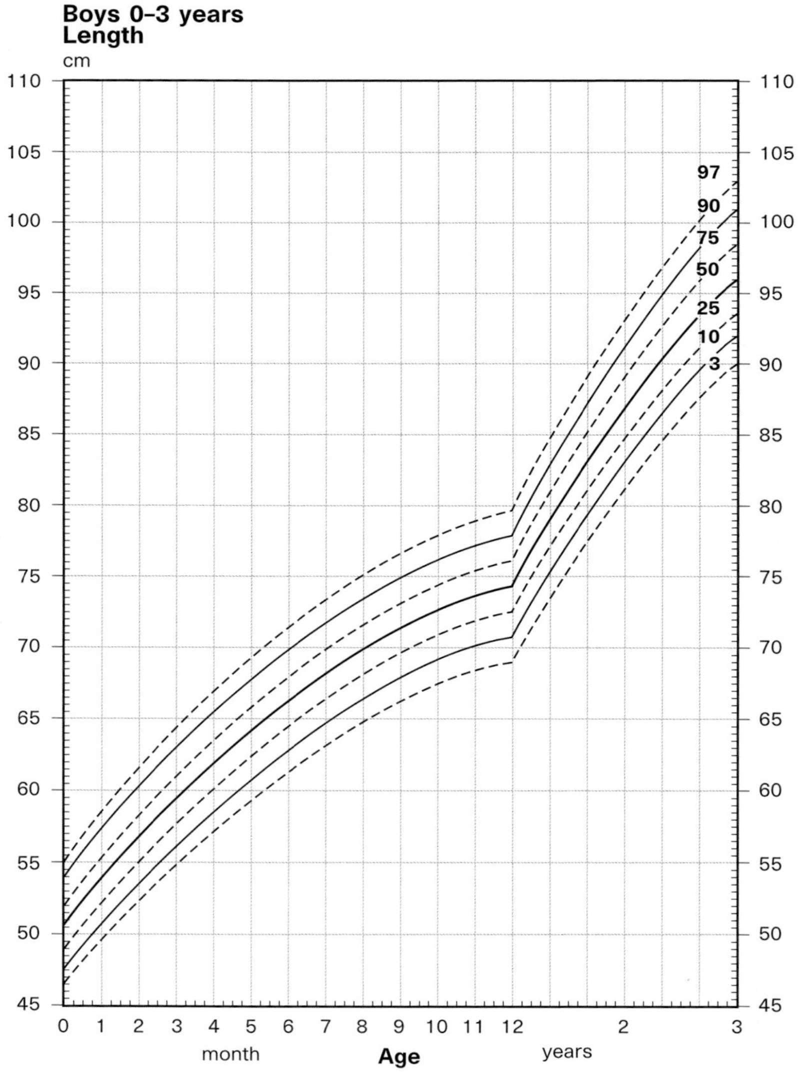
Boys 0–3 years
Length
cm
110
105
100
95
90
85
80
75
70
65
60
55
50
45
97
90
75
50
25
10
3
0 1 2 3 4 5 6 7 8 9 10 11 12
2
3
month
Age
years

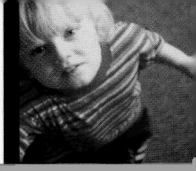

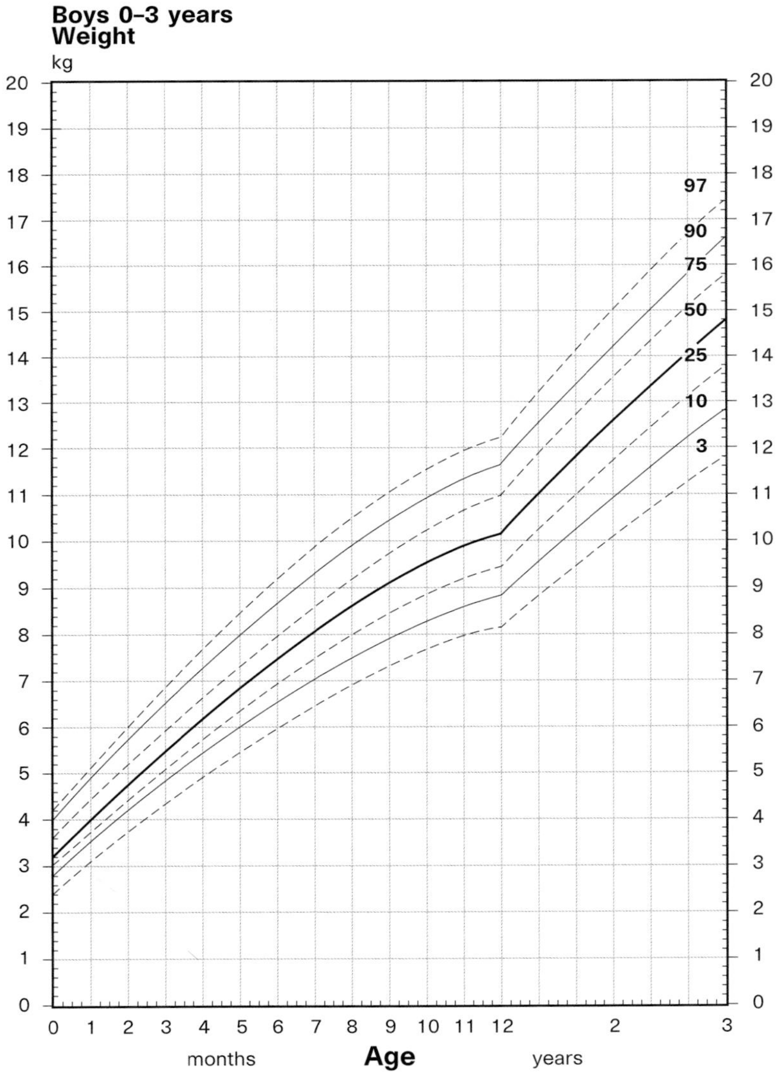
Boys 0–3 years
Weight
kg
20
19
18
17
16
15
14
13
12
11
10
9
8
7
6
5
4
3
2
1
0
97
90
75
50
25
10
3
0 1 2 3 4 5 6 7 8 9 10 11 12
2
3
months
Age
years

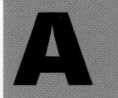

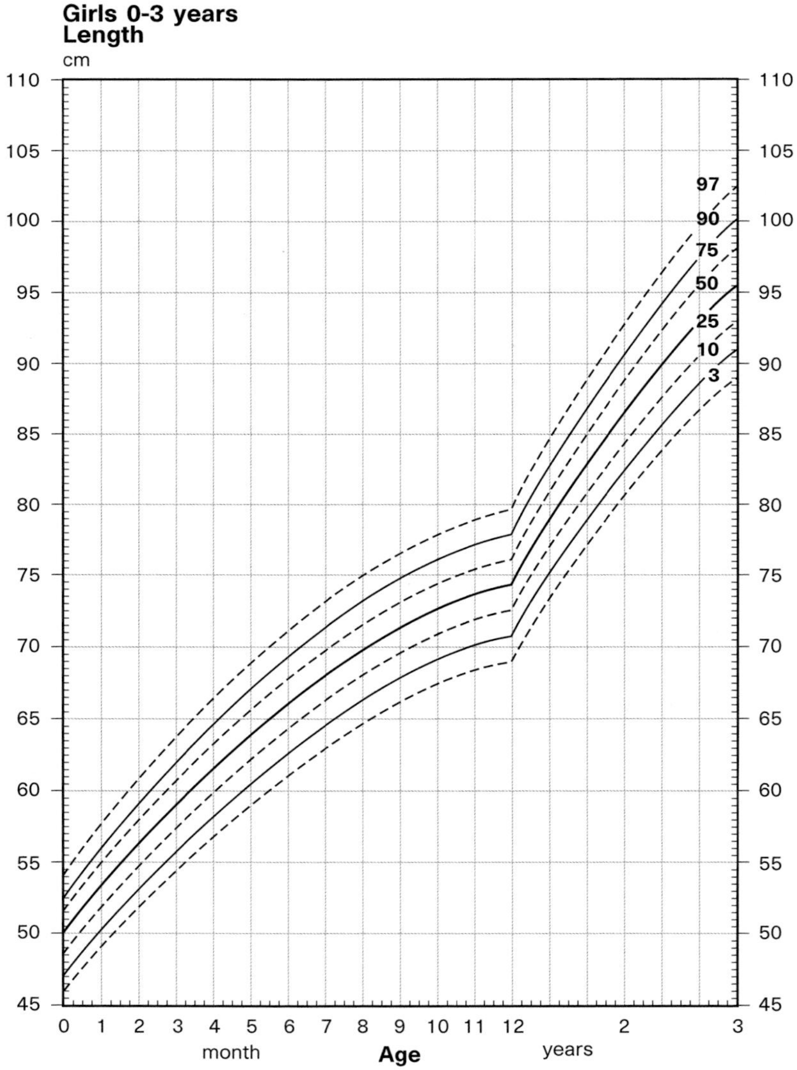
Girls 0-3 years
Length
cm
110
105
100
95
90
85
80
75
70
65
60
55
50
45
97
90
75
50
25
10
3
0 1 2 3 4 5 6 7 8 9 10 11 12
month
Age
2
years
3

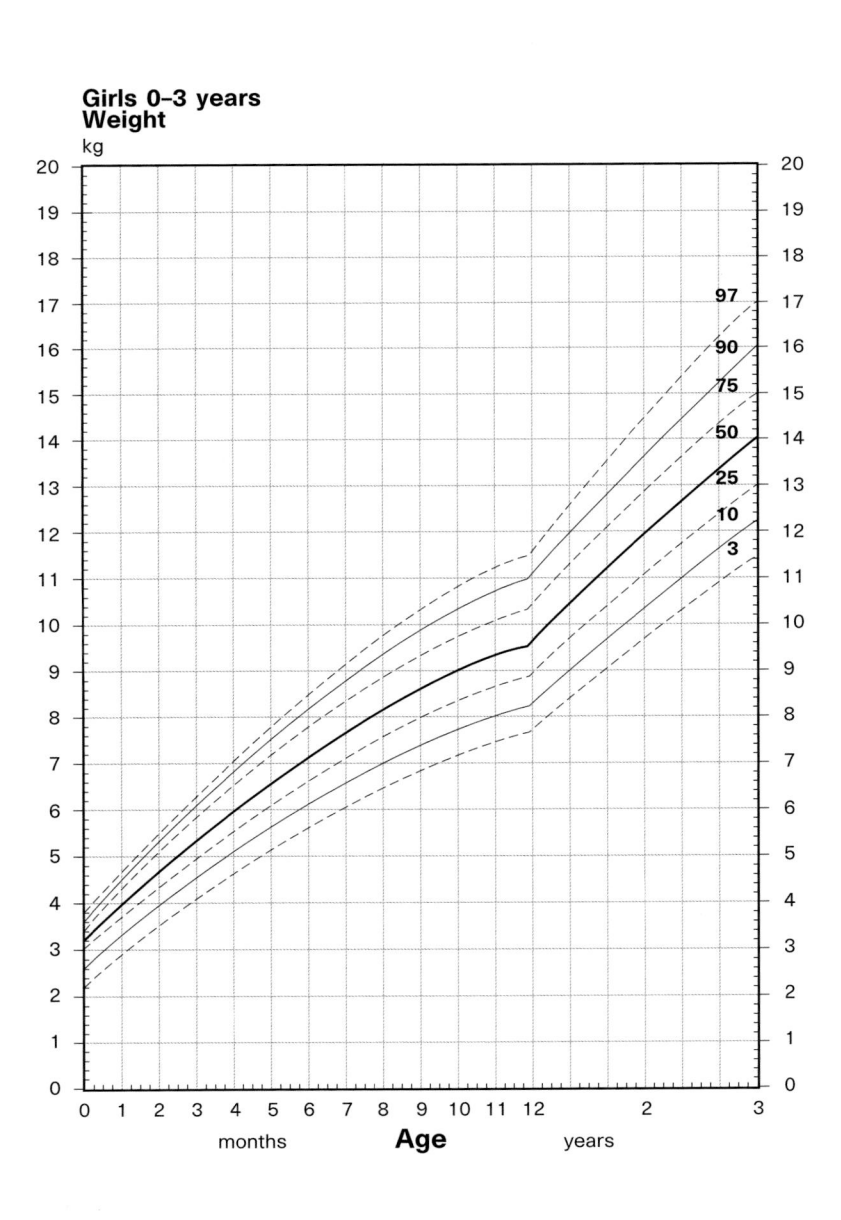

**Girls 0–3 years
Weight**

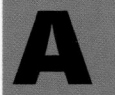
**Girls 2–19 years
Height**
cm

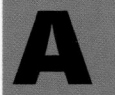

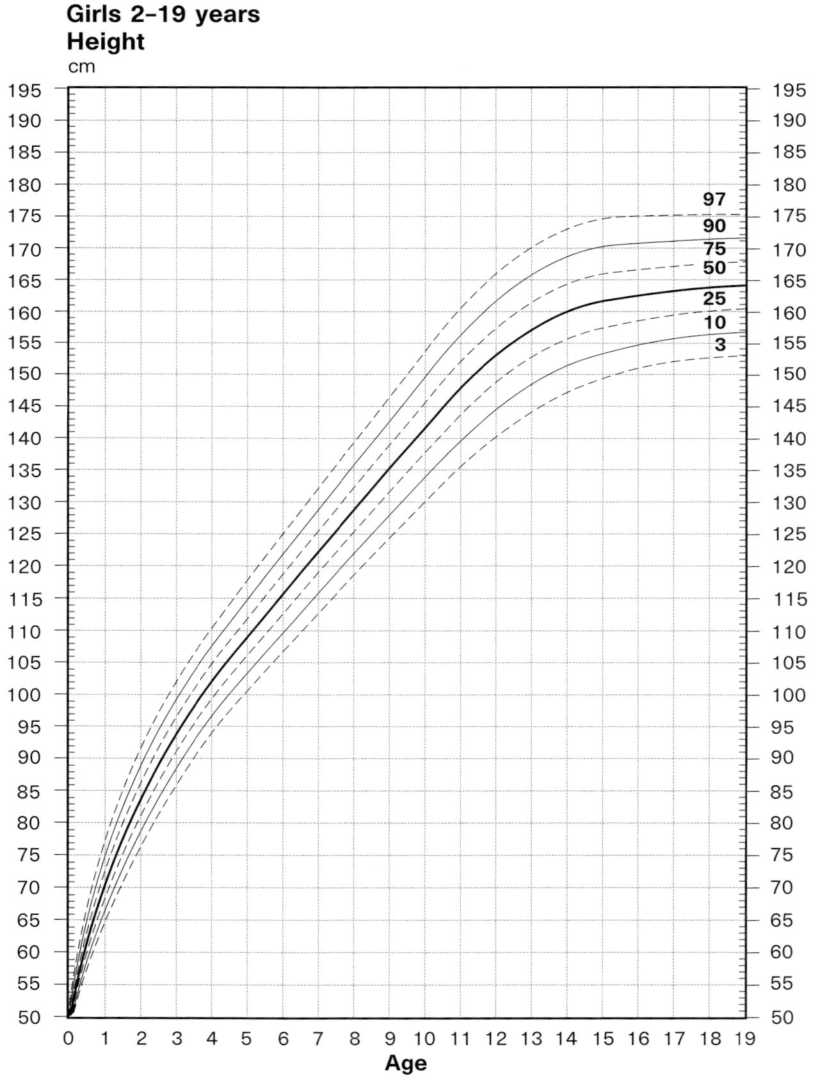

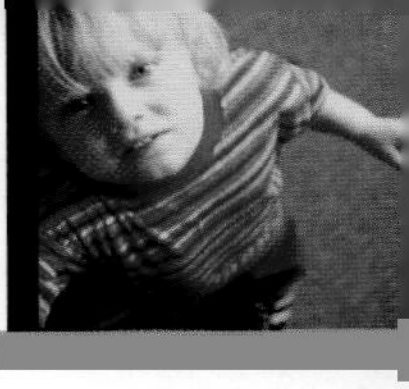

Girls 2–19 years
Weight

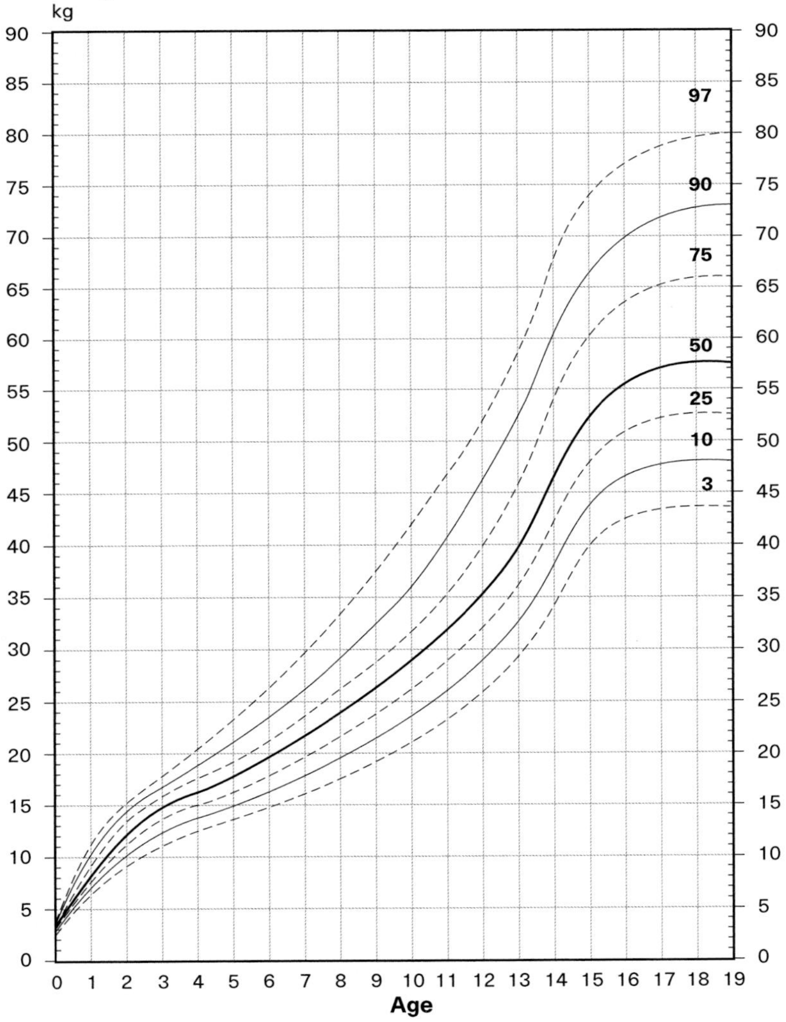

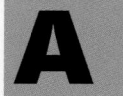
**Boys 2–19 years
Height**
cm

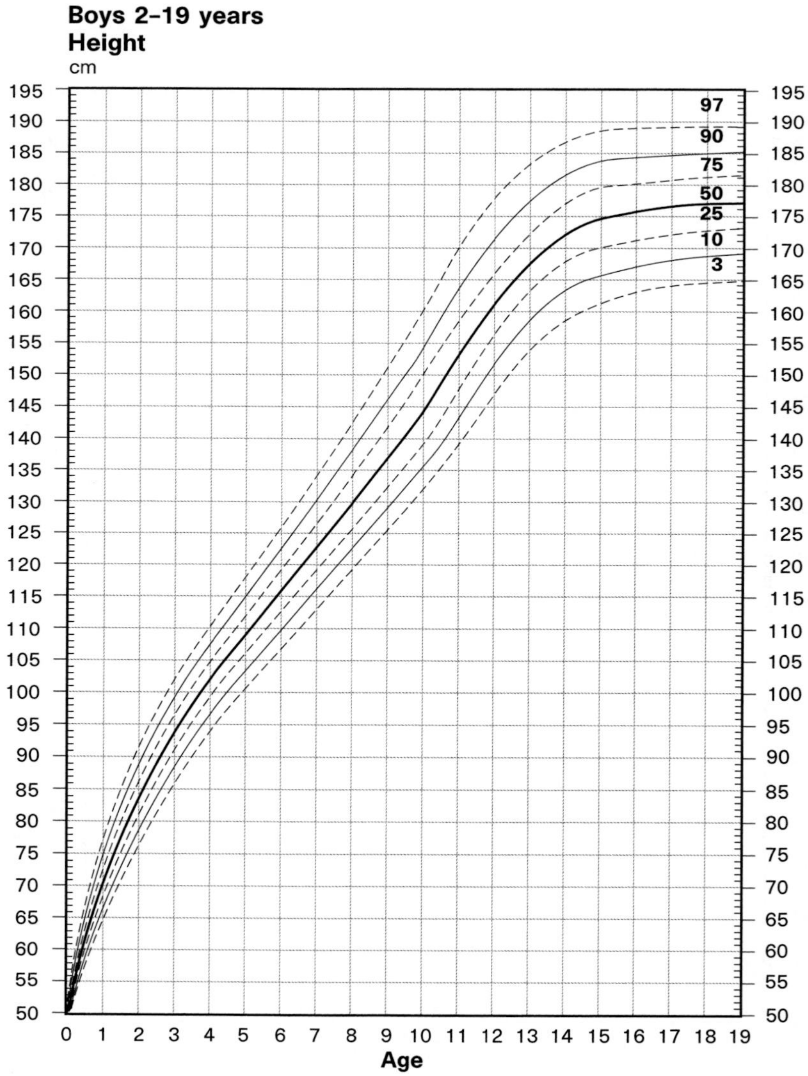

97
90
75
50
25
10
3

Age

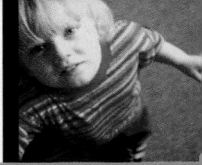

**Boys 2–19 years
Weight**
kg

Chart axes: Weight (kg) 0–90 on vertical axis, Age 0–19 on horizontal axis.

Percentile curves labeled: 97, 90, 75, 50, 25, 10, 3

Age

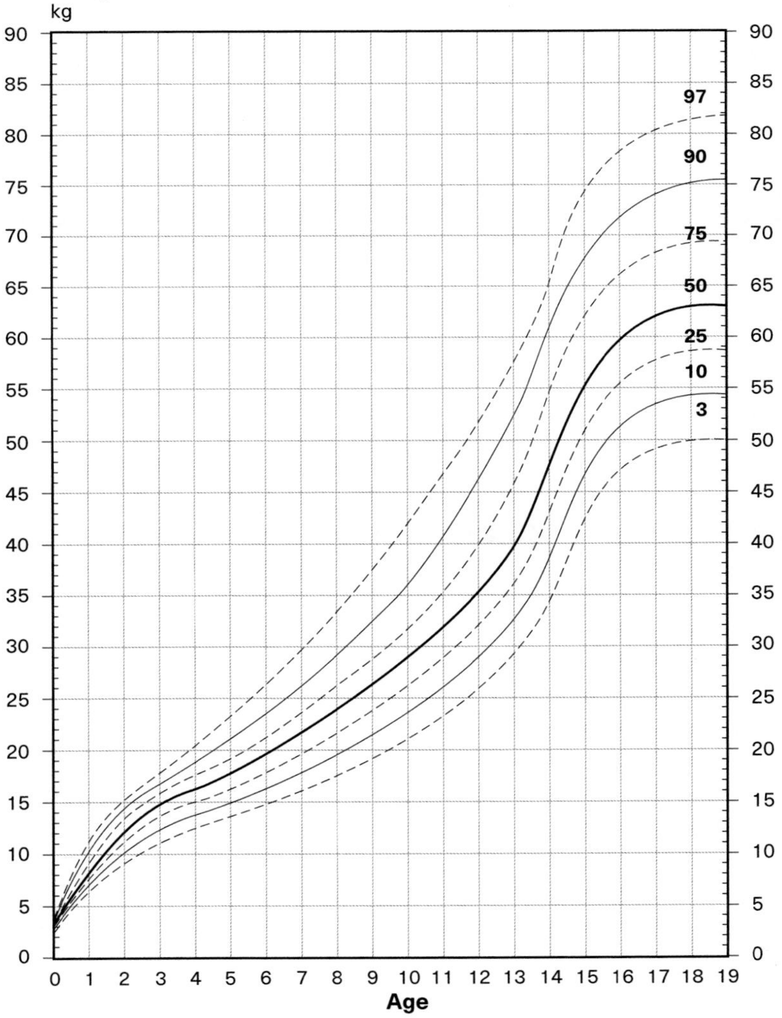

Appendix J. Differential diagnosis of radiographic pathology in children

Periapical radiolucencies

- Periapical granuloma, abscess, surgical defect, scar.
- Radicular cyst.
- Dentigerous cyst.
- Traumatic bone cyst.

Radiolucencies associated with the crowns of teeth

- Dentigerous cyst.
- Eruption cyst.
- Ameloblastic fibroma.
- Adenomatoid odontogenic tumour.
- Ossifying fibroma.
- Odontogenic keratocyst.

Separate isolated radiolucencies

- Primordial cyst.
- Traumatic bone cyst.
- Aneurysmal bone cyst.
- Odontogenic keratocyst.
- Fissural cysts.
- Median palatine cyst.
- Incisive canal cyst.
- Nasolabial cyst.
- Central giant-cell granuloma.
- Hyperparathyroidism.
- Ossifying fibroma

Multiple or multilocular radiolucencies

- Central giant-cell tumour.
- Cherubism.
- Giant-cell lesion of hyperparathyroidism.

- Langerhans' cell histiocytosis.
- Central haemangioma of bone.
- Odontogenic myxoma.
- Ewing's sarcoma.
- Desmoplastic fibroma.
- Metastatic tumours (especially rhabdomyosarcoma).

Generalized bony rarefactions

- Hyperparathyroidism.
- Thalassaemia.
- Langerhans' cell histiocytosis.
- Fibrous dysplasia.

Mixed lesions with radio-opacities and radiolucencies

- Odontoma.
- Ameloblastic fibro-odontoma.
- Calcifying odontogenic cyst.
- Odontogenic fibroma.
- Adenomatoid odontogenic tumour.
- Fibrous dysplasia.
- Garré's osteomyelitis.
- Osteogenic sarcoma.

Radio-opacities in the jaws

- Focal sclerosing osteomyelitis.
- Retained roots.
- Gardner's syndrome.
- Cleidocranial dysplasia.

Appendix K. Piaget's four stages of intellectual development

Stage one: the sensorimotor period (0–2 years)

Children in this period learn primarily through the senses of taste, touch, sight, sound, and manipulation. Mouthing of objects is a common method of learning. Intelligence is related to sensation, not reflective thought.

Stage two: the pre-operational period (2–7 years)

While children in this stage are capable of some intuitive thought, intelligence is based primarily on perception. The classic Piagetian experiment in this stage is the pouring of water into two test tubes. Children are shown that exactly the same amount of water is poured into a tall thin tube and a short wide tube. Those children between the ages of 2 and 7 years will typically argue that the taller tube contains more water, because their reasoning is tied to perception. Pre-operational children believe what they see and hear.

Stage three: the concrete operational period (7–11 years)

Children in this stage develop the ability to reverse their thinking and to employ basic logic. They begin to question whether their perceptions are true. For example, whereas a 4-year-old will believe that Santa Claus exists because they saw him in a shopping centre, the 9-year-old will question the existence of Santa Claus because actions such as flying in a sleigh defy logic.

Stage four: the formal operational period (11–15 years)

With the beginning of adolescence comes the possibility of reaching the highest level of intellectual development: the ability to think abstractly. This stage is not reached by all individuals. Intellectually, those in the formal operational period are capable of thinking in propositions. Subjects like algebra and geometry require this type of abstract thought.

Implications for dentists

Effective communication with a child or adolescent requires some understanding of their intellectual development. For example, consider how the following joking comment might differentially affect a 4-year-old and an 11-year- old: 'Sit really still so I don't accidentally drill through your head'. An 11-year-old might see the humour in what the dentist has said. At 11 years of age, the child has reached the 'concrete operational' stage and can therefore employ logic to realize that the dentist is exaggerating. The pre-operational 4-year-old, on the other hand, may become frightened by the sarcastic comment. Children at this stage often take at face value what adults tell them.

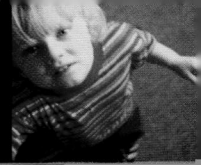

Appendix L. Glasgow Coma Scale

The Glasgow Coma Scale (GCS) is a rating score for head injury and the score gives an indication of degree of injury and level of consciousness. The table below has been modified for children, by the Adelaide Women's and Children's Hospital, as response scores are usually lower in children. Children between 6 months and 2 years of age may localize pain but not obey commands and before 6 months the best score is withdrawal from pain or abnormal extension and flexion. There is no modification of the adult eye-opening scale. Verbal responses should be consistent with age.

Outcomes

Children with GCS scores of 3 or 4 have significant mortality rates (between 20 and 70%), whereas those with scores over 5 have a low mortality and morbidity (<30%). If the child does not die within the first 24 hours the risk of death falls to between 10 and 20%. Sixty-four percent of children who do not open their eyes spontaneously within 24 hours will die or survive in a vegetative state. It is important to note that over 90% of children who are comatose initially with a GCS score greater than 3 will recover to an independent state, although 50% will have neurological impairment. If coma persists for longer than 3 months there is almost always neurological and cognitive damage.

Table A-4 Modified Glasgow Coma Scale

	Response	Response for infants	Score
Eye Opening	Spontaneously	Spontaneously	4
	To speech	To speech	3
	To pain	To pain	2
	None	None	1
Verbal	Orientated	Coos and babbles	5
	Words	Irritable cries	4
	Vocal sounds	Cries to pain	3
	Cries	Moans to pain	2
	None	None	1
Motor	Obeys commands	Normal spontaneous movements	6
	Localizes	Withdraws to touch	5
	Withdraws from pain	Withdraws from pain	4
	Abnormal flexion to pain	Abnormal flexion	3
	Extension to pain	Abnormal extension	2
	None	None	1
Best possible score			15

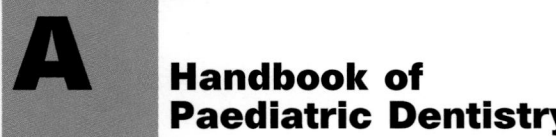
Appendix M. Use of drugs in paediatric dentistry

Drug	Route	Dose	Frequency	Notes
Antibiotics				
Amoxycillin	PO	25–50 mg/kg/day	tds	Syrup or chewable tablets for young children
	IV	100–400 mg/kg/day	tds	
	PO, IV	50 mg/kg up to adult dose 3 g	1 hour before	Endocarditis prophylaxis. For highly susceptible patients, half dose 6 hours later
Amoxycillin plus clavulanic acid	PO	20–40 mg/kg/day	tds	For beta-lactam resistant organisms only
Ampicillin	IV	50–100 mg/kg/day	qid	
	IV	50 mg/kg	stat	Endocarditis prophylaxis
Benzylpenicillin	IV	15–350 mg/kg/day 20,000–500,000 U/kg/day	qid	First IV drug of choice for odontogenic infections
Penicillin VK	PO	<5 years 500 mg/day >5 years 1–2 g/day	qid	Give 1 hour before meals
Cephalexin	PO	25–50 mg/kg/day	qid	
Cephalothin IV	IV	40–80 mg/kg/day	qid	Not in pregnancy
Cephalozin	IV	25–50 mg/kg/day		
Erythromycin	PO	25–40 mg/kg/day	qid	Ethylsuccinate is readily absorbed
Metronidazole	IV	22.5 mg/kg/day	tds	Not in pregnancy
	PO	10–15 mg/kg/day	tds	
Gentamycin	IV	2.5 mg/kg (children) up to 80 mg maximum	stat	Endocarditis prophylaxis highly susceptible patients. In conjunction with ampicillin. Follow-up dose of ampicillin or amoxicillin required 6 hours later

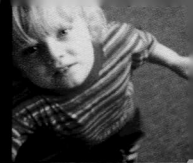

Drug	Route	Dose	Frequency	Notes
Antibiotics				
Clindamycin	PO, IV	15–40 mg/kg/day	qid	Risk of pseudo-membranous colitis
	PO, IV	10 mg/kg up to adult dose 600 mg	oral 1 hour before, IV stat	Endocarditis prophylaxis. Susceptible patients. Follow-up dose half initial dose, 6 hours later (5 mg/kg up to 300 mg)
Vancomycin	IV	20 mg/kg up to adult dose 1 g	infused over 1 hour	Endocarditis prophylaxis, susceptible patients allergic to penicillin
Antifungals				
Nystatin	Tablets	500 000 U	tds	
	Mixture	100 000 U/mL	6-hrly	Apply to affected area
Amphotericin B	Lozenges	10 mg	6-hrly	Apply to affected area
	Suspension	100 mg/mL	6-hrly	Apply to affected area
	Ointment	3%	6-hrly	Apply to affected area
Analgesics and sedatives				
Aspirin				Should not be used in children under 12 years of age because of the risk of Reye's syndrome
Paracetamol	PO, PR	15 mg/kg	4-hrly	Hepatotoxic if overdose
Codeine phosphate	PO	1–1.5 mg/kg single dose 1–3 mg/kg/day	4–6 divided doses	Similar side-effects to narcotics, including nausea and constipation
Pethidine	IV, IM	1 mg/kg	3–4 hrly	Maximum 100 mg

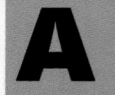

Handbook of Paediatric Dentistry

Drug	Route	Dose	Frequency	Notes
Analgesics and sedatives				
Morphine	IV, IM	0.1–0.2 mg/kg	6-hrly	Should only be used in admitted patients
Naloxone	IM, IV	1–10 µg/kg	stat	May be repeated at 2–3-minute intervals if necessary
Midazolam	IV, IM	0.1–0.2 mg/kg	single dose	Sedation, may be given intranasally
Chloral hydrate	PO	30–50 mg/kg/day, 15–20 mg/kg single dose	4–6 hourly	Sedation
Trimeprazine	PO	3–4 mg/kg	single dose	Vallergan, sedation
Metoclopramide	PO, IM	3–5 years 2 mg 5–9 years 2.5 mg 9–14 years 5 mg 15–19 years 10 mg	single dose	Single dose after narcotic if vomiting or nausea. Maxolon. Dystonic reactions may occur
Other medications				
Kenalog in Orabase	Ointment	Triamcinolone 0.1%	4–6 hrly	Recurrent severe oral ulceration in children, apply to ulcer but do not rub ointment in
ε aminocaproic acid	IV	30 mg/kg		Antifibrinolytic, loading dose of 100 mg/kg
Tranexamic acid	PO	15–20 mg/kg	qid	Antifibrinolytic
DDAVP	IV	0.3 µg/kg		Infused over 1 hour before surgery
Heparin	IV	50–100 U/kg	4–6hrly	Anticoagulant
Tetanus toxoid	IM	0.5 mL	single dose	If immunization protocol not complete, course should be given. Otherwise, a booster may be required for tetanus-prone wounds if >2 years since last booster

The table which forms Appendix M is a guide to the administration of commonly used drugs in paediatric dentistry. Medications for children should always be prescribed in relation to weight. It is of utmost importance that clinicians understand the contraindications and precautions relevant to the drugs they are prescribing and should consult prescribing information supplied by the pharmaceutical manufacturers and relevant pharmacopeia. In the table, PO = oral, IV = intravenous, IM = intramuscular, tds = ×3 daily, quid = ×4 daily and stat = immediately.

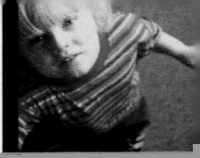

Appendix N. Eruption dates of teeth

Tooth	Initiation (*weeks in utero*)	Calcification begins (weeks *in utero*)	Crown formation at birth (38–42 wks)	Crown complete (months)	Eruption (months)
Table A-5 Primary Teeth					
Central incisor	7	13–16	5/6 maxilla 3/5 mandible	1–3	6–9
Lateral incisor	7	14–16	2/3 maxilla 3/5 mandible	2–3	7–10
Canine	7.5	15–18	1/3	9	16–20
First molar	8	14.5–17	cusps united, occlusal surface complete, 1/2 to 3/4 crown height	6	12–16
Second molar	10	16–23	cusps united, 1/4 crown height	10–12	23–30

From: Logan WHG, Kronfeld R (1933); Shour I, Massler M (1940).

Notes on eruption of teeth

All of these values are based on work that was published over 50 years ago. To this date there has been very little up-to-date work on the eruption of teeth. It should be noted that there is extreme variability within normal populations and it is of more value to compare the eruption pattern of the whole dentition rather than one particular tooth. Eruption sequence is of particular importance and may be indicative of pathology, for example a supernumerary tooth blocking the eruption of a central incisor.

References

LOGAN WHG, KRONFELD R. Development of the human jaw and surrounding structures from birth to the age of 15 years. *J Am Dent Assoc* 1933, **20**:379-427.

SHOUR I, MASSLER M. Studies in tooth development. The growth pattern of human teeth. *J Am Dent Assoc* 1940, **27**:1918-31.

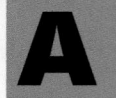
Table A-6 Permanent teeth

	Initiation	Calcification begins	Crown complete (years)	Eruption (years)
Mandible				
Central incisor	20–22 weeks IU*	3–4 months	4–5	6–7
Lateral incisor	21–22 weeks IU	3–4 months	4–5	7–8
Canine	20–26 weeks IU	4–5 months	6–7	9–11
First premolar	38–42 weeks IU	1.75–2 years	5–6	10–12
Second premolar	7.5–8 months	2.25–2.5 years	6–7	11–12
First molar	15–17 weeks IU	Birth	2.5–3	6–7
Second molar	8.5–9 months	2.5–3 years	7–8	11–13
Third molar	3.5–4 years	8–10	12–16	17–25
Maxilla				
Central incisor	20–22 weeks IU	3–4 months	4–5	7–8
Lateral incisor	21–22 weeks IU	11 months	4–5	8–9
Canine	21–26 weeks IU	4–5 months	6–7	11–12
First premolar	38–42 weeks IU	1.25–1.75 years	5–6	10–11
Second premolar	7.25–8 months	2–2.5 years	6–7	10–12
First molar	3.5–4 weeks IU	Birth	2.5–3	6–7
Second molar	8.5–9 months	2.5–3 years	7–8	12–13
Third molar	3.5–4 years	7–9 years	12–16	17–25

*IU = in utero

Appendix O. Construction of family pedigrees

Pedigrees are a useful presentation of families in clinical notes. It displays information about past generations and the transmission of genetic traits through families. The symbols used in constructing pedigrees are shown in Figure A.3. The affected individual at examination is termed the proband and an arrow is used to indicate this patient. Generations are numbered with Roman numerals and Arabic numerals are used to indicate individuals within each generation. An example of a family pedigree, displaying a sex-linked transmission, is shown in Figure A.4.

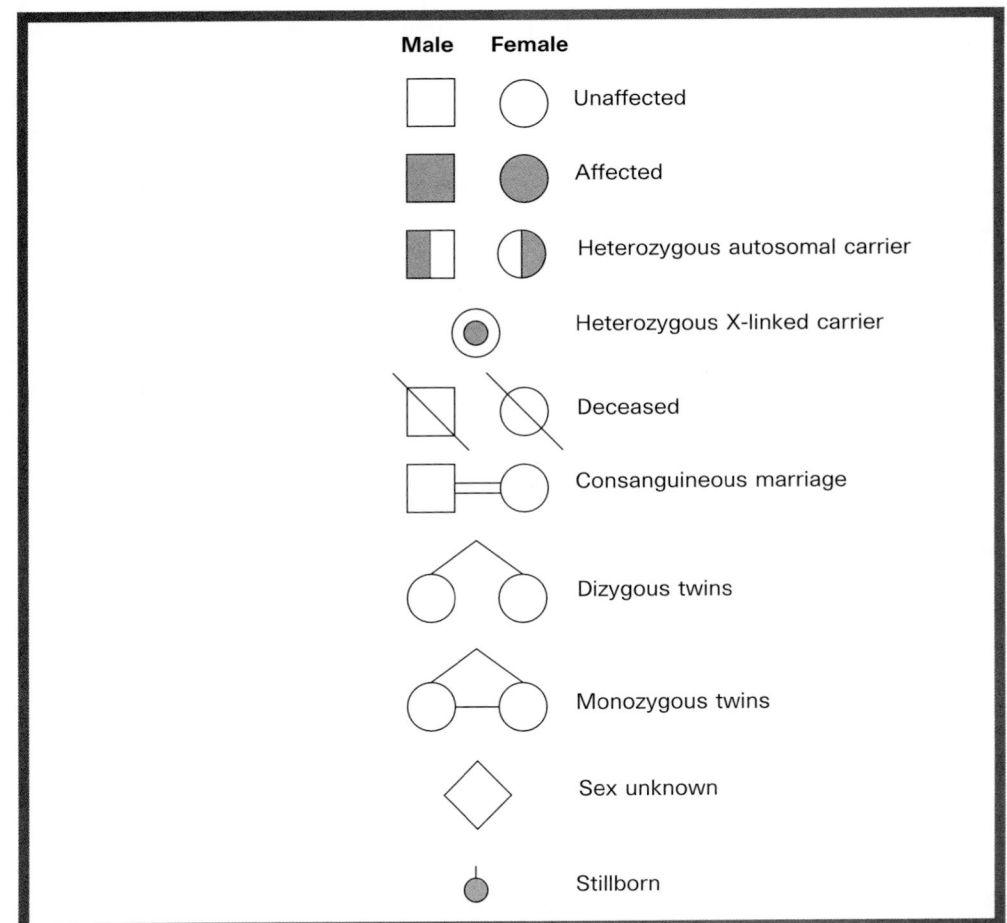

Figure A.3 Symbols used in the construction of pedigrees.

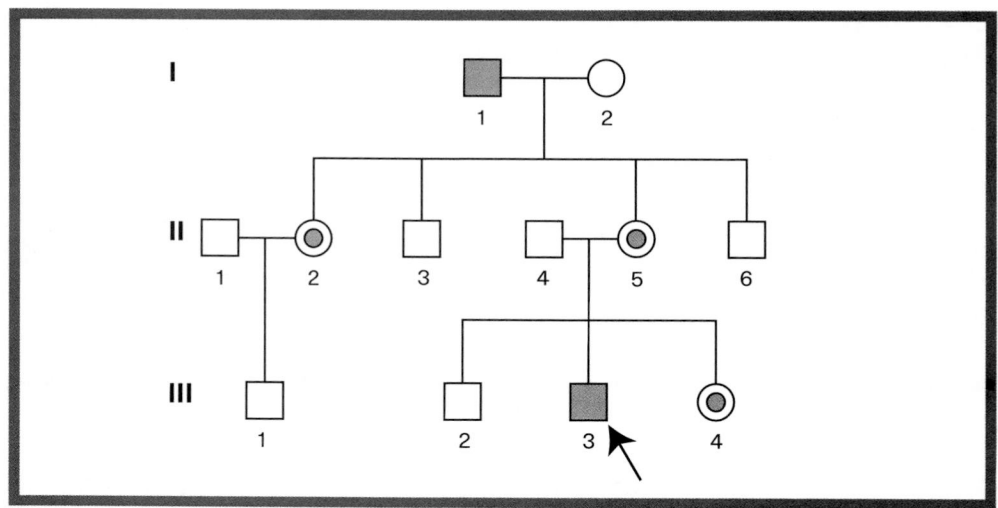

Figure A.4 A pedigree of a family with ectodermal dysplasia, demonstrating sex-linked inheritance. In the first generation, the grandfather (I1) of the proband (III3) (arrowed) had no hair, was hyperthermic and only had three permanent teeth. Of his offspring, all the females were heterozygotes (II2 and II5). The younger had sparse hair, suffered from eczema and was missing seven teeth including the lower canines. It is important to note that there is no male to male transmission. The daughter then passed the mutation to one of her sons (III3), who fully expresses the gene and one of her daughters who is a carrier.

Other Recommended Reading

GORLIN RJ, COHEN MM, LEVIN. *Syndromes of the head and neck*, 3rd ed. Oxford: Oxford University Press; 1990.

HALL RK. *Pediatric orofacial medicine and pathology*. London: Chapman and Hall Medical; 1994.

KABAN LB. *Pediatric oral and maxillofacial surgery*. Philadelphia: WB Saunders; 1987.

KOCH G, MODEER T, POULSEN S, RASMUSSEN P, eds. *Pedodontics—a clinical approach*. Copenhagen: Munksgaard; 1991.

PINKHAM JR, CASAMASSIMO PS, MCTIGUE DJ, FIELDS HW, NOWAK A. *Pediatric Dentistry. Infancy through adolescence*. Philadelphia: Saunders; 1994.

ROSE LF, KAY D, eds. *Internal medicine for dentistry*, 2nd ed. St Louis: Mosby; 1990.

WEI SHY. *Pediatric Dentistry—total patient care*. Philadelphia: Lea and Febiger; 1988.

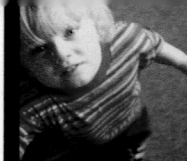

Appendix P. Charting form

Westmead Hospital Dental Clinical School

Title	Family Name	M.R.N.
Given Names		History Number
C.M.O.	Fin Class.	Address:
Date of Birth	Sex	Ward	

Postcode _____

Condition on Initial Examination

| 18 | 17 | 16 | 15 | 14 | 13 | 12 | 11 | | 21 | 22 | 23 | 24 | 25 | 26 | 27 | 28 |

| | | | 55 | 54 | 53 | 52 | 51 | | 61 | 62 | 63 | 64 | 65 |

RIGHT   LEFT

| | | | 85 | 84 | 83 | 82 | 81 | | 71 | 72 | 73 | 74 | 75 |

| 48 | 47 | 46 | 45 | 44 | 43 | 42 | 41 | | 31 | 32 | 33 | 34 | 35 | 36 | 37 | 38 |

Initial Perio Exam

17—14	13—23	24—27
47—44	43—33	34—37

Treatment Required — Perio

_____

_____

_____

Restorations Required:

| 18 | 17 | 16 | 15 | 14 | 13 | 12 | 11 | | 21 | 22 | 23 | 24 | 25 | 26 | 27 | 28 |

| | | | 55 | 54 | 53 | 52 | 51 | | 61 | 62 | 63 | 64 | 65 |

RIGHT   LEFT

| | | | 85 | 84 | 83 | 82 | 81 | | 71 | 72 | 73 | 74 | 75 |

| 48 | 47 | 46 | 45 | 44 | 43 | 42 | 41 | | 31 | 32 | 33 | 34 | 35 | 36 | 37 | 38 |

Fissure Tx _____   Endo _____

GIC _____   Inlay/Onlay _____

Composite _____   Crown/Bridge/Veneer _____

Amalgam _____   Other _____

Removable Pros _____

Treatment Sequence: _____

_____

_____

_____

_____

TREATMENT PLAN

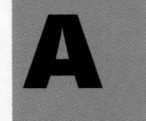
Appendix Q. Neurological observation chart

					Date																										
LEGEND		Record best responses as ●		Time																											
Eye Opening:	G L A S G O W	B E S T	Eye Opening	Spontaneously	4																										
Eyes closed by swelling = C				To speech	3																										
				To pain	2																										
				None	1																										
Verbal:	C O M A	R E S P O N S E	Verbal	Oriented	5																										
Endotracheal tube or tracheostomy				Confused	4																										
= T				Inappropriate Words	3																										
				Incomprehensible Sounds	2																										
				None	1																										
Motor:	S C A L E		Motor	Obeys Commands	6																										
Record the best arm response				Localises	5																										
				Withdrawal from pain	4																										
				Abnormal flexion to pain	3																										
				Extension to pain	2																										
				None	1																										
		COMA	Best Eye Opening																												
			Best Verbal																													
		SCORE	Best Motor																													
			TOTAL																													

Record Right (R) and Left (L) separately if there is a difference between the two sides	L I M B	A	Normal power																											
		R	Mild weakness																											
		M	Severe weakness																											
		S	No power																											
	P O W E R	L	Normal power																											
		E	Mild weakness																											
		G	Severe weakness																											
		S	No power																											

+ Brisk	PUPIL	Right	Size (mm)																			
s Sluggish			Reaction																			
– None	REACTION	Left	Size (mm)																			
o Untestable			Reaction																			

Pupil Scale
● 1 mm
● 3 mm
● 5 mm
● 7 mm

OTHER COMMENTS

Neurological Observation Chart

7/86

ANY CHANGE MUST BE REPORTED IMMEDIATELY

Index